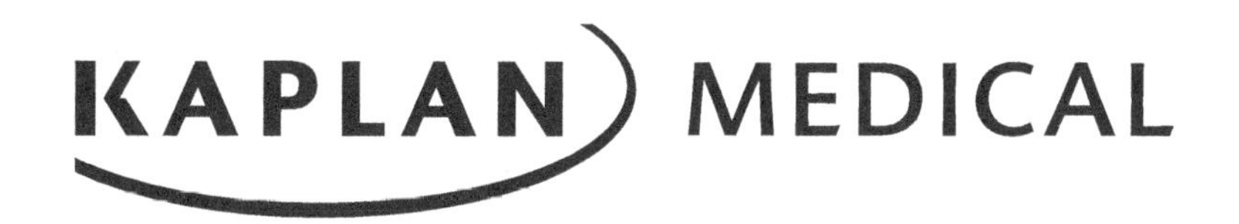

# CLINICAL MANAGEMENT REVIEW 2023–2024 VOLUME 1

## FOR USMLE® STEP 3 AND COMLEX-USA® LEVEL 3

Published by Kaplan Medical, a division of Kaplan North America, LLC.
1515 West Cypress Creek Road
Fort Lauderdale, Florida 33309



10 9 8 7 6 5 4 3 2 1

Course ISBN: 978-1-5062-8327-2
Course Kit ISBN: 978-1-5062-8333-3

Retail ISBN: 978-1-5062-8575-7
Retail Kit ISBN: 978-1-5062-8331-9

Kit items come as a set and should not be broken out and sold separately.

Kaplan Publishing print books are available at special quantity discounts to use for sales promotions, employee premiums, or educational purposes. For more information or to purchase books, please call the Simon & Schuster special sales department at 866-506-1949.

# EDITORS

## Internal Medicine

**Joseph J. Lieber, MD**
*Director of Medicine*
*Elmhurst Hospital Center*

*Associate Professor of Medicine*
*Associate Program Director of Medicine for Elmhurst Site*
*Icahn School of Medicine at Mount Sinai*
*New York, NY*

**Frank P. Noto, MD**
*Internal Medicine*
*New York, NY*

**Manuel A. Castro, MD, AAHIVS**
*Diplomate of the American Board of Internal Medicine*
*Certified by the American Academy of HIV*
*Wilton Manors, FL*

**Raj Dasgupta, MD, FACP, FCCP, FAASM**
*Associate Professor of Clinical Medicine*
*Assistant Program Director of Internal Medicine Residency*
*Associate Program Director of Sleep Medicine Fellowship*
*Department of Medicine, Division of*
*Pulmonary, Critical Care and Sleep Medicine*
*Keck School of Medicine of USC, University of Southern California*
*Los Angeles, CA*

## Psychiatry and Ethics

**Alina Gonzalez-Mayo, MD**
*Psychiatrist*
*Dept. of Veteran's Administration*
*Bay Pines, FL*

We want to hear what you think. What do you like or not like about the Notes?
Please email us at **medfeedback@kaplan.com**.

# Table of Contents

# PART I

# INTERNAL MEDICINE

# Preventive Medicine 1

## CANCER SCREENING

Regular screening is recommended for cancers of the colon, breast, cervix, and lung.

### Colon Cancer

Patients with no significant family history of colon cancer should begin screening at age 50. The choices are:

- Colonoscopy every 10 years (preferred screening modality)
- Fecal occult blood testing every year
- Sigmoidoscopy with barium enema every 5 years

Patients who have a single first-degree relative with colorectal cancer diagnosed age <60 or multiple first-degree relatives with colon cancer diagnosed at any age should undergo colonoscopy starting at one of the following, **whichever age occurs earlier**:

- Age 40
- Age that is 10 years younger than the age at which the youngest affected relative was diagnosed

In this group of high-risk patients, colonoscopy should be repeated every 5 years.

### Breast Cancer

The 3 tests used to screen for breast cancer are mammogram, manual breast exam, and self-breast exam. The American Cancer Society no longer recommends monthly self-breast exam alone as a screening tool.

- Patients age ≥50, screen with mammogram (with or without clinical breast exam) every 1–2 years
- Patients with very strong family history, consider prophylactic tamoxifen ("very strong family history" defined as multiple first-degree relatives)

### Cervical Cancer

The screening test of choice for the early detection of cervical cancer is the Papanicolaou smear ("Pap" test). In average risk women, Pap screening should be started at age 21—regardless of onset of sexual activity—and performed every 3 years until age 65.

- As an alternative, women age 30–65 who prefer to screen every 5 years can do so by co-testing with Pap and HPV.
- In higher risk women, e.g., HIV-positive, more frequent screening or screening after age 65 may be required.

### Lung Cancer

Current lung cancer screening guidelines recommend the following:

- Patients age 55–80 who have >30 pack-years of smoking (current smoker or have quit <15 years), screening with low dose CT (non-contrast) is recommended annually
- Patients age >80, have quit >15 years, or have other medical problems (e.g., severe COPD) significantly limiting life expectancy or ability to undergo surgery, no screening is recommended

## TRAVEL MEDICINE

### Hepatitis

Hepatitis A infection is travelers' most common vaccine-preventable disease. Hepatitis A infection is possible wherever fecal contamination of food or drinking water may occur. If a patient is leaving within 2 weeks of being seen, both the vaccine and immune serum globulin are recommended.

A booster shot given 6 months after the initial vaccination confers immunity for approximately 10 years.

Hepatitis B vaccination is recommended for patients who work closely with the indigenous population. Additionally, patients who plan to engage in sexual intercourse with the local populace or to receive medical or dental care, and those who plan to remain abroad for >6 months, should be vaccinated.

### Malaria

For malaria prophylaxis, mefloquine is used, although doxycycline is an acceptable alternative. For pregnant patients requiring malaria chemoprophylaxis, chloroquine is preferred.

### Rabies

Rabies vaccination is recommended for travel to areas where rabies is common among domesticated animals (India, Asia, Mexico). Chloroquine can blunt the response to the intradermal form of rabies vaccine. Therefore, when both malaria prophylaxis and rabies prophylaxis are required, the intramuscular form of the vaccine should be administered.

Rabies vaccination is not considered a routine vaccination for most travelers.

### Yellow Fever

Yellow fever vaccine is required for travel to sub-Saharan Africa and certain South American countries.

### Typhoid

Typhoid vaccination is recommended for patients who are traveling to developing countries and will have prolonged exposure to contaminated food and water.

### Polio

Adults who are traveling to developing countries and have never received a polio vaccine should receive 3 doses of the inactivated polio vaccine. Patients who have been previously immunized should receive a one-time booster. The live attenuated polio vaccine is no longer recommended because of the risk of vaccine-associated disease.

### Meningitis

Patients traveling to areas where meningococcal meningitis is endemic or epidemic (Nepal, sub-Saharan Africa, northern India) should be immunized with the polysaccharide vaccine. Additionally, Saudi Arabia requires immunization for pilgrims to Mecca. Patients with functional or actual asplenia and patients with terminal complement deficiencies should also receive the vaccine. Meningococcal vaccine is now routine to give at age 11.

### Diarrhea

To prevent traveler's diarrhea, patients should be educated regarding the advisability of avoiding salads and unwashed fruit and drinking tap/ice water. Patients who experience loose stools without fever or blood can safely take loperamide. Treatment with a fluoroquinolone or azithromycin is reserved for patients with moderate to severe symptoms (bloody diarrhea).

## IMMUNIZATIONS

### Influenza Vaccine

Influenza vaccination is recommended annually for all adults, regardless of age. Additionally, those who have a history of cardiopulmonary disease, DM, or hemoglobinopathy, or who are residents of a chronic care facility should receive an annual influenza vaccination, regardless of age.

Pregnant women who will be in their second or third trimester during the influenza season should also receive the vaccine.

### Pneumococcal Vaccine

Pneumococcal vaccination with the pneumococcal polysaccharide vaccine (PPSV23) is indicated for all adults age >65. Additionally, the following should receive the vaccine at any age:

- Those with history of sickle-cell disease or splenectomy
- Those with history of cardiopulmonary disease, alcoholism, or cirrhosis
- Alaskan natives and certain Native American populations
- Those who are immunocompromised (hematologic malignancy, chronic renal failure, nephrotic syndrome, HIV-positive; or taking immunosuppressive medications)

**Additionally:**

- Those age >65 who received PPSV23 earlier than age 65 also need a booster shot if it has been more than 5 years since being vaccinated
- Those with high risk of fatal infection (asplenic patients, immunocompromised patients, kidney disease, chemotherapy, long-term steroids, cancer including leukemia and lymphoma, organ transplant) should be revaccinated 1× after 5 years
- No one gets more than 1 booster shot per lifetime

## Varicella Vaccine

Varicella vaccine is a live, attenuated vaccine recommended for use in all adults who lack a history of childhood infection with varicella virus. Being a live, attenuated vaccine, varicella vaccine should not be given to immunocompromised patients, HIV-positive patients when symptomatic, those with <200 CD4 cells, or pregnant women.

## Shingles Vaccine

The shingles (zoster) vaccine is recommended routinely in order to reduce the risk of shingles and its associated pain in people ≥60. Only one dose of zoster vaccine is typically given. Persons who report a previous episode of zoster and persons with chronic medical condition (chronic kidney disease, diabetes) can be vaccinated.

Zoster vaccination is **not indicated** to treat acute zoster, to prevent those with acute zoster from developing post-herpetic neuralgia, or to treat ongoing post-herpetic neuralgia. Before routine administration of zoster vaccine, it is not necessary to ask patients about their history of varicella (chickenpox) or to conduct serologic testing for varicella immunity. The zoster vaccine is a lyophilized preparation of live, attenuated VZV.

## HPV Vaccine

The quadrivalent human papilloma virus (HPV) vaccine prevents against 4 types of HPV (types 6, 11, 16, 18) that are associated with genital warts and cervical cancer. It is given in 3 doses and it is recommended for those age 11–12, but can be given at age 9.

It is also recommended for those who did not complete the series or were never vaccinated from age 13–26. Males age 9–26 might get the vaccine to prevent genital warts. Cervical cancer screening with Pap smear should continue after vaccination.

## SMOKING CESSATION

Smoking cessation is the best way to prevent disease. Smoking is responsible for 1 in every 5 deaths in the United States. There are 5 steps a physician can take to help patients stop smoking:

- ASK about smoking at every visit.
- ADVISE all smokers to quit at every visit.
- ATTEMPT to identify those smokers willing to quit.
- ASSIST smokers in quitting by setting a quit date (usually within 2 weeks) and using nicotine patches/gum or the oral antidepressant bupropion as supportive therapy. Varenicline, a nicotinic receptor partial agonist, can also be used to treat nicotine addiction.
- ARRANGE follow-up. Provide positive reinforcement if the quit attempt was successful. If the quit attempt was not successful, then determine why the patient smoked and elicit a recommitment to smoking cessation. Most patients will require several attempts before being successful.

U/S should be given once in male smokers age >65 in order to screen for abdominal aortic aneurysm. There are no screening recommendations in male nonsmokers and women, regardless of smoking history.

## OSTEOPOROSIS PREVENTION

All women age >65 should be given a DEXA scan. Screening should begin at age 60 if there is low body weight or increased risk of fractures.

## PREVENTION OF ALCOHOL ABUSE

Physicians should screen for alcohol abuse by using the CAGE questionnaire:

- Have you ever felt the need to: Cut down on your drinking?
- Have you ever felt: Annoyed by criticism of your drinking?
- Have you ever felt: Guilty about your drinking?
- Have you ever taken a morning: Eye opener?

A positive screen is 2 "yes" answers. One "yes" should raise the possibility of alcohol abuse.

## PREVENTION OF VIOLENCE AND INJURY

Injuries are the most common cause of death age <65. The role of the physician is to advise patients about safety practices that can prevent injury.

- Wear seatbelts and bicycle helmets
- Do not drive after drinking alcohol
- Be aware of the risks that firearms pose in the home

Another essential role for the physician is to identify those at increased risk of physical or sexual abuse. Simply asking patients if they have been hit, kicked, or physically hurt can increase identification by more than 10%.

# Infectious Disease 2

## CASE 1

### Chief Complaint

Fever, cough, and chest pain of 5 days duration

### History and Physical Examination

A 32-year-old man comes to the emergency department with 5 days of fever, fatigue, shortness of breath, a cough productive of bloody sputum, and pleuritic chest pain. He is an active IV drug user and last used drugs yesterday. His past medical history is significant for skin abscesses. He uses no prescription drugs and has no allergies. A COVID test is performed and is negative. Blood pressure is 112/72 mm Hg, pulse 110/min, respirations 22/min, and temperature 39 C (102.2 F).

He is a thin, weak-appearing man. Examination of the head, eyes, ears, nose, and throat shows no evidence of petechiae in the mouth or on the conjunctivae. Funduscopic examination is unremarkable. On chest auscultation there are rhonchi and wheezes throughout both lung fields. A 2/6 systolic ejection murmur is audible over the lower left sternal border. There is no radiation of the murmur. The abdomen is benign, extremities have no clubbing, and the fingernails/hands appear normal.

### Differential Diagnosis

1. MRSA bacteremia
2. Infective endocarditis (IE)
3. Tuberculosis
4. Strep pneumonia

#### NOTE

Management is not yet clear for the **COVID-19** virus, an infectious disease caused by a newly discovered coronavirus. Therefore, questions about COVID are unlikely to be seen on the exam at this time.

- Symptoms can include fever, loss of taste or smell, cough, and shortness of breath, possibly leading to pneumonia.
- Testing is PCR (best) or antigen-testing; chest x-ray (will show interstitial pneumonia mostly when it affects the lungs), and inflammatory markers (very elevated).
- Treatment, while not yet definitive, should include respiratory isolation and anti-inflammatories such as steroids early in the course. Monoclonal antibody therapy has shown promise.
- Prevention is best achieved with vaccination.

**CCS NOTE**

For the CCS be organized, address the chief complaint and stabilize the patient by addressing any abnormal vital signs first. In this case, make sure the heart (with an abnormal rate) is monitored on a monitor bed or EKG.

### Initial Management

**Setting**: emergency department

### Diagnostic/Therapeutic Plan

- EKG and monitor bed
- Chest x-ray
- Blood cultures

### Test Results

- Chest x-ray: multiple nodular opacities are visible bilaterally
- Blood cultures from peripheral sites, aerobic and anaerobic: results pending

### Assessment

An IV drug user will be at increased risk of methicillin-resistant staph aureus (MRSA), which can cause skin abscess, endocarditis, pneumonia, and even osteomyelitis and septic arthritis. Suspect endocarditis in anyone with a fever and a murmur; blood cultures will be necessary. Furthermore, complaints of cough productive of bloody sputum plus fever with pleuritic chest pain in an IV drug user are suggestive of a typical pneumonia.

Due to the acute presentation here, TB and malignancies are less likely in the differential diagnosis. When pneumonia is considered, only the typical pneumonias have pleuritic chest pain (because they affect the pleura), e.g., *S. pneumoniae*, *S. aureus*, *K. pneumoniae*, *H. influenzae*. In contrast, the atypical (non-typical) pneumonias affect the interstitial space only (do not affect the pleura and are not associated with pleuritic chest pain).

Diagnosis of IE requires use of the modified Duke criteria: 2 major and 1 minor criterion **OR** 1 major and 3 minor criteria **OR** 5 minor criteria.

- **Two major criteria**: positive blood culture and imaging showing endocardial involvement with vegetations
- **Five minor criteria**
  - Major risk factor, eg, IVDU
  - Fever >38 C (100.4 F)
  - Embolic phenomena including septic pulmonary embolization, Janeway lesions, or conjunctival hemorrhages
  - Osler nodes, Roth spots, or a positive rheumatoid factor
  - Blood cultures growing organism normally not causing endocarditis

**Acute endocarditis**, as the name suggests, is usually acute in onset. It is commonly caused by MRSA and mostly affects the right side of the heart. The vegetations—caused by staph—are very large and usually only embolize to the lungs. They will not cause the typical findings of microembolization seen in subacute endocarditis.

**Subacute endocarditis** is caused by an organism such as strep, which entering the body (e.g., through a contaminated procedure such as gingival manipulation) can seed previously damaged valves (usually valves affected by conditions like rheumatic fever, which mostly involve the left-sided valves). Subacute endocarditis produces microscopic embolization, and thus you will see the typical Roth spots in the retina, Osler's nodes (pain in the palms of the hands), Janeway lesions, and splinter hemorrhage on the fingernails—none of which this patient has.

### Further Management Plan/Results

- **Lab results**: blood cultures positive for *Staphylococcus aureus*, antibiotic susceptibility pending
- **Transthoracic echocardiogram (TTE):** vegetation visible on tricuspid valve with tricuspid regurgitation
- **EKG**: sinus tachycardia is seen but otherwise is unremarkable

### Further Management

- Empiric antibiotic (something that covers MRSA such as vancomycin) until the sensitivities are back reporting any other organism; then, adjust the antibiotic at that time (take 3 sets of blood cultures before starting the antibiotics)
- TTE: if positive, nothing further needed for diagnosis but if negative, transesophageal echocardiogram (TEE) which is much more sensitive; further evaluation by TEE may be needed for those with significant valvular regurgitation (to determine need for surgery) and those with ≥1 risk factors for perivalvular abscess (including new conduction delay on EKG, aortic valve endocarditis, and persistent bacteremia/fever despite appropriate antimicrobial therapy). IV antibiotic (e.g., nafcillin or oxacillin) for 4–6 weeks, with gentamicin for first week if it is methicillin-sensitive
- Possible surgical replacement of valve if there is acute decompensation, myocardial abscess, repeated emboli, very large vegetations, fungal endocarditis, or prosthetic valve endocarditis

### Discussion

*S. aureus* accounts for 60–90% of endocarditis in IV drug abusers, and, depending on local conditions, a large percentage of this may be methicillin-resistant. A large portion of *S. aureus* endocarditis cases are attributed to health care–associated bacteremia. Empiric therapy for IE includes:

- **Community-acquired native valve IE**: vancomycin plus gentamicin
- **Nosocomial-associated IE**: vancomycin, gentamicin, rifampin, and an antipseudomonal beta-lactam (i.e., cefepime, meropenem)
- **Prosthetic valve IE**: vancomycin, gentamycin, rifampin

**Native valve subacute endocarditis** is typically caused by *Streptococci.*

- *Viridans streptococci* (normal inhabitants of the mouth) (75% of cases)
- *Streptococcus bovis* and *Clostridium septicum* (20% of cases) (associated with neoplastic diseases of the colon)
- Staphylococci (30% of cases, most *S. aureus*)
- Enterococci (5–10% of cases)

**Culture-negative endocarditis** is caused by the HACEK organisms.

- *Haemophilus* (*Haemophilus parainfluenzae*), (*Haemophilus aphrophilus*), (*Haemophilus paraphrophilus*)
- *Actinobacillus*
- *Cardiobacterium hominis*
- *Eikenella corrodens*
- *Kingella* (*Kingella kingae*)

However, studies have found that the HACEK organisms can be easily isolated with current blood culture systems when incubated for at least 5 days.

**Prosthetic valve endocarditis** is typically caused by *Staphylococci* in the early postoperative period. *Staphylococcus epidermidis* is more common in the first 2 mos after the replacement.

Complications of endocarditis include CHF (most common cause of death); embolic phenomena (seen in 25% of patients within 1 week of treatment); abscess/mycotic aneurysm/abscess; renal infarction/abscess; splenomegaly; valvular degeneration; and glomerulonephritis if not treated.

The blood culture results for this patient eventually confirm methicillin-sensitive *S. aureus* (MSSA). Treatment is nafcillin (or oxacillin or cefazolin) for 4-6 weeks. Gentamicin or another aminoglycoside is often added for the first 5 days; these are bactericidal and must be used over vancomycin if the organism is methicillin-sensitive.

- For native valve subacute endocarditis due to a sensitive *S. viridans*, penicillin G or ceftriaxone for 4 weeks alone is often sufficient. Alternatively, use gentamicin plus either aqueous crystalline penicillin G or ceftriaxone for 2 weeks, in the absence of renal insufficiency.
- For *Enterococcus*, use a beta-lactam antibiotic such as penicillin or ampicillin, plus an aminoglycoside (gentamicin or streptomycin) for the entire 4-6 weeks.
- For HACEK organisms, use ceftriaxone, ampicillin-sulbactam, or ciprofloxacin for 4 weeks.
- For Q fever endocarditis, use hydroxychloroquine plus doxycycline.
- For an urticarial rash to vancomycin or vancomycin MIC >2, use daptomycin to treat right-sided MRSA endocarditis.
- Surgery is indicated under the following conditions:
  - Evidence of uncontrolled infection (can mean persistence of positive blood cultures while already on therapy, recurrent emboli formation of myocardial or valvular ring abscesses, or spread of infection to involve the conduction system of the heart)
  - Acute heart failure (can indicate degeneration of the valves, papillary muscles, or chordae tendineae sufficient to cause evidence of CHF)
  - Valvular regurgitation
  - Recurrent embolic event while on antibiotics

Antibiotic prophylaxis is recommended for IE under the following conditions (**high-yield**):

- Prosthetic cardiac valve or prosthetic material used in valve repair
- Previous endocarditis
- Congenital heart disease
- Unrepaired cyanotic heart disease
- Cardiac transplantation with cardiac valvular disease
- Post-prosthesis surgery or surgical repair of a congenital heart disease (for 6 months, since endothelialization of prosthetic material occurs within that time period)
- Unepithelialized prosthetic patch or prosthetic device
- Manipulation of gingival tissue or periapical region of the teeth or perforation of oral mucosa
- Incision or biopsy of the respiratory tract mucosa (bronchial biopsy, tonsillectomy, and adenoidectomy)

When giving antibiotic prophylaxis, give 2 hours before the procedure (and possibly 2 hours after the procedure). Medications include amoxicillin (PO) (**preferred**) or ampicillin (IV) (alternates include clindamycin, azithromycin, and ceftriaxone/cefazolin (IM/IV).

## Final Diagnosis

Acute bacterial endocarditis

### Basic Science Correlate

- *Streptococcus viridans* (**most common organism to cause endocarditis**) is a low-virulence organism that infects previously damaged valves (MVP or chronic rheumatic heart disease because of valve scarring). Subacute endocarditis is typically associated with small vegetations that do not destroy the valve.
- *Staphylococcus aureus* is a high virulence organism associated with IV drug use. It results in large vegetations, which rapidly destroy the valve.
- *Staphylococcus epidermidis* is associated with endocarditis of prosthetic valves within 2 months after surgery.
- *Streptococcus bovis* is associated with colorectal cancer.

**CLINICAL PEARL**

Start empiric antibiotics for all presumed infections after cultures have been drawn. The best antibiotics for MSSA are oxacillin, nafcillin, and cefazolin.

**NOTE**

Q fever is a mild atypical pneumonia in patients exposed to livestock (e.g., farmers, large animal veterinarians, and slaughterhouse workers). Consider Q fever endocarditis in those who had Q fever from 2 months to 2 years after acute Q fever.

**CLINICAL PEARL**

In chronic rheumatic heart disease, the mitral valve is almost always involved. It leads to mitral stenosis, and gives patients a "fish-mouth" appearance. Patients are often immigrants from low-income countries.

**CLINICAL PEARL**

Libman-Sacks endocarditis is due to sterile vegetations, which arise in association with SLE. Vegetations are present on and under the surface of the mitral valve and result in mitral regurgitation. (Think of this in a young female with rash, joint pain, and MR without fever.)

# CASE 2

## Chief Complaint

Pain and swelling of left leg

## History and Physical Examination

A 72-year-old man with a history of prostatic cancer metastatic to bone and the lymphatic system comes to the emergency department because of a several-day history of increasing swelling and erythema of left leg from the knee down. He denies shortness of breath or chest pain. The patient feels warm. His T is 38.4 C (101.1 F).

Physical examination reveals a left leg that is swollen and erythematous below the knee, moderately tender and warm to touch; there is no palpable fluid collection or skin breakdown.

## Differential Diagnosis

1. Cellulitis
2. Deep venous thrombosis
3. Lymphangitis

## Initial Management

**Setting:** outpatient or emergency department

## Diagnostic/Therapeutic Plan

- Duplex U/S scan of venous system of the leg

## Test Results

- No evidence of thrombosis

## Assessment

With a unilateral red, tender, warm, swollen leg without evidence of deep venous thrombosis, cellulitis is the most likely possibility. No further diagnostic tests are required. The primary means of diagnosing cellulitis is by clinical examination and history.

Venography is **not the first test** to exclude a thrombosis, even though it is slightly more sensitive and specific than U/S. This is because of the risk of renal toxicity in the older adult or allergic reaction from exposure to the required contrast agent. Venogram is done if the suspicion for a clot is very high and U/S is negative.

**CCS NOTE**

A specific microbiologic diagnosis is almost never obtained in the clinical management of a skin infection. Treatment is empiric.

Specific microbiologic diagnosis is not routinely indicated. This is sometimes done in unresponsive cases by injecting a small amount of saline subcutaneously into the leading edge of the infection. Then, aspirate and send the sample for culture.

### Treatment Plan

1. IV antibiotics with oxacillin or nafcillin
2. Elevation of leg and warm soaks
3. Oral dicloxacillin (mild cases); if mild penicillin allergy such as rash, use oral cephalexin; if life-threatening penicillin allergy such as anaphylaxis, use clindamycin, macrolides, and new fluoroquinolones

### Discussion

The most likely organisms in cellulitis are group A streptococci (*S. pyogenes*) and *S. aureus*.

- Mild infections can be treated in the outpatient setting with oral dicloxacillin or oral cephalosporins.
- For moderate cellulitis or cellulitis that does not resolve with oral treatment, a first-generation IV cephalosporin such as cefazolin or cephalexin is appropriate.
- In cases of severe penicillin allergy (e.g., anaphylaxis), vancomycin or clindamycin is used.
- Rates of cross-reaction between penicillin and cephalosporins are <5%. For reactions that were originally just a rash, cephalosporins are safe to use.
- Antibiotics are continued until symptoms have resolved. Duration of treatment varies depending on how long it takes to improve.
- Vancomycin cannot be used orally to treat cellulitis because it is not absorbed.

The magnitude of CA-MRSA infections has reached epidemic proportions in the United States. Certain risk factors put some groups at higher risk:

- Household contacts of patients with proven CA-MRSA infection
- Children
- Men who have sex with men (MSM)
- Injection drug users
- Athletes engaged in contact sports
- Certain racial and ethnic groups such as Native Americans and Pacific Islanders

However, most patients with MRSA have none of these risk factors.

Surgical drainage, along with incision of abscess and deeper infection, is crucial for adequate treatment.

### CLINICAL PEARL

Cellulitis with abscess formation or purulent drainage is most likely MRSA. In recent years there has been a dramatic increase in skin and soft-tissue (and other site) infections due to community-acquired strains of MRSA. Unlike hospital-associated isolates of MRSA, patients with CA-MRSA infection are relatively young and healthy, having had no recent contact with the health care system.

Antibiotics guidelines are as follows:

- **Severe, invasive infection that requires IV antibiotics as inpatient**: vancomycin (**preferred**), daptomycin, ceftaroline, tigecycline, telavancin, or linezolid
- **Mild infection**: empiric oral antibiotic, e.g., trimethoprim-sulfamethoxazole, doxycycline, or linezolid (if cultures are sensitive, use clindamycin)
- **Small abscess with no surrounding erythema**: no antibiotics needed

Antibiotics are also indicated for the following:

- Patients who are very young/older adult or who have multiple infection sites, systemic illness/comorbidity/immunosuppression
- Infection that quickly progresses and is associated with concomitant cellulitis
- Abscess that does not respond well to incision/drainage or is too difficult to drain

### Final Diagnosis

Cellulitis

# CASE 3

## Chief Complaint

Right leg pain

## History and Physical Examination

A 45-year-old woman presents to the emergency department with 2 days of severe right lower extremity pain and swelling. The pain has been getting progressively worse and is now so intense that she cannot walk on her leg. The pain started over the shin and has now spread rapidly from the ankle to just below the knee. She is currently in extreme pain. She also complains of fevers. She has a past medical history of type 2 diabetes and is non-compliant. The diabetes is poorly controlled and her last Hb A1C about 1 year ago was 10%.

Physical examination reveals T 103° F, pulse 120/min, and BP 100/50 mm Hg. She is diaphoretic, lethargic, and toxic-appearing. The lungs are clear. Cardiac exam is normal except for tachycardia. Her right lower extremity shows tense edema with erythema and dark purple bullae expanding from the ankle to the knee. Warmth and tenderness are noted.

## Differential Diagnosis

1. Cellulitis
2. Deep venous thrombosis
3. Necrotizing fasciitis

## Clues

- History and physical exam findings are very concerning for necrotizing fasciitis.
- Extreme pain and tense edema with dark bullae with fevers and systemic toxicity on examination are very worrisome for necrotizing fasciitis.

## Initial Management

**Setting:** emergency department

## Diagnostic/Therapeutic Plan

- CBC
- Lactic acid
- Chemistry profile
- Immediate surgical debridement (consult surgery); if there is clinical suspicion and physical exam is consistent with diagnosis, patient can be sent to operating room without imaging
- Broad spectrum IV antibiotics

### Test Results

- CBC: WBC 30,000 cells/mL, segments 90%, Hb 10 mg/dL, platelets 100,000
- Lactate: 8.2 mmol/L
- Chemistry profile: bicarbonate 12 mmol/L, glucose 400 mg/dL, creatinine 2.5 mg/dL, BUN 35 mg/dL

### Assessment

This presentation is consistent with necrotizing fasciitis. The patient has poorly controlled diabetes with a very serious skin and soft tissue infection that is rapidly progressing.

Cellulitis involves the skin and subcutaneous tissue. Patients with cellulitis very rarely have high fever or leukocytosis. If a cellulitis spreads rapidly or has tense edema or discoloration or blister formation, one must consider necrotizing fasciitis. If the PE is uncertain, CT may be helpful by showing gas formation, though clinical judgment is still the most important element in diagnosis.

The gold standard for diagnosis is tissue biopsy obtained during surgical exploration. Nothing else can rule out the diagnosis.

- Best initial management is early aggressive surgical exploration and debridement of necrotic tissue, together with broad spectrum empiric antibiotic therapy and hemodynamic support
- Surgery is indicated in the setting of severe pain, toxicity, fever, and elevated serum creatine kinase, with or without radiographic evidence of fasciitis
- Antibiotic therapy without debridement is associated with mortality rate approaching 100%
- Aggressive supportive care with IV fluids and vasopressors may be needed for hemodynamic instability

### Further Diagnostic Testing

- CT (or plain x-ray) shows gas formation in different areas of the right leg, as well as swelling and necrosis of various muscle groups

#### Basic Science Correlate

Necrotizing fasciitis is a destruction of the fascia and muscle through the release of toxins (virulence factors), which include streptococcal pyogenic exotoxins. Most cases are polymicrobial including anaerobes and aerobes. Common organisms include group A streptococcus (*Streptococcus pyogenes*), *staphylococcus aureus*, *clostridium perfringens*, *Bacteroides fragilis*, and *Aeromonas*.

- Clindamycin inhibits production of exotoxins by binding to and inhibiting the 50S subunit of the bacterial ribosome.
- Penicillin inhibits the formation of peptidoglycan cross-links in the bacterial cell wall. Its 4-membered $\beta$-lactam ring binds to the enzyme DD-transpeptidase. As a consequence, DD-transpeptidase cannot catalyze formation of these cross-links, and an imbalance between cell wall production and degradation develops, causing the cell to rapidly die.

### Discussion

Necrotizing fasciitis has a high mortality. Clinical judgment is still the most important element in diagnosis. Signs include:

- Tense edema
- Grayish, purplish, or other discolored wound drainage
- Vesicles or bullae
- Necrosis
- Ulcers
- Crepitus

Pain may be out of proportion to findings.

CT or MRI finding may be helpful but may be non specific. Leukocytosis, thrombocytopenia, and elevated creatinine with lactic acidosis may also be seen. CT may show fascia edema and subcutaneous gas.

If the suspicion is there, immediate surgical exploration is the correct answer. The gold standard for diagnosis is tissue biopsy obtained during surgical exploration. Nothing else can rule out the diagnosis. Time-to-first-debridement and its adequacy are predictors of survival.

### Final Diagnosis

Necrotizing fasciitis

### CLINICAL PEARL

Any serious skin and soft tissue infection caused by group A streptococcus–specifically necrotizing fasciitis–is treated with immediate surgical debridement and penicillin with clindamycin. Most cases are caused by a mixed flora and require one of the following in addition to surgical debridement:

- Vancomycin, daptomycin, tigecycline, ceftaroline, or linezolid (to cover MRSA) **plus** (coverage for gram-negative, including pseudomonas **plus** anaerobes)
- Imipenem/meropenem
- Piperacillin/tazobactam
- Ticarcillin/clavulanate **plus** clindamycin for toxin production

*Clostridium perfringens* is a rare cause from deep stab wounds or black tar heroin abuse (skin popping is when people inject heroin into subcutaneous tissue). Treat with penicillin **plus** clindamycin.

# CASE 4

## Chief Complaint

Fever, headache, and neck stiffness for 3 days

## History and Physical Examination

A 34-year-old man HIV positive is brought to the emergency department by his roommate because of high fever, headache, and neck stiffness for the last 3 days. Since yesterday he has started to become confused. Currently his medications are bictegravir, tenofovir alafenamide and emtricitabine. His last CD4 count was 945 cells/mm3.

The patient appears muscular, lying on the stretcher with his hands over his eyes. His temperature is 38 C (104 F). Examination of head, eyes, ears, nose, and throat shows no papilledema. There is moderate nuchal rigidity and marked photophobia. Heart, lung, and abdominal examination are normal. He is oriented to place but gets confused with the time. He knows his own name and can recognize his roommate. There are no focal motor or sensory deficits. The Babinski reflex shows toes that are down-going.

## Differential Diagnosis

1. Cryptococcal meningitis
2. Tuberculous meningitis
3. *Neisseria meningitidis*
4. *Streptococcus pneumoniae*
5. Viral meningitis

## Initial Management

**Setting:** emergency department

## Diagnostic/Therapeutic Plan

- Empiric antibiotic and dexamethasone
- CT of the brain
- CSF culture

## Test Results

- CT of the brain: unremarkable with no evidence of mass-occupying lesions
- WBC 3,500/$mm^3$ with 95% neutrophils, negative Gram stain, elevated protein, decreased glucose
- CSF culture: *Streptococcus pneumoniae*

### Assessment

Looking at the presenting symptoms, it takes very little time to realize that headache, nuchal rigidity, and photophobia are classic signs of meningitis. In the differential diagnosis we have viral meningitis, bacterial meningitis, fungal meningitis, and tuberculous meningitis. Because of the duration of symptoms here of only 3 days, the patient has either bacterial or viral meningitis; these can be differentiated with a lumbar puncture (LP).

If the meningitis had lasted more than 10-14 days or was subacute, then conditions such as fungal or tuberculous meningitis should be considered. So the differential diagnosis can be narrowed down to *N. meningitidis* and *S. pneumoniae*.

Brain abscess is unlikely here. That usually presents with only focal neurological signs and symptoms, but because this patient is confused a brain CT is needed before an LP. (Brain CT is always needed with focal neurological deficits, immunocompromised patients, altered mental status, new onset of seizures, history of CNS disease, and papilledema.)

### Further Management Plan/Results

- Lumbar puncture

### Discussion

The timing of this patient's symptoms (only lasting 3 days) points toward a viral or bacterial origin to his meningitis. The only concerning symptom is his confusion, which required a CR of the brain to rule out mass-occupying lesions prior to doing an LP. Once the LP is done, focus on the nature of the liquid:

- Cloudy liquid indicates a high WBC >1000, and likely means a bacterial cause to the meningitis; in these cases, the differential will show mostly neutrophils (as in our case here).
- When WBC <1000 (especially when <500), the cause is a likely virus, fungus, or mycobacterial infection.

Next, look at the blood glucose. In this case the glucose is decreased, which means the process is consuming glucose. Viruses are the only organisms whose process does not lead to the consumption of glucose.

### CCS NOTE

Body fluid infections such as urine, CSF, and pleural effusion are initially diagnosed based on cell count, but because cultures are never available at the time a treatment decision must be made empiric therapy must be started. Because of the severe symptoms here plus a high CSF WBC count (most likely neutrophils), give ceftriaxone and vancomycin until the culture results are known.

## Follow-up Management and Prevention

1. Initial empiric therapy is ceftriaxone and vancomycin until results of the sensitivities are known
2. If organism is penicillin-sensitive, change the antibiotic to penicillin or ampicillin
   - Corticosteroid (dexamethasone) therapy is now considered standard empiric therapy for most cases of bacterial meningitis; benefits are greatest in patients with pneumococcal meningitis, resulting in decreased morbidity (deafness) and mortality
   - Dexamethasone should be given immediately before, or with, the first dose of antibiotic and continued for 4 days
   - Steroids can be discontinued if etiology of meningitis turns out to be non-pneumococcal
3. Repeat lumbar puncture after a few days to ensure that infection has cleared; necessary only if prompt clinical resolution does not occur
4. Examine for otitis, mastoiditis, and sinusitis to try to identify the origin of the meningitis
5. For brain abscess, do surgical drainage PLUS empiric coverage with metronidazole AND ceftriaxone with or without vancomycin (polymicrobial, including anaerobes, most importantly, *B. fragilis*)
6. For post-neurosurgical or post-head traumatic patients, give vancomycin PLUS cefepime or meropenem or ceftazidime to cover MRSA and pseudomonas

## Final Diagnosis

Pneumococcal meningitis

### CLINICAL PEARL

Consider other types of meningitis:

**Cryptococcal Meningitis**

- History of HIV with $<100$ CD4 cells. India ink positive in 50–70%, antigen test positive in $>90\%$
- More gradual in onset, less severe
- Initial therapy with amphotericin and flucytosine, followed by 3 months of fluconazole until CD4 count $>100$/mm

**Rocky Mountain Spotted Fever**

- Rash on wrists and ankles that moves toward the body
- Confirm with serology specific for *Rickettsia*; treat with doxycycline until results of testing are known

**Lyme Disease**

- Endemic area such as the Northeast; history of rash
- Diagnose with positive enzyme-linked immunosorbent assay or Western blot; treat with ceftriaxone

# CASE 5

## Chief Complaint

"My belly is swollen, and it hurts."

## History and Physical Examination

A 59-year-old woman comes to the emergency room with 2 days of increasing abdominal pain and distension. She has a history of alcoholism and biopsy-proven cirrhosis of the liver. Her ascites had been controlled in the past with a low-sodium diet and spironolactone, but she has been noncompliant with her medications recently.

Vital signs are T 38.4 C (101.1 F), BP 105/70 mm Hg, and pulse 120/min. Physical examination shows a few spider angiomata visible on the face. Her extremities have a 2+ pitting edema in the legs to the mid-thigh. Her abdomen is moderately distended with the presence of a fluid wave; it is diffusely tender but soft. There is no guarding or rebound tenderness. The liver and spleen are not palpable secondary to the ascites. There are normal bowel sounds. The remainder of the physical examination is unremarkable.

## Differential Diagnosis

1. Spontaneous bacterial peritonitis
2. Secondary peritonitis (bowel perforation)
3. Pancreatitis
4. Cholangitis
5. Diverticulitis

## Initial Management

**Setting:** emergency department

| Initial Diagnostic Plan | Results |
|---|---|
| CBC | WBC 14,500/mm$^3$ with 77% polymorphonuclear leukocytes, platelets 118,000/mm$^3$ |
| Prothrombin time | 14.7 seconds (normal: <13 seconds) |
| Albumin | 2.7 g/dL (normal: 3.5–5 g/dL) |
| AST/ALT | Normal |
| Abdominal x-ray | No obstruction, no air-fluid levels |
| Chest x-ray | No infiltrates, no air under the diaphragm |

### Assessment

The ascites that accumulates from alcoholic cirrhosis is especially predisposed to spontaneous peritonitis. Spontaneous peritonitis presumably occurs from hematologic seeding in the absence of perforation of an abdominal organ or trauma, such as a knife wound. Although this patient's complaints (pain and distension) and physical exam (fever, tenderness) are clearly indicative of peritonitis, these findings do not have to be present for spontaneous bacterial peritonitis to occur. Ultimately, the only certain diagnostic method is a paracentesis of the ascitic fluid. Patients may also present with hepatic encephalopathy.

**CLINICAL PEARL**

The Gram stain is relatively specific if it is positive, but it lacks sensitivity and cannot exclude infection if it is negative. This is also true for the culture of the paracentesis fluid.

A paracentesis must be performed in new-onset ascites even in the absence of symptoms because spontaneous bacterial peritonitis can still be present. Criteria for diagnosis are a polymorphonuclear leukocyte count of >250/mm$^3$ or total WBC count >500/mm$^3$ in the ascitic fluid. The elevation of the prothrombin time and the decreased albumin are indicative of the decreased synthetic function of the liver with far advanced cirrhosis. The transaminases are normal because eventually the liver becomes so destroyed that the transaminases return to normal. If the ascitic fluid has very low glucose (<50 mg/dL), very high LDH or neutrophil count >10,000, or is polymicrobial, suspect secondary peritonitis and proceed to imaging.

| Further Diagnostic Plan | Results |
|---|---|
| Paracentesis | WBC count 750/mm$^3$ with 90% polymorphonuclear leukocytes<br>Culture yields *E. coli*<br>Fluid albumin 2.2 mg/dL |

### Treatment Plan

1. Antibiotics for gram-negative bacilli and *S. pneumoniae* (cefotaxime or ceftriaxone) **plus** infusion of IV albumin; in this case we know the cause is *E. coli*, but most cases are culture-negative, thus the need to cover *S. pneumoniae* with cephalosporins
2. Diuretics and repeated abdominal paracenteses to remove larger volumes of fluid if patient becomes uncomfortable or respiratory function is compromised

### Discussion

Although spontaneous bacterial peritonitis implies that all abdominal organs are intact, the most common organisms are the bowel flora. Most often it is caused by a single agent. Polymicrobial infections generally indicate perforation of a viscus. Aerobic gram-negative bacilli (*Enterobacteriaceae*) such as *E. coli* are the most common. Gram positives such as *S. pneumoniae*, group A streptococci (pyogenes), and enterococci are also common. It is caused by translocation of enteric bacteria across the bowel wall.

Studies have shown that giving IV albumin infusion on days 1 and 3 of antibiotic treatment increases the effective arterial circulating volume and renal perfusion, thus decreasing the incidence of hepatorenal syndrome and improving mortality.

IV cefotaxime has evolved as the drug of choice, however. Cefotaxime will cover *E. coli* as well as *S. pneumoniae*. Anaerobes are rarely the causative organism in spontaneous bacterial peritonitis. When a specific organism is identified, as with this patient, the choice depends upon the specific sensitivities of the organism.

### Prevention

Around 70% of patients who survive spontaneous bacterial peritonitis will have another episode within 1 year. Oral norfloxacin, ciprofloxacin, and trimethoprim-sulfamethoxazole have been shown to reduce the rate of recurrent infections to <20%. Therefore, any patient with a history of spontaneous bacterial peritonitis should take one of these agents for prophylaxis indefinitely.

When patients with cirrhosis have bleeding esophageal varices, they are at an increased risk of developing spontaneous bacterial peritonitis. Studies show that giving these patients ceftriaxone or ciprofloxacin for 1 week during the bleed reduces the risk. Therefore, during a variceal bleed, patients with cirrhosis should receive antibiotics, even if they do not have clinically apparent ascites.

### Final Diagnosis

Spontaneous bacterial peritonitis

## CASE 6

### Chief Complaint

"I'm here to see what medications I need."

### History and Physical Examination

A 47-year-old woman who has recently found that she is HIV-positive comes to your office for an initial evaluation. She has always been healthy and took the test only because an old boyfriend died of AIDS. She has no other medical problems and is currently on no medications.

Her only tests done so far are CD4 (T-cell) count 47 cells/mL (normal 600–1,200 cells/mL), polymerase chain reaction-RNA viral load 180,000 (normal <50 to >750,000), a genotype resistance test (pending), and PPD skin test with 8 mm in duration. She has no symptoms. Her last Pap smear was 4 years ago. Vital signs and examination, including pelvic examination, are normal.

**NOTE**

Genotype resistance testing is done at initial diagnosis to determine if resistance to antiviral therapy exists. It is used to select treatment medications.

### Initial Management

**Setting:** outpatient

### Diagnostic/Therapeutic Plan

- Rapid plasma reagin or venereal disease; normal research laboratory tests for syphilis
- *Toxoplasmosis* antibody test
- CBC
- Chemistries
- Pap smear
- Chest x-ray
- Hepatitis A, B, and C serology

### Test Results

- Rapid plasma reagin or venereal disease: normal
- *Toxoplasmosis* antibody test: normal
- CBC: normal
- Chemistries: normal
- Pap smear: normal
- Chest x-ray: normal
- Hepatitis A, B, and C serology: negative

### Assessment

All patients who present for initial evaluation of HIV should have a set of routine lab evaluation tests to determine the need for prophylactic medications and determine prognosis. T-cell subsets (CD4 count) are the primary indicator for the need to initiate antiretroviral therapy and for making decisions about prophylactic medications. CD4 count tells us what diseases the patient is at risk for now, and it is the major clinical marker of the immunocompetence of the patient.

Viral load testing tells us how aggressive a person's disease is, i.e., the magnitude of replication of the virus in the body. A high viral load implies a more aggressive disease in which the CD4 count will drop more rapidly. Viral load testing gives a numerical value to the amount of HIV in the patient's blood. Viral load is like a glucose level in a diabetic patient: Higher viral load implies the need for more medication. The viral load is the most important test to monitor response to therapy. The aim of therapy is to have an undetectable HIV viral load in the serum after 6–12 mos of therapy (<50 copies/μL).

The other routine tests in HIV—syphilis serology, toxoplasmosis serology, TB skin testing with PPD, and Pap smear—determine the likelihood of common opportunistic infections. This patient's PPD is considered positive because the induration is >5 mm in diameter (erythema without induration is not considered a positive test).

- Induration of ≥15 mm is considered positive for the general population that is at low risk of developing active TB
- Cutoff ≥5mm is considered for those patients at the highest risk of disease, e.g., HIV-positive patients, recent contact of TB patients, patients with fibrotic changes on chest x-ray consistent with prior disease, and organ transplant recipients or immunosuppressed patients.
- Cutoff ≥10 mm is used for those at intermediate risk of the disease, e.g., recent immigrants from endemic countries (within 5 years), health care personnel, injection drug users, mycobacteriology laboratory personnel, children age <4, and infants/children/adolescents exposed to adults with active TB

| **Further Diagnostic Plan** | **Results** |
|---|---|
| Repeat viral load testing | 150,000 |

Guidelines recommend Tb screening be repeated in those with HIV, when CD4 count >200.

### Treatment Plan

1. *Pneumocystis jirovecii* (formerly *carinii*) pneumonia prophylaxis with trimethoprim/sulfamethoxazole
2. Antiretroviral therapy with 2 nucleosides and either 1 protease inhibitor (PI) or a non-nucleoside reverse transcriptase inhibitor (NNRTI)
3. Isoniazid plus rifampin or rifapentine for 3 months for latent TB; vitamin B6 only for high-risk patients (DM, alcoholics, malnourished, CKD, HIV)
4. Pneumococcal pneumonia vaccination
5. Hepatitis A and B vaccination
6. Influenza vaccination yearly

*Mycobacterium avium complex* (MAC) prophylaxis is no longer recommended.

### Discussion

Pneumocystis pneumonia prophylaxis must be initiated in all patients with <200 CD4 cells/mL. The most effective therapy is trimethoprim/sulfamethoxazole. If the patient is allergic to sulfa drugs, dapsone or atovaquone may be used as an alternative. Aerosolized pentamidine is only used in patients who cannot tolerate either trimethoprim/sulfamethoxazole or dapsone. Pentamidine is less efficacious than trimethoprim/sulfamethoxazole, dapsone, or atovaquone and is rarely used. For treatment of pneumocystis in patients with sulfa allergy, the options include IV pentamidine, clindamycin with primaquine, or atovaquone. Pentamidine has many side effects, including hypoglycemia, hyperglycemia, acute pancreatitis, ATN, and hepatotoxicity.

MAC prophylaxis is indicated in all patients with <50 CD4 cells/mL, using azithromycin or clarithromycin. (Azithromycin is taken only 1x/week so is easier than clarithromycin, which is taken 2x/day.) Rifabutin is the least effective option and has many side effects, such as uveitis. Additionally, rifabutin has numerous interactions with other medications that are metabolized through the hepatic p450 system. MAC treatment is a macrolide with ethambutol, with or without rifabutin.

- Antiretroviral therapy initiation is now recommended with the diagnosis of HIV irrespective of CD4 count.
- In pregnancy, always treat with combination therapy, even if CD4 >500, to prevent perinatal transmission. Start treatment immediately, i.e., do not wait for second trimester, and always use at least 3 drugs.
- Never use efavirenz in pregnancy.
- Give the baby zidovudine during delivery and for 6 weeks after.

The starting regimen is a combination of 2 nucleoside medications and at least 1 protease inhibitor **or** a non-nucleoside reverse transcriptase inhibitor (NNRTI).

- Nucleoside medications: zidovudine, lamivudine, abacavir, didanosine, emtricitabine, stavudine, DDC, tenofovir
- Protease inhibitors: indinavir, ritonavir, nelfinavir, saquinavir, amprenavir, lopinavir/ritonavir, fosamprenavir, atazanavir, tipranavir, darunavir
- NNRTIs: efavirenz, etravirine rilpivirine, nevirapine

**NOTE**

All of the protease inhibitors end in *-navir.*

**CLINICAL PEARL**

HIV patients with CD4 count >200 can get any vaccination.

The **most common regimen** for therapy today is emtricitabine-tenofovir or abacavir-lamivudine + an integrase inhibitor.

If there is resistance to first-line agents, use a second-line agent: integrase inhibitor raltegravir, entry inhibitors, enfuvirtide (penetration), or maraviroc (attachment).

Most **protease inhibitors** are now **boosted** with ritonavir, another protease inhibitor. Ritonavir by itself is not an effective antiretroviral because of poor efficacy and side effects. However, when given in low doses with other protease inhibitors, it boosts serum levels by inhibiting patients' metabolism by inhibiting on the cytochrome P450 system. This allows for higher serum levels of the boosted protease inhibitor, which decreases the probability of the HIV virus developing resistance. In addition, a lower dose of the boosted protease inhibitor can be given, which decreases adverse effects and improves compliance, also contributing to the decreased likelihood of developing resistance.

HIV-positive patients should be treated at any age if their PPD is >5 mm in size. The usual length of therapy in an HIV-negative patient is 9 months. Patients with HIV are treated for 9 months as well. Pneumococcal vaccination is indicated for most patients with significantly compromised immune systems, such as HIV-positive patients. Vaccination is indicated whenever you encounter the patient, regardless of T-cell count.

Let's say a 19-year-old man is evaluated in the emergency department for a 10-day history of fever, cervical lymphadenopathy, malaise and fatigue, sore throat, headache, and nausea, but no vomiting, diarrhea, abdominal pain, nasal congestion, or cough. He had a rash a few days ago that has resolved. He is sexually active with both men and women and does not use condoms. What is the next step?

The next step is the HIV nucleic acid amplification test. These symptoms may represent infectious mononucleosis or syphilis, but this may also be acute HIV syndrome. It presents within 2–4 wks of infection and lasts for a few weeks. Symptoms usually resolve without treatment.

HIV nucleic acid amplification test is the test of choice. The ELISA/Western blot will be false negative at this point because antibodies have not yet formed.

### CCS NOTE

On the CCS, knowledge of preventive medicine in an ambulatory setting is more important than knowledge of complex exotic diseases. Similarly, knowing when to start prophylaxis in HIV is more important than knowing specific antiretrovirals.

### Final Diagnosis

Acquired immunodeficiency syndrome (AIDS)

#### Basic Science Correlate

Presumptive diagnosis is made with ELISA (sensitive, high false-positive rate and low threshold, **rule out** test); results are then confirmed with Western blot assay (specific, high false-negative rate and high threshold, **rule in** test).

- HIV PCR/viral load tests determine the amount of viral RNA in the plasma.
- ELISA/Western blot tests look for antibodies to viral proteins; these tests often are falsely negative in the first 1–2 months of HIV infection.

# CASE 7

## Chief Complaint

Elevated liver enzymes

## History and Physical Examination

A 39-year-old man with a history of IV drug use 20 years ago presents for evaluation of elevated liver enzymes. He offers no complaints and feels well. He has no history of anorexia, nausea or vomiting, malaise, fatigue, dark urine, or upper abdominal discomfort. He denies blood transfusions or alcohol intake. He denies light-colored stools. He is taking isoniazid for treatment of positive PPD.

During recent routine screening, the patient was told that he had elevated liver enzymes. His temperature is 37.4° C and BP 150/80 mm Hg. Physical examination shows no scleral icterus or jaundiced skin. The liver is non-palpable and non-tender; the spleen is not palpable. There is no right upper quadrant tenderness.

## Differential Diagnosis

1. Chronic viral hepatitis (B or C)
2. Drug-induced hepatitis
3. Autoimmune hepatitis
4. Choledocholithiasis
5. Fatty liver

| Initial Diagnostic Plan | Test Results |
| --- | --- |
| • LFTs | Bilirubin (total) 1.0 mg/dL;<br>AST (SGOT) 50 u/L (normal: 5–45 units);<br>ALT (SGPT) 150 u/L (normal: 5–45 units);<br>albumin 2.7 mg/dL (normal: 3.5–5.5 mg/dL) |
| • PT | 13.2 seconds (normal: <13 seconds) |
| • CBC | Normal |

### Assessment

This patient has elevated liver enzymes, which have many causes. Alcohol is not a likely factor because the ratio of AST:ALT is not 2:1.

Acute hepatitis is not likely because the patient is asymptomatic and has mildly elevated transaminases. Symptoms of acute hepatitis include malaise, anorexia, jaundice, abdominal pain/tenderness (they are all identical). In acute viral hepatitis, transaminases would be very high (1000-3000 u/L).

Hepatitis B and C are characterized occasionally by extrahepatic manifestations such as rash, arthralgias, glomerulonephritis, cryoglobulinemia (hepatitis C), and polyarteritis nodosa (hepatitis B) in a small number of cases.

Drug-induced or toxin-induced hepatic injury, such as from the patient's isoniazid or other medications, is also indistinguishable from acute viral hepatitis. Acetaminophen, halothane, alpha-methyldopa, erythromycin, and allopurinol are among the most common causes of drug-induced hepatitis, but in those cases the transaminases would be >3000 u/L. Wilson disease, hemochromatosis, primary biliary cirrhosis, and autoimmune hepatitis are other forms that can often only be distinguished by a liver biopsy, and the transaminases are much higher in autoimmune hepatitis.

The initial step for determining the cause is to check hepatitis serologies. CT scan offers little help. MRI scan shows increased iron, and sonography shows fat infiltration.

This patient needs a workup for chronic hepatitis that includes transferrin saturation for hemochromatosis, hepatitis serologies, anti-smooth muscle, and anti-LKM for autoimmune hepatitis. Wilson's is less likely due to the absence of CNS symptoms.

### Further Diagnostic Plan/Results

Hepatitis serologies:

- **Hepatitis A**: IgM and IgG negative
- **Hepatitis B**: anti-HB core: IgM negative anti-HB core: IgG positive: HBsAg positive; HBe Ag-positive; anti-HBs antibody-negative
- **Hepatitis C**: Ab negative
- **HBV DNA**: high

### Treatment Plan

Tenofovir. (Lamivudine is no longer used first line, due to high rates of resistance. Tenofovir and entecavir are newer, preferred agents with lower rates of resistance.)

Because patients with chronic hepatitis B can progress to cirrhosis, assess for liver fibrosis; if cirrhosis develops, assess for hepatocellular carcinoma.

## Discussion

This patient has chronic active hepatitis B.

- **Hepatitis A** is diagnosed with serology; a positive serology indicates acute or past infection. Acute hepatitis A is diagnosed with a positive HAV IgM positive, and chronic hepatitis A is diagnosed with a positive HAV IgG, neither of which this patient had positive therefore hepatitis A can be ruled out.
- **Hepatitis B (HB)** is slightly more complex. There are 3 antigens to consider.
    - **HBsAg (surface antigen)** which, if present, indicates active disease. The presence of antibodies to HBsAg or HBsAb indicates that the patient is immune.
    - **HBcAg (core antigen)** is used to determine the timing of the disease; the patient will always develop antibodies to this antigen. The presence of IgM antibodies indicates a recent or acute hepatitis B, but the presence of IgG indicates chronic or remote hepatitis B.
    - **HBeAg (envelop antigen)** indicates that the virus can easily invade other cells of the liver and can progress to cirrhosis or hepatocellular carcinoma.
    - The goal of treatment is to convert patients who are HBeAg-positive to HBe antibody-positive which confers the patient protection from cirrhosis or hepatocellular carcinoma. Now having antibodies to the envelope does not mean that the patient is less infectious to others, as others do not have antibodies to the envelope and the virus and easily replicate on them and cause hepatitis B infection.
- **Hepatitis C** treatment no longer involves interferon as a first line agent, as there are good nucleoside/nucleotide analogs that work well for hepatitis B such as tenofovir and entecavir.

Hepatitis A differs from hepatitis B in that it is acquired via oral ingestion of contaminated food or water, and only causes acute infection in the immunocompetent host. Hepatitis B is spread via sexual contact and blood-borne through contaminated needles and close contact with a hepatitis B patient. Hepatitis B also can be chronic, not usually the case for hepatitis A.

Treatment for chronic hepatitis B is indicated under either of the following conditions:

- Hep Be Ag is positive and ALT is elevated and DNA viral load >20,000 IU/mL
- Hep Be Ag is negative and ALT is elevated and DNA viral load >2,000 IU/mL

Never treat if ALT is normal. Treatment is tenofovir or entecavir, with interferon only as a second-line choice.

Chronic hepatitis C is the most common cause of cirrhosis and hepatoma in the United States. It is transmitted via exposure to blood and blood products. Diagnosis is done with a positive HC antibody test. Once an antibody test is positive, the next step in management is to obtain an HC viral load. If the viral load is positive, then obtain a genotype and resistant panel. (The genotype will help in selecting the appropriate antiviral.)

Many antivirals exist now that obviate the need for interferon; the antivirals are combination drugs, which used together, produce a cure rate of over 90%. Many regimens exist, and they are chosen based on the patient's genotype; they are available usually for patients without prior treatment for hepatitis C.

For treatment-naïve patients, the most recent recommended regimen is combglecaprevir/ pibrentasvir or sofosbuvir/velpatasvir for 8-12 weeks, sufficient to obtain a cure in most patients. Other regimens exist for patients who have cirrhosis, and these regimens vary on the genotype of the patient but all genotypes can use the combination regimen of glecaprevir/ pibrentasvir for 8 weeks.

- If PCR-RNA viral load is elevated, patients should be treated.
- If the liver biopsy shows fibrosis, patients should receive immediate treatment to prevent progression to (irreversible) cirrhosis.

Acute hepatitis E is found mostly in Asia. It is particularly associated with increased severity in pregnant women. It has the same acute presentation as acute hepatitis A and B.

### CCS NOTE

As you advance the clock, you can use the "INTERVAL HISTORY" button at the top of the physical examination screen to give you a progress report on the patient.

### Final Diagnosis

Chronic hepatitis B

# CASE 8

## Chief Complaint

"I've had a pain in my leg for the last several weeks."

## History and Physical Examination

A 54-year-old man with a history of diabetes mellitus and peripheral vascular disease comes to your office with an ulcer on his left leg below the knee for the last week. He has been on aspirin alone as treatment for his peripheral vascular disease for several years and has a stable pattern of leg claudication after he walks more than several blocks or a few flights of stairs. He has had ulcerations of the skin on his legs intermittently for several years, which have all resolved with local care. Generally, these ulcerations have not been painful. The area at the site of the ulcer has been painful for the last 2 weeks.

Vital signs are T 37.4 C (99.3 F), BP 130/80 mm Hg, and pulse 72/min. He appears to be pleasant and in no distress. Examination of the extremities shows a 3-cm ulceration on the medial surface of proximal left tibia. The area is erythematous, mildly swollen, and tender with a small sinus tract that drains a tiny amount of purulent material. The remainder of the physical examination is normal.

## Differential Diagnosis

1. Aseptic ulceration
2. Osteomyelitis
3. Cellulitis
4. Skin abscess

### CCS NOTE

The CCS values an orderly and sequential evaluation over a jump straight to a single most accurate diagnostic test.

- When patient is short of breath, do chest x-ray before chest CT.
- When patient has leg ulcer, do x-ray before bone scan or MRI, even if the x-ray comes back negative.

## Initial Management

**Setting**: outpatient; emergency department if symptoms are severe

## Diagnostic/Therapeutic Plan

- Plain x-rays of leg
- ESR
- CBC

### Test Results

- X-rays of leg normal
- ESR elevated at 90 mm/h (normal <20 mm/h)
- CBC normal

### Assessment

This patient is at increased risk of infection because of the poor circulation from his peripheral vascular disease. Diabetes gives a similar risk. Other risks for osteomyelitis also include bacteremia from any source with seeding of the bone, although this is more common in children, and the presence of a prosthetic device (e.g., total knee replacement).

An overlying ulceration and cellulitis can often be difficult to tell apart from an underlying osteomyelitis. This patient's symptoms are worse than usual with his ulcers in the past. In addition, the area is tender with a draining sinus tract, which is more consistent with osteomyelitis. The ESR is also quite elevated, which is consistent with osteomyelitis as well.

A normal x-ray of the bone does not rule out osteomyelitis; it can take many weeks for it to become abnormal because >50% of the bone must become demineralized first. A technetium bone scan is more sensitive and will detect an osteomyelitis after several days. However, an overlying infection can obscure the definitive diagnosis, and CT or MRI is superior for localizing the infection to the bone itself. CT or MRI is also superior for identifying the precise amount of bony destruction. MRI is superior to CT in terms of sensitivity. The MRI becomes abnormal within 2 days after the onset of osteomyelitis. This is equal in sensitivity to bone scan but with far greater specificity. MRI is excellent at distinguishing bone involvement from overlying soft tissue infection. Bone biopsy prior to starting antibiotics is mandatory to identify a specific organism.

#### CCS NOTE

The status of your patient can come up spontaneously as a "nurse's note," telling you how the patient is doing. You can't predict when this will happen. These notes come up spontaneously as the clock is moved forward.

| Further Diagnostic Plan | Results |
|---|---|
| MRI scan of the leg | Mild bony destruction of the proximal tibia |
| Biopsy of the tibia | Neutrophils visible on Gram stain, *S. aureus* grows in culture |

### Treatment Plan

1. IV antibiotics for 6–12 wks; oxacillin or nafcillin if the organism is sensitive, vancomycin if it is MRSA
2. Surgical debridement as necessary

## Discussion

The most common organism causing osteomyelitis is still *S. aureus*. In diabetics or in osteomyelitis contiguous to decubitus ulcers, gram-negative bacilli such as *E. coli* or *Pseudomonas* are also common.

Bone biopsy is essential because there is no other definitive way to know the specific agent causing the infection. Culture of the wound or draining sinus tract does not correlate well with the organism causing the bone infection. Empiric treatment should be discouraged.

Oxacillin (or nafcillin) and ciprofloxacin or oxacillin and a third-generation cephalosporin are adequate empiric treatment before knowing the results of the bone biopsy. Vancomycin to cover the gram-positive organisms can be used if the patient has had an anaphylactic reaction to penicillin. Cephalosporins can be used if the penicillin allergy is only a rash. Other options for empiric osteomyelitis therapy before knowing the results of bone biopsy are carbapenems or the beta lactam/beta lactamase combinations, such as piperacillin/tazobactam or ampicillin/sulbactam.

Biopsy is essential because gram-negative osteomyelitis can be treated with oral ciprofloxacin. You cannot adequately treat the patient without the biopsy.

## Final Diagnosis

Acute osteomyelitis

# CASE 9

## Chief Complaint

Fever, cough, body aches, and chest pain

## History and Physical Examination

A 77-year-old man comes to the emergency department complaining of an episode of shaking chills earlier that night. He has since developed right-sided pleuritic chest pain, fever, sweats, malaise, and purulent sputum with mild hemoptysis. He has osteoarthritis, but his past medical history is otherwise unremarkable. He has smoked 1 pack of cigarettes per day for 30 years.

Vital signs are T 39.8 C (103.6 F), BP 90/60 mm Hg, pulse 106/min, and respirations 32/min. The patient is diaphoretic but alert. Lung examination reveals right basilar rales. Examination of skin, heart, joints, and nervous system are normal.

## Differential Diagnosis

1. Pneumococcal pneumonia (*Streptococcus* pneumonia)
2. *Legionella* pneumonia
3. *Haemophilus* pneumonia
4. Aspiration pneumonia
5. Tuberculosis
6. Postobstructive pneumonia from lung cancer
7. Bronchitis
8. *Mycoplasma* pneumonia

## Initial Management

**Setting**: emergency department

## Diagnostic/Therapeutic Plan

- Chest x-ray
- Sputum Gram stain
- Sputum culture
- Pulse oximeter
- CBC
- Blood culture (due to shaking chills, which suggest bacteremia)

### Test Results

- Chest x-ray: Right lower lobe, infiltrate with blunting of right costophrenic angle
- Sputum Gram stain: abundant polymorphonuclear leukocytes with gram-positive, lancet-shaped diplococci in pairs and chains
- Sputum culture: grows pneumococcus
- Pulse oximeter: 92% saturation
- CBC: WBCs 23,000/mm$^3$
- Blood culture: negative

**CCS NOTE**

For dyspneic patients, an oximeter is very accurate in the assessment of hypoxia. ABG is necessary when $CO_2$ retention is a possibility, as in COPD.

### Assessment

The history, physical examination, and chest x-ray confirm that this is pneumonia. To evaluate pneumonia, do the following:

- First, try to determine the most likely pathogen, and whether it is caused by a typical or nontypical organism. Typical organisms cause cough that is productive, oftentimes accompanied by pleuritic chest pain, while nontypical organisms do not. So that excludes a lot of organisms from our list of differential diagnosis, e.g., mycoplasma and legionella which are nontypical organisms.
- If the sputum does not reveal a specific organism, then bronchoscopy with biopsy can be done to confirm a specific bacteriologic diagnosis (but bronchoscopy is only necessary if there is no response to empiric therapy and the patient is worsening).

**CLINICAL PEARL**

Clinical improvement in pneumonia may not be apparent for up to 72 hours after the initiation of antibiotics. If there is no improvement after that time, potential issues include resistant organisms, metastatic foci, effusions, or non-infectious etiology. In this case, chest CT and possible bronchoscopy should be considered.

| Further Diagnostic Plan | Results |
|---|---|
| Decubitus x-rays of chest | Fluid in chest is free-flowing (i.e., presence of an effusion) |

### Treatment Plan

1. Ceftriaxone plus azithromycin or moxifloxacin or levofloxacin

### Discussion

Outpatient treatment of CAP is as follows:

- **Young and healthy with no comorbidities**: amoxicillin or doxycycline or macrolide (if local pneumococcal resistance to macrolides <25%)
- **Older adult or with comorbidities** (chronic heart, lung, liver, kidney disease, DM, alcoholism, asplenia, malignancy, immunosuppression, history of smoking): oral beta lactam (amoxicillin-clavulanate, cefuroxime, or cefpodoxime) plus macrolide or doxycycline OR monotherapy plus a respiratory fluoroquinolone
- **All patients with pneumonia**: check a nasal swab for influenza PCR in the winter and if positive, add oseltamivir to antibiotics (even after 48 hours of symptoms)

Inpatient treatment of CAP is as follows:

- Levofloxacin, moxifloxacin, or gatifloxacin
- Second- or third-generation cephalosporin such as cefotaxime or ceftriaxone plus a macrolide antibiotic, e.g., azithromycin, clarithromycin, doxycycline

**CCS NOTE**

- Admission criteria for pneumonia are based on the severity of the illness, not the x-ray findings. Culture results will not be given at the time you must make this triage decision.
- The regular hospital ward is the location for most pneumonia patients who are admitted. Choose the ICU only for the persistently hypoxic or hypotensive.

The Pneumonia Severity Index (PSI) (**preferred**) and CURB-65 are good prognostic tools for predicting mortality in those with CAP. They determine where a patient should be managed, i.e., outpatient, inpatient, or in the ICU. You will not have to calculate these scores on the exam.

- **PSI** score, calculated by medical apps, looks at factors such as comorbidities, vital signs, hypoxia, altered mental status, and labs. Patients with low risk factors (risk class I or II) are managed as outpatient. Risk class III is left up to the clinical team. Risk class IV or higher should be admitted.
- **CURB-65** gives 1 point for each positive indicator: confusion, BUN >19.6 mg/dL (7.0 mmol/L), RR ≥30/min, systolic BP <90 mm Hg or diastolic BP ≤60 mm Hg, and age ≥65. Score 0–1 likely indicates outpatient management; score ≥2 likely indicates hospitalization; and score ≥3 likely indicates the need for the ICU.

All older patients (age >70) with serious co-morbid conditions such as CHF or liver/renal disease should be strongly considered for hospital admission. Other criteria include an inability to take oral medications; confusion, tachycardia, hypoxia, high fever, leukocytosis, and hypotension.

MRSA is increasingly recognized as a cause of CAP. Think of it in preceding influenza infection, hospitalization, IV drug use, or parenteral antibiotics in the last 90 days. Empiric coverage should be given to these patients or anyone with gram-positive cocci in clusters on the Gram stain, necrotizing pneumonia (multiple cavities), or MRSA growth on previous sputum vultures.

- Use vancomycin, linezolid, or ceftaroline.
- Daptomycin cannot be used because it binds to surfactants and is not effective.
- If blood and sputum cultures are negative, antibiotics should be deescalated.

Consider *Pseudomonas* in those who are immunocompromised, those with bronchiectasis or cystic fibrosis, and those with recent hospitalization or parental antibiotics in the last 90 days. Treatment should include an antipseudomonal beta-lactam (piperacillin-tazobactam, cefepime, ceftazidime, aztreonam, or meropenem) plus a fluoroquinolone. If the patient was hospitalized in the preceding 3 months, MRSA and *Pseudomonas* should be covered.

Empiric coverage for hospital or ventilator-associated pneumonia should include coverage for MRSA and 2 agents for *Pseudomonas* in patients with IV antibiotics within 90 days, septic shock, ARDS, hospitalization ≥5 days, or on dialysis. One example would be ceftazidime, ciprofloxacin, and vancomycin.

### Final Diagnosis

Community-acquired pneumonia

#### CLINICAL PEARL

Consider community-acquired MRSA in IV drug users, concurrent or recent influenza (**high yield**), severe pneumonia requiring intubation and ICU admission, and necrotizing (cavitary) pneumonia.

#### CLINICAL PEARL

Make sure you know what covers *Pseudomonas* and when you need to cover it:

- Hot tub folliculitis
- Malignant otitis externa in diabetics
- Septicemia
- Burn victims
- Cystic fibrosis
- Severe neutropenia (<500 neutrophils/mm$^3$) presenting with fever (usually those on chemotherapy)
- Ventilator-associated pneumonia

Beta-lactams that cover *Pseudomonas* include cefepime; ceftazidime; piperacillin/tazobactam; ticarcillin/clavulanate; imipenem/meropenem (**not** ertapenem); and aztreonam (**no** gram-positive coverage). Non-beta-lactams include aminoglycosides and ciprofloxacin.

# CASE 10

## Chief Complaint

"I have a burning sensation in my penis when I urinate."

## History and Physical Examination

A 28-year-old man comes to your office with several days of burning on urination and a yellowish penile discharge. He reports a history of a similar illness a year ago for which he received some medication but cannot describe. He is otherwise healthy and uses no medications. He is sexually active but denies HIV risk factors. He is adamant that all of his sexual partners have been completely healthy because he hates using condoms and makes sure his partners have no symptoms.

He is afebrile, and there is no adenopathy. Except for a yellow discharge coming from the urethra, the remainder of the examination is normal.

## Differential Diagnosis

1. Gonococcal urethritis
2. Nongonococcal urethritis (chlamydia, herpes, *Mycoplasma hominis, Ureaplasma*)
3. Trichomoniasis
4. Reiter syndrome

## Initial Management

**Setting:** outpatient

## Diagnostic/Therapeutic Plan

- Urine nucleic acid amplification test (NAAT) for gonorrhea and chlamydia

## Test Results

- NAAT: negative for organism

### Assessment

NAAT of the urine (or urethra, cervix, pharyngeal, and possibly anal sample) is the best test to work up urethritis. NAAT of both chlamydia and gonorrhea should be sent to the lab; if the chlamydia NAAT is negative, it should NOT be treated. (The chlamydia NAAT has excellent sensitivity and negates the need to treat chlamydia if it is negative.)

A thorough sexual history must be taken and if the patient had oral or anal intercourse, those areas should be tested with NAAT.

### Further Management Plan/Results

| | |
|---|---|
| 1. Culture of urethral swab on Thayer-Martin medium | Positive for *N. gonorrhoeae* |
| 2. DNA probe for both chlamydia and gonorrhea | Positive for gonorrhea |
| 3. VDRL test | Negative |
| 4. HIV test | Negative |
| 5. NAAT for chlamydia | Negative |

### Treatment Plan

1. Ceftriaxone 125 mg intramuscularly once plus single-dose azithromycin
2. Cefixime if ceftriaxone not available
3. If allergic to ceftriaxone, use gentamycin plus azithromycin

### Discussion

Treatment for chlamydia is azithromycin 1 gm po single dose or doxycycline for 7 days. Treatment for disseminated gonorrhea is 7-10 days of ceftriaxone. After 48 hours of improvement, transition to an oral cephalosporin.

An increasing amount of gonorrhea is resistant to penicillin, so ceftriaxone is now the treatment of choice. A single dose is effective. Azithromycin or doxycycline is used to treat *C. trachomatis*. Other effective regimens for gonorrhea are spectinomycin, and third-generation cephalosporins such as cefotaxime, ceftizoxime, and cefixime.

### CLINICAL PEARL

**Classic findings of DGI:**

- Migratory polyarthralgia evolving into frank arthritis (consider *N. gonorrhoeae* infection in the differential of monoarticular septic arthritis in a sexually active patient)
- Tenosynovitis in $\geq 1$ joints
- Skin lesions (common), classically a few necrotic vesicopustules on an erythematous base
- Negative blood and synovial fluid cultures (common); a high index of clinical suspicion for DGI should prompt the collection of specimens from the cervix/urethra, pharynx, and rectum for culture to make a presumptive diagnosis

### CLINICAL PEARL

Terminal complement deficiency (C5 to C9) can cause recurrent *Neisseria* infection.

### CLINICAL PEARL

**Pelvic Inflammatory Disease (PID)**

PID, a group of infections involving the fallopian tubes, uterus, ovaries, or ligaments of the uterus, is caused by *N. gonorrhoeae*, *Chlamydia*, *Mycoplasma*, anaerobic bacteria, or gram-negative bacteria. IUDs predispose to PID. Symptoms include lower abdominal/pelvic pain on palpation of the cervix, uterus, or adnexa. Fever, leukocytosis, and discharge are common, and cervical discharge may be present. Uterine, adnexal or cervical motion tenderness is key. Complications of PID include infertility and ectopic pregnancy.

To diagnose *N. gonorrhoeae* and chlamydia trachomatis, order an NAAT:

- If there is fluid in the retrouterine cul-de-sac, perform a culdocentesis (rare).
- Do a pregnancy test.

Treatment is as follows:

- **Inpatient**: doxycycline and cefoxitin (or cefotetan); indications for treating inpatient include no improvement in 48-72 hours; nausea/vomiting; high fever; pregnancy; or abscess OR clindamycin plus gentamycin
- **Outpatient**: single-dose ceftriaxone intramuscularly and doxycycline (with or without metronidazole) orally for 2 weeks; due to resistance, fluoroquinolones should be avoided unless there is a cephalosporin allergy; use metronidazole as a second-line agent

If there no response to antibiotics, U/S of the pelvis may exclude other pathology, such as an ovarian cyst or tubo-ovarian abscess.

*Neisseria* bacteria, including *Neisseria gonorrhoeae* and *Neisseria meningitidis*, will grow on a **Thayer-Martin agar**, which is 5% chocolate sheep blood and antibiotics.

- It contains vancomycin, which is able to kill most gram-positive organisms
- Colistin, which is added to kill most gram-negative organisms except *Neisseria*
- Nystatin, which can kill most fungi
- Trimethoprim, which inhibits gram-negative organisms, especially swarming *Proteus*

## Treatment

Ceftriaxone

## Final Diagnosis

Gonococcal urethritis

# CASE 11

## Chief Complaint

"I've got some blisters on my penis."

## History and Physical Examination

A 37-year-old ambitious executive for a local health maintenance organization comes to your office because he developed multiple blister-like lesions on his penis over the last 1–2 days. They are somewhat painful, and he is worried that he has AIDS. He denies unprotected sex and IV drug abuse and had an HIV test before his marriage 3 years ago. He reports several similar episodes several years ago when he worked as a photographer in Nepal. He was never told what they were, and they resolved over several days without any treatment.

He is afebrile, is pleasant, and does not appear to be in distress. Heart, lung, and abdomen are normal. Examination of genitals shows 6–8 vesicular lesions 3–4 mm in diameter on the glans of the penis. There is no crusting, drainage, or bleeding. They are moderately tender. There is also mild inguinal adenopathy bilaterally.

## Differential Diagnosis

1. Herpes simplex type 1
2. Herpes simplex type 2

## Initial Management

**Setting**: outpatient

## Diagnostic/Therapeutic Plan

- Polymerase chain reaction (PCR) testing of the specimens obtained from ulcers (will detect early infection by identifying whether the HSV DNA is present)
- HSV-2 antibody test only for previous infection (not very useful)

Tzanck smear (Wright or Giemsa stain of an unroofed lesion) is no longer used.

## Test Results

- Stain: multinucleated giant cells visible lesion (Tzanck prep)

## Assessment

Multiple small, tender vesicular lesions of the genitals or mouth are very characteristic of herpes simplex, and the differential diagnosis is small. Occasionally, if the lesions have unroofed or become confluent, they may be confused with chancroid, which is also painful. Most often herpetic lesions have such a characteristic appearance that no further diagnostic tests are required. If there is any doubt of the diagnosis, however, perform an HSV PCR, as that is the most sensitive and specific test.

**NOTE**

Recurrent erythema multiforme is most commonly caused by recurrent HSV infection.

The Tzanck prep has low sensitivity and specificity and would not be the correct test. Viral culture may also be used. Serology on blood testing is not useful in confirming the diagnosis because 85–90% of the population is positive. Herpes simplex 1 is found in 70% of the population, and herpes simplex 2 in 20%.

### Further Management Plan/Results

- Viral culture or HSV PCR: herpes simplex grows after 72 hours

### Treatment Plan

Acyclovir; famciclovir and valacyclovir are also acceptable alternatives.

### Discussion

This patient should be reassured that a recurrent episode of genital herpes is not indicative of AIDS. A confirmatory clue that this patient's infection is a recurrence and not a primary infection is the absence of systemic symptoms. Initial infections of both oral and genital herpes are often associated with fever, headache, malaise, and adenopathy. These symptoms are generally absent from recurrences. Recurrent herpetic lesions only need 5 days of treatment, though primary lesions may need 10 days.

Topical acyclovir is worthless for oral lesions and of very limited use in genital lesions. As with this man's original episodes several yrs ago, most episodes resolve spontaneously anyway, and the acyclovir treatment is solely to shorten the duration of the outbreak. Although oral lesions are more often caused by type 1 virus and genital lesions by type 2 virus, either one may cause oral or genital lesions. There is a clinical benefit of distinguishing between the two because viral shedding and recurrent ulcers are less likely with HSV-1 than HSV-2.

**CCS NOTE**

The options to move the clock forward also include an "as needed" option. This is for patients like this one, in which there is a brief, self-inflicted problem. See them once after the initial visit to make sure the lesions have resolved. Then click on "RETURN AS NEEDED." This is done for patients in whom the problem has resolved.

Herpes encephalitis is the most common cause of viral encephalitis.

Herpetic infections can recur at any time and with any frequency after the original infection from as infrequent as several yrs apart to as short as several wks apart. Any form of physical or emotional stress, intercurrent infection, or immunosuppression (such as with AIDS or steroid use) can cause recurrences.

Frequent recurrences of genital herpes can be suppressed with a regular dose of acyclovir 400 mg 2x/day, valacyclovir 1x/day, or famciclovir 2x/day on a chronic basis.

### Final Diagnosis

Herpes simplex of the genitals

# CASE 12

## Chief Complaint

Diarrhea for the past 2 days

## History and Physical Examination

Eighteen fellows and attending doctors from the department of medicine have come unexpectedly to the employee health service over the past 36 hours with a history of 1–2 days of diarrhea. All of them were present at a large dinner party given by one of the hospital's gastroenterologists several days ago. They all complain of multiple episodes of watery diarrhea. Some have blood visible in their stool, and some have profound abdominal cramping and fever. They all ate multiple dishes at the party including chicken, lamb, beef, salads, sauces, and an excellent tiramisu (sponge cake with eggs, espresso, wine, sugar, melted chocolate, and cheese).

Their temperatures range from 37.6 to 38.6 C (99.7 to 101.5 F). Chest, heart, head, eyes, ears, nose, and throat are all normal. Abdominal examination shows some distention with generalized, mild tenderness.

## Differential Diagnosis

1. *Salmonella*
2. *Campylobacter*
3. *Shigella*
4. Norwalk virus
5. *Yersinia*
6. Enteroinvasive *E. coli*

## Initial Management

**Setting**: outpatient

## Diagnostic/Therapeutic Plan

- Stool examination for blood and leukocytes
- Blood culture
- Stool culture

## Test Results

- Stool exam: positive blood in the stool; positive leukocytes with methylene blue staining of the stool
- Blood culture: positive for *Campylobacter*
- Stool culture: positive for *Campylobacter*

### Assessment

*Salmonella, Shigella, Campylobacter, Yersinia,* and *E. coli* can all present with a dysentery syndrome of multiple watery bowel movements, fever, abdominal pain, and blood in the stool. It is generally not possible to distinguish the causative agents on the basis of the history alone. *S. aureus* and *Bacillus cereus* tend to present with a more acute onset of 2–6 hours after ingestion of the contaminated food with more upper GI symptoms. Viral diarrhea is seldom accompanied by blood or WBCs in the stool. Almost all of them are benign and self-limited.

The definitive diagnosis of bacteria-related food poisoning depends upon stool culture. *Campylobacter* and *Salmonella* are the most common causes of bacterial food poisoning. *Giardia* and cryptosporidiosis are uncommon in this setting in which the water supply is presumably safe. In addition, *Giardia* and cryptosporidiosis do not give red or white cells in the stool. *Giardia* is treated with metronidazole.

### Treatment Plan

1. Supportive with hydration alone in the majority of cases
2. Spontaneous resolution expected in 3–7 days
3. Avoidance of antimotility agents such as diphenoxylate and loperamide
4. Severe cases of infectious diarrhea with signs of sepsis, such as hypotension, fever, and tachycardia, are treated empirically with ciprofloxacin.

### Discussion

Gastrointestinal infections are an enormous source of illness worldwide and rank second only to respiratory infections as a cause of death. They are the leading cause of death in children worldwide, with >12,000 deaths per day.

The vast majority of cases of food poisoning resolve spontaneously without antibiotics and with the use of hydration alone. The rehydration solutions are a combination of water, salt, potassium, and sugar. Antimotility agents are avoided because they may lead to toxic megacolon and buildup of the infectious agent. For instance, when diphenoxylate is used in *Shigella*, there can be prolonged fever and shedding of the organism. In *Salmonella*, they can increase the risk of bacteremia.

If a patient is extremely ill or if the diarrhea is not resolving, antibiotics may be used. In the absence of a specific etiology, ciprofloxacin is a good choice. Trimethoprim/sulfa may also be adequate. However, due to high resistance to fluoroquinolones, macrolides are now the agents of choice if antibiotics are needed.

Although almost all food poisoning in the United States is self-limited, there are some occasional complications. In cases where the diarrhea is <24 hrs, there is no need to send stool studies.

### Final Diagnosis

Infectious diarrhea secondary to *Campylobacter*

# CASE 13

## Chief Complaint

Dyspnea and dizziness

## History and Physical Examination

A 45-year-old man presents to the emergency department with 3 days of dizziness and dyspnea. He denies chest pain or palpitations. He has no cough or fever. His past medical history is unremarkable. He lives in Massachusetts and works as a lawyer. He goes camping on the weekends with his children, but has not noticed any tick bites or rashes.

On physical examination he appears well. Temperature is normal, BP is 100/60 mm Hg, and pulse 35/min. Other than bradycardia, the remaining physical examination findings are unremarkable. Results of initial lab studies show a normal CBC, metabolic panel, and cardiac enzyme measurements.

EKG is shown. Relevant findings are complete heart block.

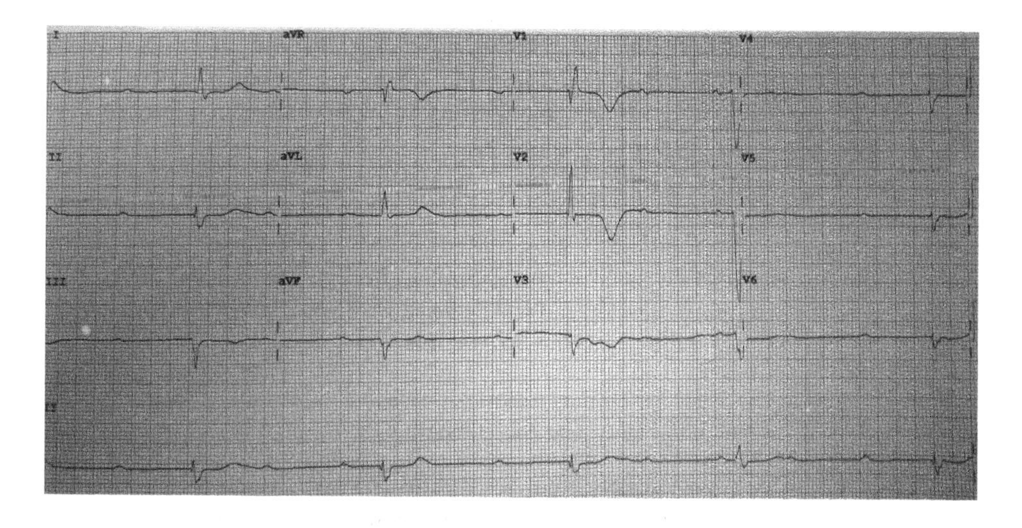


## Differential Diagnosis

Bradycardia with heart block can be due to:

1. Hypothyroidism
2. Lyme disease
3. Beta-blocker or calcium channel blocker use
4. Ischemic heart disease

### CLINICAL PEARL

With patients from the northeast United States, camping/tick exposure, and bradycardia, always consider Lyme disease.

## Initial Management

**Setting:** emergency department

## Diagnostic/Therapeutic Plan

- Immediate treatment with IV ceftriaxone
- Serologic testing for *Borrelia burgdorferi*; enzyme-linked immunosorbent assay is the initial test and a Western blot assay is used for confirmation

## Discussion

Lyme disease is the most common arthropod-borne infection in the United States, with around 26,000 confirmed cases reported in 2014. The incidence varies geographically, and hyperendemic areas in the northeast and north central United States reflect the geographic density of the vector deer tick, *Ixodes scapularis*, in these areas. The causative spirochete is *Borrelia burgdorferi* sensu stricto, which is transmitted to humans following vector tick attachment and feeding. Deer ticks may also serve as vectors for other tick-borne infection, and coinfection may occur.

The clinical manifestations of Lyme disease depend on the stage of infection.

- Early localized Lyme disease typically occurs 1–2 wks following infection.
- The initial clinical manifestation is erythema migrans, an erythematous skin lesion at the site of tick attachment (noted in 70–80% of patients with confirmed infection).
- Classically, the border of erythema migrans expands over several days, and the lesion develops central clearing, leading to the description of a "target" or "bull's-eye" appearance.

If erythema migrans is seen, there is no need to send serology because a measurable antibody response may not have had time to develop and will be negative. If you're given erythema migrans on the exam, the answer is to treat with doxycycline.

Neurologic manifestations of early disseminated Lyme disease include cranial nerve palsy (unilateral or bilateral), aseptic meningitis, and radiculopathy.

Late-stage Lyme occurs in as many as 60% of untreated patients. Lyme arthritis is characterized by migratory monoarticular or oligoarticular inflammation, which often improves spontaneously and then recurs in the same joint or another joint months to year later. The knee is involved in 85% of patients.

The finding of *B. burgdorferi* antibodies in patients who have nonspecific symptoms of fatigue or myalgia or who are unlikely to have been exposed to a vector tick likely represents a false-positive test result for Lyme disease.

Therefore, serologic testing for Lyme disease should be restricted to patients with clinically suggestive signs or symptoms who either reside in or have traveled to an endemic area.

Patients who have nonspecific symptoms such as fatigue, myalgia, or arthralgia but a low pretest probability for Lyme disease should not be tested for this disease.

Patients with erythema migrans, Bell's palsy, or joint involvement should be treated with doxycycline or amoxicillin. Although amoxicillin covers Lyme disease, doxycycline is also active against *Anaplasma phagocytophilum* and is the preferred agent for patients age $\geq$8 who are not pregnant or breast-feeding. *Anaplasma phagocytophilum* is also transmitted via the *Ixodes scapularis* and there is commonly coinfection.

IV ceftriaxone is the recommended therapy for patients with Lyme myocarditis associated with second- or third-degree heart block or Lyme meningitis or encephalitis.

## Final Diagnosis

Lyme disease

# CASE 14

## Chief Complaint

Fever, urgency, and dysuria

## History and Physical Examination

A 25-year-old woman comes to the office with a 3-day history of lower abdominal pain that is beginning to radiate to her right flank. She denies nausea or vomiting, but states she feels feverish and is worried that she may have the flu. She denies diarrhea; her last bowel movement was this morning, and she has been drinking a lot of fluids. She has noticed an increase in her urinary frequency.

Vital signs are T 39.2 C (102.6 F), BP 120/70 mm Hg, pulse 95/min, and respirations 16/min. Physical examination shows tenderness in the suprapubic region, hyperactive bowel sounds, and no peritoneal signs or masses. Her right flank is tender to light percussion. The remainder of the physical examination is within normal limits.

## Differential Diagnosis

1. Pyelonephritis
2. Cystitis
3. Pelvic inflammatory disease
4. Perinephric abscess

## Initial Management

**Setting:** outpatient or emergency department

## Initial Diagnostic Plan

- Urinalysis

## Test Results

- 50–100 WBC per high-power field; trace proteinuria; many bacteria; nitrate-positive

## Assessment

A febrile person with complaints of fever and dysuria clearly has an infection of the urinary system. The high fever and flank pain point to an upper urinary site. Pyelonephritis and perinephric abscess are most likely. Perinephric abscess is less common with such a short duration of illness of only 3 days. Perinephric abscess most often arises from a preexisting pyelonephritis that has been present for several wks, particularly in association with stones.

| Further Diagnostic Plan | Results |
|---|---|
| Urine culture | >100,000 colonies of *Escherichia coli* |
| Blood culture | negative |

### Treatment Plan

IV antibiotics active against gram-negative bacilli (fluoroquinolones or cephalosporins)

### Discussion

In healthy individuals with uncomplicated UTI or mild pyelonephritis, numerous medications are effective, e.g., all quinolones (though they can be expensive).

- UTI: trimethoprim-sulfamethoxazole (TMP/SMZ)
- Cystitis: TMP/SMZ or ciprofloxacin

Note: Due to increasing resistance among the gram-negative bacilli, TMP/SMZ is becoming less useful as empiric therapy for UTI, and it should not be used as empiric therapy for pyelonephritis. For empiric therapy prior to knowing the susceptibility data on an individual organism, consider antibiotics that are effective against the gram-negative bacilli.

- When there is high fever, shaking chills, or other evidence of bacteremia, IV antibiotics are indicated.
- When there is significant nausea/vomiting or any other inability to take oral antibiotics, hospital admission and IV antibiotics are indicated.

If IV medication were required, the medications of choice would be the drugs just described (in IV form):

- Third-generation cephalosporins
- Aztreonam
- Ticarcillin-clavulanic acid
- Piperacillin (possibly in combination with an aminoglycoside, depending upon severity of infection)

Do not use aminoglycosides alone for the treatment of any serious infection. In addition, use the culture and sensitivity to guide modification of antibiotic therapy. IV ceftriaxone has become the first-line agent for empiric treatment of pyelonephritis.

It is very important to narrow the coverage as soon as culture results have returned.

No predetermined length of treatment can be given for pyelonephritis. Treatment is usually continued for 7–14 days; however, it may need to be continued longer, depending upon the severity of the illness and how long it takes for the person to become afebrile.

Additional testing such as renal U/S or IV pyelography is indicated only if a complication such as a stone, stricture, or tumor is suspected to be causing the pyelonephritis. Otherwise, those tests are not part of routine management of a simple, uncomplicated pyelonephritis. If symptoms persist beyond 3–5 days of effective treatment, obtain U/S or CT scan of the kidney to exclude a perinephric abscess or other drainable collection of fluid.

### Final Diagnosis

Pyelonephritis

# Cardiology 3

## CASE 1

### Chief Complaint

Severe pain in the chest

### History and Physical Examination

A 68-year-old man comes to the emergency department with 30 min of severe, dull, substernal chest pain. There is no radiation of the pain. He is somewhat short of breath but is not diaphoretic or nauseated. The pain occurred while he was helping his son move furniture into his new apartment. He is a nonsmoker whose father died at 67 of "heart trouble."

Vital signs are T 37.4 C (99.3 F), BP 130/80 mm Hg, and respirations 22/min. Head, eyes, ears, neck, and throat examination is normal. The chest is clear bilaterally, and the pain is not reproduced by palpation. Cardiovascular exam shows tachycardia with no murmurs or gallops. The liver is not enlarged, and the extremities are not edematous.

### Differential Diagnosis

1. Unstable angina
2. Acute myocardial infarction (MI)
3. Dissecting aortic aneurysm
4. Pericarditis
5. Esophageal spasm
6. Pulmonary embolism
7. Musculoskeletal pain
8. Pancreatitis
9. Pneumothorax
10. GERD

#### CCS NOTE

Exertional chest pain is very specific for ischemia.

**CCS NOTE**

When deciding how much physical examination to choose for the CCS, choose those parts of the exam that you think might be abnormal. Do not worry if they are all normal; what matters is that they might have been abnormal.

**CCS NOTE**

When the presentation is consistent with ischemic pain, order aspirin, morphine, and nitroglycerin at the same time that you order the EKG.

### Initial Management

**Setting:** emergency department

### Diagnostic/Therapeutic Plan

- Aspirin oral; nitroglycerin sublingual or paste to chest wall; morphine
- EKG
- CK-MB and troponin
- Chest x-ray
- Pulse oximetry

### Test Results

- EKG: sinus tachycardia with 2 mm of ST elevation in leads V2–V4
- CK-MB and troponin: normal
- Chest x-ray: normal
- Pulse oximetry: 98% saturation on room air

### Assessment

Determining the etiology of chest pain depends on the following:

- Quality of the pain
- Where it radiates
- Risk factors present
- Whether pain develops during exertion

Pain that is pleuritic (i.e., changes with respiration) occurs with pulmonary emboli, pneumothorax, pneumonia, and pericarditis. Aortic aneurysmal pain typically radiates to the back and is described as "tearing" quality. Acute MI is often preceded by escalating episodes of exertional chest pain, often accompanied by nausea, vomiting, and diaphoresis, and may radiate to the jaw, arms, or back.

Until the EKG or cardiac enzymes are performed, however, it is impossible to distinguish between unstable angina and infarction.

Infarction may occur with only a single millimeter of ST elevation. Infarction typically causes ST segment elevation, while ischemia typically causes ST segment depression. It is possible to have an MI with ST segment depression. This **distinction is critical**, since ST elevation MI (STEMI) is treated with urgent percutaneous coronary intervention (PCI) or thrombolytic agents, while non-STEMI is not.

A benign physical examination does not include or exclude an infarction.

- The initially normal CK-MB is expected because it only elevates 4–6 hrs after the start of the infarction and peaks 12–18 hrs later.
- Troponin, another cardiac enzyme with a very high specificity for the heart, may elevate earlier than CK-MB. Virtually any elevation in troponin is an indication of myocardial damage. (Troponin elevation lasts for 1–2 wks, whereas CK-MB elevation lasts for just 2–3 days.)
- Myoglobin, another cardiac enzyme with a very high sensitivity for myocardial damage, is the only cardiac enzyme that can elevate within 4 hrs of damage. Unfortunately, it is very nonspecific.

### Further Management Plan

- Clopidogrel oral (or ticagrelor)
- Metoprolol PO, statin such as atorvastatin oral, ACE inhibitor (e.g., lisinopril) oral
- Angioplasty or thrombolytic
- Cardiology consultation
- Repeat CK-MB and troponin in 4 hrs
- Repeat EKG in 15 min

### Discussion

This patient is having an acute MI. The primary objectives in management are to **decrease oxygen demand** and **reestablish perfusion**. Regardless of whether the MI is STEMI or NSTEMI, all acute MI patients are given pain control, oxygen (if needed), nitrates, aspirin, a beta-blocker such as metoprolol, clopidogrel, and heparin (either systemic or enoxaparin). Heparin is always used unless there are contraindications to anticoagulation.

Because this patient has a STEMI, he should also receive one of the following:

- Urgent PCI intervention (cardiology consult)
- tPA, streptokinase (do not use streptokinase in those who have had streptokinase before)
- Another thrombolytic, i.e., alteplase, APSAC, reteplase
  - Indications include symptom onset within 12 hrs and unavailability of primary PCI within 120 minutes of first medical contact
  - Most effective within first 3-6 hours of symptom onset
  - Contraindications include (**absolute contraindications**) severe GI bleed, intracranial hemorrhage, recent surgery, aortic dissection, and any active internal bleed, and (**relative contraindications**) BP >180/110 mm Hg [in this case, start a labetalol drip to lower and then give tPA], active ulcer, recent head trauma, and pregnancy
- Beta-blocker (if no contraindications, conduction defect, hypotension, or markedly decreased ejection fraction) to decrease heart rate/myocardial contractility and thus lower myocardial work and oxygen consumption

Thrombolytics, aspirin, and nitrates all directly contribute to increasing blood flow.

Primary PCI remains the preferred strategy. Guidelines for the use of PCI are as follows:

- If a PCI lab is on-site at the hospital, PCI should be done within 90 minutes of presentation.
- If there is not a lab on-site and the patient must be transferred, the "door to balloon time" is <120 min. If that can be done, transfer.
- If <120 min is not possible, give thrombolytics and then transfer.
- Give patients who are undergoing PCI the following: aspirin, IV unfractionated heparin or bivalirudin (direct thrombin inhibitor), and a loading dose of P2Y12 inhibitors (clopidogrel or ticagrelor).

#### CCS NOTE

All consultations will ask for a 10-word explanation clarifying the need for the consultation. Explain why you called.

#### CLINICAL PEARL

Oxygen during an MI can actually be harmful, so should be used only if oxygen saturation <90% (usually in cases with pulmonary edema).

#### CLINICAL PEARL

- In the past, the timing for "first medical contact to balloon time" had been **<90 min**, but has now been changed to **<120 min**. So "transfer to a PCI center for primary PCI" is the correct answer if the door to balloon time is <120 min. If a patient gets thrombolytics, then transfer to a PCI center.
- Use reperfusion treatment for symptoms <12 hrs.

### Further Management Plan/Results

| Repeat CK-MB or troponin | Elevated at 12 and 18 hrs after presentation with 5.8% MB fraction and elevated troponin level |
|---|---|

### Discussion

The most common complication of an acute MI in the first 3 days is arrhythmia. This is why patients are placed in a monitored setting in the critical care unit. Other complications of MI include:

- Valvular dysfunction
- Cardiogenic shock
- Aneurysm formation
- Mural thrombus
- Myocardial rupture
- Conduction defects such as atrioventricular (AV) dissociation (complete heart block) and left bundle branch block and pericarditis ("Dressler syndrome")

### Follow-up Management and Prevention

- Admit to critical care unit.
- Aspirin for all patients, continued indefinitely
- Oxygen (only if oxygen saturation <90%)
- Primary angioplasty has superior efficacy compared with thrombolytics. It should be performed within 90 min of coming to the door (120 minutes if you must transfer). Primary angioplasty is also preferred if there are any contraindications to thrombolytics or if pain >2 hrs.
- Beta blockers (metoprolol ) and statins reduce mortality. Do not give beta blockers if there is evidence of cardiogenic shock, bradycardia, or hypotension. Calcium-channel blockers can be used if there is a major contraindication to the use of beta-blockers. Calcium blockers do not lower mortality.
  - If beta blockers are contraindicated, calcium-channel blockers (CCBs) can be used.
  - CCBs do not lower mortality.
- Thrombolytic therapy (tPA or streptokinase) should be followed by heparin use within 12 hrs of chest pain.
- ACE inhibitor when ejection fraction is low (<40%) or for any large anterior infarction (ACE inhibitor can be started in any MI but should be stopped at 6 wks if there is normal left ventricular function)
- P2Y12 inhibitor (clopidogrel, prasugrel, ticagrelor) continued for several months whether there is a stent or not
- DAPT for 3 months following a drug-eluting stent in patients with high bleeding risk (CKD, anemia, history of GI bleed, advanced age)
- Intra-aortic balloon pump (IABP) if valve rupture is involved
- High intensity statin, started within 24 hours and continued indefinitely (atorvastatin or rosuvastatin)

In long-term management, ACE inhibitors also decrease mortality by improving myocardial remodeling. This is particularly true in the presence of left ventricular dysfunction, as evidenced by signs of decreased cardiac output or decreased ejection fraction on echocardiogram.

- A decreased ejection fraction or large anterior infarction is an indication to start ACE inhibitors.
- Primary angioplasty is superior in efficacy to thrombolytics (and is always indicated if there is a reason not to use thrombolytics, i.e., a predisposition to bleeding). It is also superior when there is evidence of cardiogenic shock or if the patient's condition is worsening in spite of thrombolytics.

If there is still evidence of ongoing ischemia even after thrombolytics and angioplasty, emergency coronary bypass is performed.

### Final Diagnosis

Acute ST elevation MI

**CCS NOTE**

On the exam, the generic or brand name of a medication can be ordered, e.g., metoprolol or Toprol. However, the generic names are more reliably useful for questions.

# CASE 2

## Chief Complaint

Rapid drop in blood pressure

## History and Physical Examination

A 68-year-old man was recently admitted through the emergency department to your ICU for chest pain and electrocardiogram abnormalities consistent with an acute inferior wall myocardial infarction. The chest pain resolved, and he has been stable. You are called by the nurse to see the patient because of a sudden drop of blood pressure from 130/90 mm Hg to 70/50. The patient denies chest pain, though he is somewhat confused.

Vital signs are T 37.0 C (98.6 F), BP 70/50 mm Hg, and pulse 40/min. Physical examination shows visible "cannon" a-waves. Chest is clear bilaterally, and cardiovascular examination shows a 2/6 systolic murmur. His abdomen is benign. The patient is confused as to time and place, but the neurologic examination is otherwise nonfocal.

## Differential Diagnosis

1. Hypovolemia
2. Cardiogenic shock from extension of the MI
3. Valvular or chordae tendineae rupture
4. Papillary muscle rupture
5. Jarisch-Bezold reflex
6. Complete heart block
7. Ventricular tachycardia
8. Sinus bradycardia
9. Ventricular rupture
10. Ventricular septal defect

## Initial Management

**Setting:** emergency department

## Diagnostic/Therapeutic Plan

- EKG
- Atropine
- IV fluids (normal saline or Ringer's lactate)
- Discontinue beta blockers, nitrates, and calcium channel blockers while hypotensive

### Test Results

- EKG: complete heart block with ventricular rate 40/min

### Assessment

This case is meant to illustrate all the main complications of myocardial infarction (MI). All the disorders listed in the differential can result in sudden hypotension in a patient with an acute MI. Inferior wall MI usually carries the lowest mortality (5% after 1 year). However, extension to the other walls or the valves is always possible. Jarisch-Bezold reflex is a vagally mediated reflex, resulting in bradycardia, hypotension, nausea, and vomiting. This is particular to inferior wall MI because of the inferior wall's proximity to the diaphragm.

All of the arrhythmias can be excluded first because an EKG is generally much easier to obtain than an echocardiogram. In addition, all of the valvular abnormalities severe enough to give this presentation would certainly result in an audible murmur.

Anatomic defects such as ventricular septal defect, valve rupture, and free wall rupture usually occur several days after an infarction. They usually need several days for sufficient necrosis to occur.

The most essential feature of this case is the bradycardia. All the complications of MI described here—besides AV block—should cause tachycardia. Valve rupture and ventricular septal defect should give rales on lung examination. The most common cause of third-degree AV block is idiopathic fibrosis.

The cannon a-waves visible on the physical exam are exaggerated pulsations from the atria contracting out of sync with the ventricles and, hence, against a closed AV valve. This produces a backflow of blood into the neck veins, resulting in the cannon a-waves. The cannon a-waves are the main way to clinically distinguish this case from simple sinus bradycardia. Complete heart block is a well-known complication of MI. It is particularly associated with inferior wall infarction because in most people the right coronary artery supplies the blood to both the inferior wall and the AV node.

### Further Management Plan

- Pacemaker placement, transcutaneous; of ineffective, consider dopamine to support BP
- Transvenous pacemaker
- Cardiology consult
- Keep in ICU

### Discussion

Although large volumes of IV fluid are generally the initial treatment for hypotension, atropine should be the primary, specific treatment for complete heart block. Atropine can accelerate the heart rate instantly and restore BP that way. If it does not work, give fluids. (On the exam, if you see isoproterenol in the answer choice, it is always wrong.)

#### CCS NOTE

In an unstable patient with bradycardia, atropine can be ordered at the same time as the EKG and bolus of saline. All symptomatic bradycardias should be treated with atropine, so the specific etiology is not as important as stabilization.

Pacemaker placement is central to treatment because it is the only modality that can continually keep the heart rate adequate. Complete heart block can also occur as a form of toxicity with any medication that is negatively dromotropic, e.g., a beta-blocker or digoxin. Myocarditis resulting from a virus or Lyme disease can also cause complete heart block, although this is rare. Besides the acute MI described in this case, the most common cause of AV block is aging and fibrosis of the conduction system. Treatment of third-degree AV block from digoxin overdose is with digoxin-binding antibodies (digoxin immune Fab, or Digibind).

Simple hypovolemia is treated with fluids and dopamine. Wall and valve rupture and ventricular septal defects require emergent operative repair. Ventricular tachycardia with the hypotension described in this case needs immediate electrical cardioversion. Right ventricular infarction could cause hypotension and is often associated with an inferior wall myocardial infarction. This is because the right ventricle has the same arterial supply as the inferior wall. Right ventricular infarction should give tachycardia and would not give the cannon a-waves. Right ventricular infarction is treated with fluid administration.

### Follow-up Management and Prevention

- Keep patient in ICU until pacemaker placed and hemodynamically stable
- Continue ACE inhibitor, statin, aspirin, and second anti-platelet agent (clopidogrel)
- Consider angiography and angioplasty/stenting (relieving ischemia improves many arrhythmias)
- Administer GP IIb/IIIa agent if patient gets stented (e.g., eptifibatide, tirofiban)
- Educate patient on smoking cessation and exercise when he is stable

### Final Diagnosis

Complete heart block

#### CCS NOTE

Consultants will see the patient in 20 min. They will never give specific advice or direction.

#### CLINICAL PEARL

Prasugrel or ticagrelor is used as a second anti-platelet agent in conjunction with stenting.

#### CLINICAL PEARL

In the setting of an MI, other causes of a rapid drop in BP include:

- **Valvular rupture and septal rupture**: occur 5–10 days after an MI with sudden dyspnea, rales, tachycardia; prominent new murmur confirmed with echocardiography; afterload reduction with ACE inhibitors and immediate surgery
- **Ventricular rupture/tamponade**: sudden hypotension, tachycardia, clear lungs; jugulovenous distension and pulsus paradoxus; confirm with echocardiogram and treat with an emergent pericardiocentesis and surgical correction
- **Cardiogenic shock**: tachycardia, hypotension, and prominent rales on examination

#### CCS NOTE

Always bolus the patient with normal saline or the initial set of orders in a hypotensive patient.

# CASE 3

## Chief Complaint

"I have a funny sensation in my chest."

## History and Physical Examination

A 72-year-old man comes to the emergency department suffering from chest discomfort for less than 1 hour. He states that he has a history of arrhythmia but is taking no medications. He has had similar episodes in the past. The chest discomfort does not radiate and does not cause dyspnea but is associated with diaphoresis.

Vital signs are BP 80/60 mm Hg, pulse 180/min, and respirations 24/min. Physical examination shows jugular venous distention. Breath sounds are diminished at the bases, and heart sounds are distant. The remainder of the examination is unremarkable.

## Differential Diagnosis

1. Ventricular tachycardia
2. Supraventricular tachycardia
3. Atrial fibrillation
4. Atrial flutter
5. Myocardial infarction
6. Myocardial ischemia

## Initial Management

**Setting:** emergency department

## Diagnostic/Therapeutic Plan

- EKG
- Oxygen, normal saline bolus
- Oximeter

## Test Results

- EKG: ventricular tachycardia at rate 180/min
- Oximeter: 98% saturation on room air

### CLINICAL PEARL

Although you cannot determine a specific etiology from the physical examination, the heart rate in this patient means that there has to be a rhythm disturbance. Sinus rates maximize at 220/min minus the age. Thus, in this patient, any rate >150/min would indicate an arrhythmia.

### Patient Safety Note

Check oximeter and give oxygen to anyone who is dyspneic or hyperventilating.

## Assessment

Ventricular tachycardia is characterized electrocardiographically by a rapid rhythm with a widened QRS complex and evidence of atrial-ventricular dissociation.

- Often associated with underlying heart disease, which is often ischemic
- Often deteriorates into ventricular fibrillation; stroke volume will be markedly decreased because of loss of filling time for the ventricles, resulting in cardiovascular collapse
- Arises from a focus of irritability in the ventricle due to ischemia or scar; heart rate is usually 100–180/min

Electrolyte abnormalities such as hypomagnesemia, hypocalcemia, hyperkalemia, and hypokalemia can also lead to ventricular tachycardia. Tricyclic antidepressant overdose can lead to ventricular tachycardia as well.

Torsades de Pointes is a particular type of ventricular tachycardia with an undulating baseline. Torsades is particularly associated with hypomagnesemia, drugs that widen the QT interval, and a congenital prolonged QT syndrome. Drugs that prolong the QT are quinidine, procainamide, and tricyclic overdose.

## Further Management Plan

- DC cardioversion
- Lidocaine or amiodarone
- Check and treat underlying potassium, calcium, or magnesium abnormalities
- Electrolytes: normal

### CCS NOTE

Any patient with a ventricular rhythm disturbance should be placed in the ICU at the end of the case.

## Discussion

Ventricular tachycardia can be confused with supraventricular tachycardia with a bundle branch block; SVT with aberrant conduction or Wolff-Parkinson-White. Because of the risk of deterioration into ventricular fibrillation, ventricular tachycardia is a serious arrhythmia, even in the asymptomatic patient with adequate cardiac output.

Treatment of ventricular tachycardia, in the presence of significant hemodynamic compromise, is cardioversion, and the decision has to be made at bedside. Cardioversion should be done with systolic BP <90 mm Hg, mental status changes, CHF, and/or chest pain.

- Amiodarone should be used first in an acute episode of ventricular tachycardia.
- Lidocaine is the agent of choice for ventricular tachycardia when the myocardium is ischemic and the patient is hemodynamically stable to prevent recurrence after cardioversion.
- Procainamide and amiodarone can be used instead of lidocaine to convert the rhythm in a hemodynamically stable patient.
- Amiodarone is the better agent when there is an abnormal left ventricle.

### CLINICAL PEARL

Any wide-complex tachycardia in a patient with ischemic heart disease is ventricular tachycardia until proven otherwise.

Treatment, in the presence of hemodynamic stability and a pulse, is as follows:

1. Oxygen, IV access
2. Amiodarone
3. Lidocaine
4. Procainamide

(Amiodarone is the preferred drug when the ejection fraction is $<$40%.)

If unstable (defined as systolic BP $<$90 mm Hg, confusion, chest pain, or CHF):

1. Synchronized cardioversion 100 J
2. Synchronized cardioversion 200 J
3. Synchronized cardioversion 360 J
4. Synchronized cardioversion 360 J
5. If persistent, use amiodarone followed by lidocaine or procainamide

While electrical cardioversion must be performed immediately if the patient is unstable, premedication is still preferable when possible. A sedative such as diazepam or midazolam should be used prior to the cardioversion when time allows.

Pulseless ventricular tachycardia is managed the same way as ventricular fibrillation.

The most common side effect of lidocaine is confusion, particularly among the older adult. In the short term, amiodarone has few adverse effects when used on a regular basis. Amiodarone can lead to pulmonary fibrosis, thyroid disorders, and corneal deposits.

In those patients with a wide complex tachycardia of unknown type, procainamide or amiodarone can be used; these agents are effective for both atrial and ventricular arrhythmias. When ejection fraction is $<$40%, amiodarone is preferred.

Anyone with cardiac rhythm disturbances should have an echocardiogram. Cardiomyopathy is often associated with arrhythmia. Ischemia should be excluded as a cause of ventricular arrhythmias.

**CCS NOTE**

A cardiology consult should be ordered with any serious rhythm disorder. In this case, you will need cardiology to place an implantable defibrillator. Do not expect them to actually say anything.

## Follow-up Management and Prevention

- Keep patient in ICU
- Continue amiodarone
- Do stress (exercise-tolerance) test once patient is stable
  - If stress test or catheterization is normal, arrange electrophysiology studies
- Do echocardiography
- Arrange cardiology consult
- Consider automatic implantable cardioverter defibrillator (AICD) placement
- Metoprolol

## Final Diagnosis

Ventricular tachycardia

# CASE 4

## Chief Complaint

"My chest and stomach began to hurt as I was eating."

## History and Physical Examination

A 56-year-old man with diabetes mellitus and hypertension is brought to the emergency department because of a 30-minute history of chest and epigastric pain, which developed while eating. He has had similar episodes that occur after walking for 1 to 2 blocks and which are relieved by rest. He denies a history of myocardial infarction. He takes diltiazem to control his BP. After arriving in the emergency department, the pain starts again.

Vital signs are T 37.2 C (99.0 F), BP 140/90 mm Hg, and pulse 110/min. Physical examination shows no jugular venous distension, a clear chest bilaterally, and a benign abdomen. Cardiovascular examination shows tachycardia with no murmurs or gallops. The extremities are not edematous.

## Differential Diagnosis

1. Unstable angina
2. Myocardial infarction
3. Dissecting aortic aneurysm
4. Pericarditis
5. Peptic ulcer disease
6. Esophageal spasm

## Initial Management

**Setting:** emergency department

## Diagnostic/Therapeutic Plan

- Aspirin oral, nitroglycerin sublingual, morphine
- EKG
- Chest x-ray
- CK-MB and troponin

## Test Results

- EKG: 1 mm ST segment depression in leads II, III, and aVF
- Chest x-ray: normal
- CK-MB and troponin: elevated

### Assessment

This patient has non ST elevation MI (non-STEMI). Unstable angina is chest pain at rest or worsening of stable angina. The difference between non-STEMI and unstable angina is the production of troponins.

### Further Management Plan

- Admit to ICU (coronary/intensive)
- Repeat EKG and CPK-MB or troponin at 6-hr intervals (but do not delay treatment pending results of any test with this type of anginal pattern)
- Enoxaparin (low molecular weight heparin)
- Oxygen (only if hypoxic)
- Clopidogrel or ticagrelor prior to angiogram (prasugrel prior to angioplasty and a stent)
- Metoprolol PO, statin oral
- Glycoprotein IIb/IIIa inhibitor (eptifibatide, tirofiban) (very rarely used now)
- Repeat EKG every 15 min while pain is present

### Further Test Results

- EKG: ST depression in II, III, and aVF persists
- CKMB and troponin: elevated

### CCS NOTE

The order in which you type the medication or treatment names does not matter, as long as they are written on the same screen.

### Discussion

Acute coronary syndrome (ACS) is caused by acute plaque rupture and a clot that forms upon an underlying atheromatous plaque. It can be STEMI, NSTEMI, or unstable angina. The EKG and troponins give you the diagnosis.

The goal of acute treatment is to prevent further clotting with aspirin and heparin. Low molecular weight heparin has a superior efficacy compared with IV heparin. **Thrombolytics do not reduce mortality in unstable angina or NSTEMI**, and so are never used.

Risk assessment should be done with the TIMI score. Do not memorize it, but know the following:

- **Low risk 0-2** is treated medically with predischarge stress testing and angiography is positive
- **High risk 3-7** requires early revascularization (24 hours)

Treat all patients with NSTEMI as follows:

- Dual antiplatelet therapy (DAPT) regardless of reperfusion strategy: aspirin plus a P2Y12 inhibitor
  - If patient needs elective surgery, the P2Y12 inhibitor can be stopped after 1 month for bare metal stent and after 3 months for DES.
  - Surgery should be done with aspirin to prevent pre-op MI.
- Early loading with clopidogrel or ticagrelor (before PCI) done at presentation
- Early invasive angiography within 24 hours of presentation (if angiography cannot be done or stent cannot be placed due to anatomy, use clopidogrel or ticagrelor for 1 year and aspirin indefinitely)
- Prasugrel (very effective)
  - Use only after coronary stent placement and not at presentation
  - Use only in those who have stent; use clopidogrel or ticagrelor in those who had ACS without stent
  - Contraindicated when age >75, weight <60 kg, or history of previous stroke/TIA
- Glycoprotein IIb/IIIa inhibitors (e.g., abciximab) only for use during PCI in patients with evident
- Drug-eluting stent (sirolimus and paclitaxel) to reduce the rate of restenosis (from 30% frequency to <5%); those with stent must take aspirin and a second anti-platelet drug (e.g., clopidogrel, prasugrel)

**CLINICAL PEARL**

- Ticagrelor is associated with higher rates of bleeding and increased incidence of dyspnea and bradycardia.
- In patients tolerant of DAPT, upfront administration of GP IIB/IIIA inhibitors in the ED has no proven benefit and poses an increased bleeding risk; thus, there is no role for initiation following PCI.

### Follow-up Management and Prevention

- ICU monitoring in those patients producing enzymes consistent with MI
- Telemetry monitoring
- Aspirin and a second anti-platelet agent for those undergoing angioplasty or with MI
- One year (ideally) of DAPT in all patients with ASC (for high-risk bleeding, can reduce to aspirin only after 1 month for bare metal stent or 3 months for DES)
- High intensity statin, beta blocker, and ACE inhibitor (can stop ACE inhibitor at 6 wks if echocardiogram shows normal wall motion and ejection fraction >40%)

### Final Diagnosis

Non-ST elevation MI

# CASE 5

## Chief Complaint

Hyperlipidemia management

## History

A 58-year-old man has been referred to the office by his vascular surgeon for preoperative evaluation prior to undergoing a femoral-popliteal bypass graft. He denies a history of angina, though he does have a history of diabetes mellitus and hypertension. There is no family history of coronary artery disease. He stopped smoking 6 months ago. The initial electrocardiogram is normal.

Because of his multiple risk factors, you decide to perform a stress test. A dipyridamole thallium test is performed because his claudication leaves him unable to exercise. The stress test shows an area of reversible ischemia in the inferior wall. The surgeon is concerned because the total cholesterol is elevated at 212 mg/dL. Vital signs are T 36.8 (98.2 F), BP 124/82 mm Hg, pulse 82/min, and respirations 14/min. Examination of the head, eyes, ears, nose, and throat is normal except for arcus senilis. Peripheral pulses in his extremities, which are smooth and shiny, are diminished.

## Differential Diagnosis

1. No specific differential diagnosis
2. Patient is evaluated for PVD, HTN, diabetes, and hyperlipidemia before surgery to exclude subclinical CAD and for the management of dyslipidemia

## Initial Management

**Setting:** outpatient

## Diagnostic/Therapeutic Plan

- Total cholesterol
- LDL
- Triglycerides
- HDL

## Test Results

- Total cholesterol: 212 mg/dL (normal <200 mg/dL)
- LDL: 138 mg/dL
- Triglycerides: 125 mg/dL (normal <150 mg/dL)
- HDL: 52 mg/dL (normal 40–60 mg/dL)

### CCS NOTE

Don't forget to order the proper diet for each patient based on diabetes, hypertension, hyperlipidemia, or obesity.

### Assessment

This patient has an elevated LDL cholesterol in the presence of coronary artery disease (CAD). Although he has no history of angina, he does have multiple risk factors for CAD. Even in the absence of symptoms, preoperative evaluation with a stress test may reveal ischemic heart disease. (Remember, up to 25% of patients who have sudden death from an acute MI have no history of chest pain.)

The major risk factors for CAD are diabetes, hypertension, tobacco smoking, hyperlipidemia, HDL <40 mg/dL, and a family history of premature coronary disease in a first-degree relative. In fact, even in the absence of these traditional risk factors, the peripheral vascular disease itself could be considered evidence of probable coronary disease until proven otherwise.

The other clear problem here is that our patient has elevated LDL with cardiovascular disease. The most recent cholesterol guidelines recommend an approach which focuses primarily on risk level and intensity of statin therapy. In essence, there was a switch from treating lab tests to treating patients.

**NOTE**

The ASCVD Risk Score will be provided for you on the exam, so there is no need to memorize.

The 10-year Atherosclerotic Cardiovascular Disease (ASCVD) Risk Score should be calculated on all patients age >40, to calculate one's 10-year risk of having a cardiovascular problem, such as a heart. Things it takes into account include the patient's age, blood pressure, total cholesterol, HDL, diabetic status, hypertension, and smoking status.

- **Low risk**: <5%
- **Borderline risk**: 5–7.5%
- **Intermediate risk**: 7.5–20%
- **High risk**: ≥20%

Based on extensive research, there are 4 groups of people for whom statin therapy seems to reduce cardiovascular events with a good margin of safety:

- Those with clinical cardiovascular disease
- Those age 20–75 with primary elevation of LDL ≥190 mg/dL
- Those age 40–75 without clinical cardiovascular disease with diabetes with LDL 70–189 mg/dL and with an estimated 10-year cardiovascular disease risk ≥7.5% OR those who have had type 2 DM ≥10 years OR those who have had type 1 DM for ≥20 years OR those with complications of diabetes (e.g., albuminuria [≥30 µg of albumin per mg of creatinine]) OR estimated glomerular filtration rate <60 mL/min per 1.73 m2 OR retinopathy OR neuropathy
- 10-year ASCVD risk score ≥20%

Guidelines for statin therapy are as follows. Before initiation of a statin, aminotransferases should be checked. (In the absence of symptoms of liver injury, do not repeat this measurement during statin therapy.) Repeat lipids 4-12 weeks to assess adherence and response.

- **Patients age 40–75 with low risk diabetes (see above for high risk) and those age >40 with ASCVD risk score 7.5-20%**: moderate intensity statin
- **Patients age >75**: high intensity statins not recommended, due to risk of rhabdomyolysis
- **Patients in whom statins have not reduced LDL (or in whom statins are contraindicated)**: non-statin drug to lower LDL (possibly in combination with a statin); ezetimibe has been shown to reduce risk of cardiovascular disease and should be added to statin in patient with IHD if LDL is still >70 mg/dL

- **Patients who are intolerant to statins or high-risk patients who need additional LDL reduction**: proprotein convertase subtilisin/kexin type 9 (PCSK9) inhibitors
  - Evolocumab and alirocumab significantly reduce LDL (nearly 60% and even more when added to a statin) and have a cardiovascular risk reduction benefit.
  - Inclisiran is a small interfering RNA that binds to and degrades mRNA for PCSK9. It is a 2x/yearly injection that interferes with the transcription of and translation of PCSK9.

The guidelines also stress that lifestyle modification (heart-healthy diet, regular exercise, avoidance of tobacco, and maintenance of a healthy weight) is critically important for everyone—both before and during treatment.

Therefore, in our patient the target LDL should be <70 mg/dL, given that he has a positive stress test, peripheral vascular disease, and diabetes.

## Further Management Plan

1. Dietary modification to limit the intake of saturated fats
2. High intensity statin HMG CoA reductase inhibitors (rosuvastatin, atorvastatin)
3. Exercise
4. Liver function tests (AST, ALT, bilirubin)

### CLINICAL PEARL

PCSK9 is a protease that degrades LDL receptors in the membrane of liver cells. PCSK9 inhibitors are monoclonal antibodies that bind to PCSK9, inhibit the degradation of LDL receptors, and increase clearance of LDL from the serum.

## Discussion

This patient has an LDL >130 mg/dL in the presence of CAD. In addition, the diabetes and peripheral vascular disease should be considered the equivalent of CAD. Peripheral vascular disease is clinical cardiovascular disease, and this patient should be started on a high intensity statin.

Statins are generally the initial drug of choice because they have the greatest demonstrated effect upon mortality and the incidence of serious cardiac events such as myocardial infarction. The most common adverse effects of statins are elevated LFTs and myositis, leading to elevated creatinine phosphokinase (CPK). There is no routine recommendation to monitor CPK levels. Additionally:

- Start dietary modification and exercise
- Repeat LDL level in 4-12 weeks; if not <70 mg/dL, add ezetimibe
- Repeat LDL in an additional 4-12 weeks; if still >70, add evolocumab or alirocumab

## Follow-up Management and Prevention

- Repeat LDL cholesterol level in 6 wks (lipid levels no more than every 6–12 mos)
- Patient counseling about lifestyle modification (the CCS also accepts the terms "educate" and "advise")

## Final Diagnosis

Hyperlipidemia

## CASE 6

### Chief Complaint

"I can't breathe!"

### History and Physical Examination

A 68-year-old woman is brought to the emergency department by ambulance because of acute shortness of breath. She has a history of multiple myocardial infarctions and is normally on a diuretic, metoprolol, digoxin, and enalapril. She is normally somewhat edematous but not dyspneic.

She has become more short of breath over the past several days, even worsening over the past few hours. Vital signs are T 36.8 C (98.2 F), BP 140/90 mm Hg, pulse 120/min, and respirations 32/min. Physical examination shows marked jugular venous distention and bilateral rales to the apices. Her abdomen is soft and nontender. Cardiovascular examination shows tachycardia with a 3/6 systolic murmur at the apex and S3 gallop. There is also evidence of a bilateral lower extremity edema to the mid-thigh.

### Differential Diagnosis

1. Acute pulmonary edema
2. Noncompliance with medications
3. Arrhythmia
4. Ischemia
5. Acute myocardial infarction
6. Valvular rupture
7. Papillary muscle rupture

### Initial Management

**Setting**: emergency department

### Diagnostic/Therapeutic Plan

- Sit patient upright
- EKG
- Oxygen
- Furosemide IV (or bumetanide)
- Nitroglycerin IV or paste to chest wall
- Morphine IV
- Chest x-ray
- Arterial blood gases
- Echocardiogram
- Non-invasive ventilation if no response to loop diuretics

**NOTE**

Physical exam findings for volume overload are specific but not sensitive. A patient can have pulmonary edema without rales or even edema. Symptoms, especially paroxysmal nocturnal dyspnea (PND), are more specific for decompensated heart failure.

### Test Results

- EKG: sinus tachycardia, Q-waves in V2–V4
- Chest x-ray: cardiomegaly, bilateral pleural effusions, and pulmonary vascular redistribution with cephalization of flow; Kerley B lines are present
- Arterial blood gases: pH 7.42, $pCO_2$ 34 mm Hg, $pO_2$ 72, saturation 93%
- Echocardiogram: ejection fraction 36%

### Assessment

This patient has multiple signs of fluid overload and CHF; most importantly, dyspnea, rales, hypoxia, and an S3 gallop. The EKG shows signs of an old anterior wall myocardial infarction, and the chest x-ray is consistent with a dilated cardiomyopathy and poor left ventricular function.

Pulmonary edema is most commonly due to acute systolic or diastolic left ventricular dysfunction or to arrhythmia. Ischemia, arrhythmia, infarction, noncompliance with medication/diet, insufficient medications, or infection can all precipitate acute left ventricular dysfunction in this patient. Less common causes are the "high-output" types of failure, such as with anemia, thyrotoxicosis, and pregnancy. Fluid overload from renal failure could also be a cause.

Brain natriuretic peptide (BNP) (blood test) is elevated when there is acute congestive failure.

- Most useful for excluding a diagnosis of dyspnea caused by CHF when the diagnosis is not clear (example: use if patient is short of breath and you are not sure if the cause is CHF, COPD, or pneumonia)
- Not useful with renal failure because it is renally excreted
- Older age increases BNP
- BNP may be falsely low and is not reliable in obesity because adipose tissue has BNP clearance receptors

Remember, 100% of patients with decompensated heart failure have elevated BNP, unless they are obese.

It is important to get a thorough history from the patient and look for cause of pulmonary edema. EKG and troponins should be checked to evaluate for ischemia. Pneumonia can lead to heart failure exacerbation. Increased heart rate in patients with atrial fibrillation is a common cause and the patient should be monitored on telemetry and heart rate control should be the primary goal if needed. Compliance with salt restriction and diuretics should be assessed.

Always ask patients with volume overload about the use of NSAIDs. NSAIDs can often lead to volume overload by inhibiting prostaglandin production, causing vasoconstriction of the afferent arterioles and decreased GFR. Alcohol use and illicit drug use should also be evaluated.

#### CCS NOTE

Pulmonary edema is a perfect CCS case. Order everything together—oxygen, furosemide, morphine, nitrates, EKG, chest x-ray, oximeter, and CK-MB—all on the same screen.

#### NOTE

Non-invasive ventilation (BIPAP) has been proven to help in the treatment of pulmonary edema. It reduces all of the following: venous return, the need for mechanical ventilation, and morbidity/mortality.

### Basic Science Correlate

**Aside from just 'not taking medications,' why would a person with CHF suddenly go into acute pulmonary edema?**

- **Ischemia:** Oxygen is needed to detach actin and myosin filaments from each other. Hypoxic myocardium does not relax or contract normally. Hypoxia induces wall motion abnormalities.
- **Arrhythmia:** The usually small atrial contribution of 10–15% to cardiac output can become as large as 40–50% in a diseased heart. This is why normally benign rhythms like atrial fibrillation can result in pulmonary edema.

**Mechanism of S3 gallop:** rapid ventricular filling in diastole

**Mechanism of furosemide:** inhibition of $2Cl^-/K^+/Na^+$ pumps in the thick ascending limb of the loop of Henle; loop diuretics do not work at the tip of the loop of Henle, but rather at the thick ascending limb

**Mechanism of nitroglycerin:** nitrates are venous dilators, i.e., they increase the size of the capacitance vessels and decrease the amount of blood in the lungs; preload reducers like nitrates, morphine, and diuretics all decrease hydrostatic pressure in pulmonary veins and lessen transudation of fluid across pulmonary vessels

## Further Management Plan

- Repeat doses of furosemide
- Continue oxygen
- Transfer patient to intensive care
- Consult critical care team
- CK-MB
- Brain natriuretic peptide when diagnosis not clear (used only as a rule-out test)

## Discussion

Pulmonary edema results from fluid overload, causing death by hypoxia. The cause is increased pulmonary capillary wedge pressure from back-up of pressures due to left heart failure. Treatment is based on reducing the excess of fluid in the lungs:

- Diuresis, as rapidly as possible to decrease preload; furosemide is given in double doses every 20 min until sufficient urine is produced
- Morphine, which dilates pulmonary vasculature and also decreases preload
- Nitrates, which dilate the venous system and reduce blood return to the lungs
- Positive inotropes (useful only for impaired left ventricular function; the entire class has not shown mortality benefit); dobutamine, an IV positive inotrope, will increase contractility and empty the lungs by causing the heart to pump better; use only for cardiogenic shock
- Milrinone, a phosphodiesterase (PDE) inhibitor that works in a similar fashion to dobutamine (rarely indicated)
- Afterload reduction: enalaprilat or nitroprusside can only be given intravenously in an ICU and will rapidly reduce afterload and allow more blood to be squeezed out of the heart with each beat (has same effect as an ACE inhibitor such as captopril and enalapril). Reducing the afterload allows for an increase in stroke volume. Always continue the ACE inhibitor later.

- Spironolactone, which helps inhibit the renin-angiotensin system and lowers mortality in systolic dysfunction; use when ejection fraction <30%
- Non-invasive ventilation reduces venous return and improves oxygenation by preventing atelectasis

### Basic Science Correlate

Why do beta blockers help CHF?

- Most common cause of death in CHF is sudden death
- Ischemia leads to arrhythmia, and arrhythmia leads to sudden death
- Beta blockers are antiarrhythmic and anti-ischemic

If beta blockers are negative inotropes, why do they increase cardiac output?

- Beta blockers slow the heart rate
- Slow heart rate increases preload and ventricular filling
- More preload and filling of the heart increase stroke volume
- Beta blockers decrease aldosterone by inhibiting renin production

## Follow-up Management and Prevention

- ICU monitoring for 24–48 hrs
- Transfer to floor when MI excluded and hypoxia improved
- Echocardiography
- Dobutamine or milrinone if still symptomatic after repeat doses of preload reduction (nitrates, furosemide, morphine) and in shock
- Swan-Ganz catheter placement if still critical after initial treatment and diagnosis is not clear
  - A high PCWP is the most accurate indicator of cardiogenic pulmonary edema, due to elevated left sided pressure from left heart.
  - High pulmonary artery pressure and normal PCWP indicate a pulmonary source such as a PE or primary pulmonary hypertension.
  - If there is pulmonary edema and the PCWP pressure is normal, that is non-cardiogenic pulmonary edema (ARDS) caused by capillary leak from inflammation as in sepsis (cytokine surge, IL-1, IL-6, TNF-alfa)
- Beta-blockers, only if patient euvolemic; start with a low dose and increase slowly
- Digoxin after stabilization if still symptomatic on beta-blockers, diuretics, ACE inhibitors and spironolactone
- ACE inhibitor or ARB for all patients with heart failure unless contraindicated; sacubitril-valsartan now preferred

## Final Diagnosis

Pulmonary edema

# CASE 7

## Chief Complaint

"My breath is short and my vision is blurry. I can't think straight."

## History and Physical Examination

A 47-year-old man comes to the emergency department complaining of several hours of dyspnea, blurry vision, and difficulty thinking. He has never had symptoms like this before. They came on while he was at his sedentary office job. He also has a worsening headache, dizziness, and mild palpitations. The patient has never had a myocardial infarction in the past, but he has high BP for which he is on a thiazide diuretic.

Vital signs are T 36.9 C (98.4 F), BP 230/150 mm Hg, pulse 88/min, and respirations 18/min. Physical examination of the head, eyes, ears, nose, and throat shows arteriolar narrowing and AV nicking. A few hemorrhages are visible, and there is no jugular venous distention. Upon auscultation, there are very few scattered rales. He has a regular heart rate and rhythm, with an audible S4 gallop. His abdomen is soft and nontender, and his extremities are not edematous.

## Differential Diagnosis

1. Hypertensive emergency
2. Acute myocardial infarction
3. Intraparenchymal brain hemorrhage
4. Subarachnoid hemorrhage

## Initial Management

**Setting**: emergency department

## Diagnostic/Therapeutic Plan

- EKG
- BUN/creatinine
- CBC
- IV labetalol, nitroprusside, or enalaprilat
- Oxygen
- Oximeter

## Test Results

- EKG: sinus rhythm, S in V1 + R in V5 = 42 mm, mild down-sloping of ST segment in V2–V4
- BUN/creatinine: mildly elevated
- Hematocrit: 37%, few schistocytes visible, platelets: 110,000/$mm^3$
- Oximeter: 98% saturation on room air

### Assessment

The patient's most obvious problem on physical examination is a profoundly high BP; the dyspnea, blurring of vision, dizziness, and headache can all be the result of that. Often, these complaints can be hard to differentiate from the headache and dizziness that accompany an intracranial bleed such as a subarachnoid hemorrhage. We know that it can be characterized by disseminated intravascular coagulation, fibrinoid necrosis of arteriolar walls, microangiopathic hemolytic anemia, and dilation of cerebral blood vessels, but the root cause is unknown.

### Further Management Plan/Results

1. Head CT scan
2. Chest x-ray
3. Continue IV antihypertensive: labetalol, nitroprusside, or enalaprilat
4. Transfer to ICU for critical care consult
5. Reduction of BP by approximately 1/3, but not <95 mm Hg diastolic

### Test Results

- Head CT normal
- Cardiomegaly with clear lung fields

### Discussion

Various medications can be used to treat a hypertensive emergency. Because of the emergent nature of the crisis and the potential for myocardial infarction, stroke, and blindness, an IV agent that works in minutes is preferable. The best agents are as follows:

- **Labetalol** works through the nonspecific beta-1 and -2 blockade and is also an alpha-blocking agent. It has the added advantage of being available intravenously and orally. There are few serious side effects with emergent use. Safe in pregnancy.
- **Nitroprusside** is both an arterial and venous dilator, and has the most rapid onset of action (seconds) and shortest duration of action (minutes). Because of its potency, it should be given only in an ICU setting where an arterial line can establish very direct monitoring of pressure. Cyanide poisoning, however, may develop from its metabolites.
- **Nitroglycerin** works predominantly through venous dilation. This agent is ideal for those patients in hypertensive crisis in whom an MI may be occurring.
- Other agents are **enalaprilat** (IV ACE inhibitor), **nicardipine, fenoldopam**, and **hydralazine**. About 1% of patients with hypertension will develop a hypertensive crisis at some point, and very rarely is it the first manifestation of hypertensive disease.
- The calcium blocker **nicardipine** can also be used to lower pressure acutely.

### CCS NOTE

- For an unstable patient, move the clock forward just 15 min at a time.
- In a hypertensive emergency, the most important thing is to use an IV medication.
- On the exam you will not be asked for doses. The specific agent is not as important as the route of administration.

Hypertensive emergency (or "malignant" or "accelerated" hypertension or "crisis") is not defined on the basis of any specific blood-pressure number; it describes the development of end organ damage. The most common causes of death from hypertensive emergency are stroke, renal failure, and CHF. Other manifestations of the syndrome include retinal changes (such as in this patient) and confusion from altered cerebral blood flow. In this case the EKG abnormalities are the findings consistent with left ventricular hypertrophy (SV2 + RV5 >35 mm). ST segment depression can also result from hypertrophic cardiomyopathy.

Scleroderma-induced malignant hypertension is preferentially treated with ACE inhibitors. Cocaine-induced hypertensive crisis is treated with the alpha blocker phentolamine.

**CCS NOTE**

Patients with BP problems severe enough to cause chest pain or altered mental status should go to the ICU.

### Follow-up Management and Prevention

- When symptoms resolve, transfer patient to floor
- Stop IV medication, start oral medication
- Labetalol or enalapril orally is acceptable
- Expect to use 2–3 oral medications

### Final Diagnosis

Hypertensive emergency

# CASE 8

## Chief Complaint

"I fainted in ballet class."

## History and Physical Examination

A 17-year-old girl comes to the office for evaluation of recurrent syncope. Each episode occurred following vigorous exertional activity. The day before she came in, she had been jogging around the school track and suddenly passed out. She was reportedly unconscious for less than a minute and felt fine afterward. She had no associated palpitations, seizure-like movements, or incontinence. She reports regular menses since age 12 and has noted no association between the syncopal episodes and her menstrual cycle.

Vital signs are T 36.7 C (98.1 F), BP 110/60 mm Hg, pulse 80/min, and respirations 16/min. Cardiovascular examination shows prominent apical impulse, S4 gallop, and a 2/6 systolic murmur at the lower left sternal border. The murmur worsens with Valsalva and improves with squatting. The rest of the physical examination is unremarkable.

## Differential Diagnosis

1. Vasovagal syncopal episode
2. Seizure disorder
3. Cardiac arrhythmia
4. Hypertrophic obstructive cardiomyopathy (HOCM)
5. Aortic stenosis
6. Hypoglycemia
7. Electrolyte disorder
8. Pulmonary hypertension

### CLINICAL PEARL

The most important feature of a case of syncope is whether the **loss of consciousness occurred suddenly or gradually.** A sudden loss of consciousness is caused by cardiac and neurologic problems.

## Initial Management

**Setting:** emergency department

## Diagnostic/Therapeutic Plan

- EKG
- Telemetry

## Test Results

- EKG: left ventricular hypertrophy; nonspecific ST- and T-wave abnormalities; small Q-waves in inferior and lateral leads
- Telemetry: normal; no arrhythmias detected

## Assessment

The differential diagnosis of syncope in a young patient is quite broad. In this patient, the prominent findings on physical examination point to a cardiac etiology. Although dyspnea is the most common presenting complaint with hypertrophic obstructive cardiomyopathy, it's possible for patients to have angina or syncope. Most commonly, these symptoms are related to exertion. Characteristic findings on physical exam include sustained left ventricular apical impulse, prominent S4 gallop, and harsh systolic ejection murmur, loudest at the left lower sternal border and often associated with a thrill. A brisk carotid upstroke is often present.

Valsalva maneuver results in augmentation of the murmur, whereas squatting diminishes it. The Valsalva maneuver decreases venous return to the heart, which results in a smaller ventricular-chamber size. Anything that decreases ventricular-chamber size increases the outflow tract obstruction and therefore increases the murmur. Echocardiogram is the diagnostic procedure of choice.

## Further Management Plan

- Echocardiogram
- Troponin

## Test Results

- Thickened ventricular septum, which is hypertrophied disproportionately to the posterior wall of the left ventricle. Anterior displacement of the mitral valve apparatus during systole. Diastolic dysfunction
- Troponin normal

### Patient Safety Note

Patients with syncope should be placed on continuous cardiac monitoring. The most important aspect of a syncope case is to exclude a cardiac etiology; 80–85% of the mortality has a cardiac etiology.

## Discussion

Although HOCM may present in young adults, it does not often become clinically apparent until later in life. Asymmetric septal hypertrophy leads to outflow tract obstruction. Diastolic abnormalities with decreased compliance and delayed relaxation are not uncommon.

When symptomatic, the most common symptom of HOCM is dyspnea. Life-threatening arrhythmias, myocardial ischemia, and sudden death are all complications. Initial management usually involves giving a beta-blocker or calcium-channel blocker to enhance diastolic filling. Verapamil is preferable because of its negative inotropic effects. (In general, positive inotropes including digitalis and beta-agonists should be avoided.)

The major concern with treatment in HOCM is the associated risk of malignant arrhythmia and sudden death. Beta-blocker therapy helps to reduce this risk, though amiodarone is an option. Surgical therapy is reserved for those refractory to medical therapy.

Diuretics should be avoided, as should digoxin, nitrates, vasodilators, and ACE inhibitors. They all help reduce the left ventricular-chamber size and therefore worsen the obstruction.

HOCM is the best example of diastolic dysfunction. With diastolic dysfunction, the mainstay of therapy is beta blockers. Digoxin has no value here, and in fact may worsen symptoms.

### Follow-up Management and Prevention

- Oral beta blocker, e.g., metoprolol
- Telemetry monitoring for 24–48 hrs in hospital
- Electrophysiology evaluation
- Cardiology consult to evaluate patient for implantable defibrillator
- Avoidance of extreme exertional activity and volume depletion
- Alcohol infusion via a catheter into myometrium of the septum to cause microinfarctions of septal perforator arteries
- Surgical myomectomy when not responsive to medical management
- Possible defibrillator placement

### Final Diagnosis

Syncope due to hypertrophic obstructive cardiomyopathy (HOCM)

## CASE 9

### Chief Complaint

"I'm having a hard time breathing."

### History and Physical Examination

A 36-year-old woman from Ecuador comes to the office because of progressive dyspnea on exertion over the last several months. Although she has been symptomatic for several months, she now comes at the insistence of her employer because she is starting to cough up blood on a regular basis. The dyspnea is occurring with progressively smaller amounts of exercise. She also complains of occasional palpitations.

Vital signs are T 37 C (98.6 F), BP 110/70 mm Hg, and pulse 90/min. Examination shows jugular venous distension with prominent a-waves. Mild bibasilar rales are present upon auscultation. She has a regular heart rate and rhythm with a 2/6 diastolic murmur at the lower left sternal border and a loud S1 and snap after S2. The rest of the physical examination is unremarkable.

**CLINICAL PEARL**

Although EKG and chest x-ray should be part of any initial evaluation in shortness of breath, do not expect them to show much on valvular disorders.

### Differential Diagnosis

1. Mitral stenosis
2. Left atrial myxoma
3. Atrial septal defect
4. Primary pulmonary hypertension
5. Tuberculosis

### Initial Management

**Setting**: outpatient

### Diagnostic/Therapeutic Plan

- Chest x-ray
- EKG
- Oximeter
- Echocardiogram

### Test Results

- Chest x-ray: straightening of left heart border, some elevation of left main stem bronchus, and a density is visible behind the heart; prominent pulmonary arteries are seen
- EKG: normal sinus rhythm with biphasic P waves in V1
- Oximeter: 94% saturation on room air
- Echocardiogram: left atrial enlargement with moderate mitral stenosis

## Assessment

Although there are numerous possibilities for the cause of hemoptysis, a young patient with the physical findings above suggests a cardiac etiology. The patient is young for aortic stenosis, and the cardiac exam does not support this form of lesion in which you would expect to find a systolic murmur at the right second intercostal space.

In addition, the patient has a snap after S2, which is characteristic of the opening snap of mitral stenosis. The patient is from Ecuador and may have a history of rheumatic fever. Mitral stenosis is the most common valvular abnormality after rheumatic fever. The EKG shows the biphasic P wave in V1, characteristic of left atrial hypertrophy, and the chest x-ray shows the same.

The symptoms imply that the stenosis is becoming severe, but only cardiac catheterization from the arterial side can give a precise estimate.

All left-sided valvular disorders increase in intensity and become louder with squatting and leg-raises. Squatting and leg-raising increase the amount of venous return to the heart. Valsalva will decrease their intensity. The opposite happens with mitral valve prolapse and obstructive cardiomyopathy.

- Mechanism of hemoptysis: pulmonary hypertension
- Mechanism of atrial fibrillation: dilation of left atrium
- Mechanism of opening snap: mitral valve leaflets suddenly stopping

### Basic Science Correlate

Rheumatic fever causes fibrosis of the mitral valve.

**Mechanism of opening snap happening earlier in worsening disease:**

- Mitral valve opens when left atrial pressure exceeds left ventricular pressure
- When stenosis worsens, left atrial pressure increases

**Why does dysphagia occur in MS?**

- Most posterior structure in the heart is left atrium
- Left atrial enlargement presses against the esophagus

## Further Management Plan

- Left heart catheterization
- Salt restriction
- Diuretics

## Test Results

- Left heart catheterization: mitral stenosis with 1.3 $cm^2$ outlet

## Discussion

Symptoms of mitral stenosis usually develop in middle age, but this is usually about 20 years after an episode of acute rheumatic fever. Symptoms are based on an inability to handle the forward flow of blood through a narrowed orifice.

- Anything that elevates the amount of blood that has to flow through (i.e., exertion, excitement, infection, pregnancy, or thyrotoxicosis) will increase symptoms.
- Any cause of tachycardia will also increase symptoms because the atria empty only during diastole, and tachycardia shortens diastole.
- Anything that reduces the amount of plasma volume—salt restriction, diuretics—will decrease symptoms.

Endocarditis prophylaxis before dental or surgical procedure is not indicated. Atrial fibrillation is very common in mitral stenosis because of the dilation of the atria. Control of the rate of atrial fibrillation and anticoagulation to prevent thrombus formation is usually central to the management of mitral stenosis because a rapid rate worsens symptoms of pulmonary congestion. Digoxin is generally used for its effect on heart rate. If the rate is not sufficiently controlled with digoxin, a small dose of a beta-blocker is useful.

When the orifice of the mitral valve becomes severely narrow (<1.0 $cm^2$), surgical repair will reduce both symptoms and mortality.

Surgical therapy should be implemented before the onset of pulmonary hypertension.

- Mechanism of frequent stroke in MS: dilated left atrium, frequent atrial fibrillation
- Mechanism of hoarseness: left atrial pressure on recurrent laryngeal nerve
- Mechanism of metoprolol improving symptoms: slowing heart rate allows greater time for ventricular filling

## Follow-up Management and Prevention

- Salt-restriction and diuretics first
- Balloon valvuloplasty or commissurotomy if symptoms persist; if that fails, consider valvular replacement
- Oral metoprolol if there are symptoms of dyspnea
- Warfarin for clot prevention if atrial fibrillation develops

### Basic Science Correlate

- **Transesophageal echo is better than transthoracic echo for mitral stenosis** because the mitral valve is the most posterior valve in the heart.
- You can **balloon mitral stenosis (MS) but not aortic stenosis (AS)**; that is because the mechanism of MS is fibrosis while the mechanism of AS is calcification (you cannot balloon open calcification).

## Final Diagnosis

Mitral stenosis

# CASE 10

## Chief Complaint

"I have cramping pain in my right calf while walking."

## History and Physical Examination

A 71-year-old man with a long history of cardiovascular disease comes to your office complaining of cramping pain in the right calf while walking. In recent months he has had increased difficulty walking because of pain in the right calf, which starts after walking approximately 2 blocks. When he stops, the pain goes away, and then it begins again if he continues another 3 blocks. He experiences no pain while at rest. He had a myocardial infarction 20 years ago. He is a 40-pack-year smoker. Current medications include oral nitrates and a beta-blocker.

Vital signs are stable. Examination of the extremities shows left leg with strong pulses throughout. Right leg has diminished femoral pulse compared with the left, and there are no popliteal or pedal pulses palpable. There is an absence of hair with smooth, shiny skin in the right lower leg. Motor and sensory examination is equal bilaterally in both extremities.

## Differential Diagnosis

1. Leg claudication
2. Spinal stenosis
3. Peripheral neuropathy

## Initial Management

**Setting**: outpatient

## Diagnostic/Therapeutic Plan

- Ankle/brachial arterial pressure index (ABI)

## Test Results

- ABI: 0.5 on right, 1 on left (normal 1.0-1.4)

## Assessment

Most often, no further diagnostic evaluation is necessary. This patient's history is quite characteristic of peripheral arterial disease (PAD), a narrowing of the limb arteries. He has a history of myocardial infarction, which already indicates arterial disease, and he is a long-term smoker. Atrophic changes such as diminished peripheral pulses on the side of the pain and the absence of hair with smooth, shiny skin also contribute to the diagnosis.

Normally, the ratio of the ankle-brachial arterial pressures should be 1.0 to 1.4. The femoral and popliteal arteries are the most commonly involved in atherosclerosis of the extremities.

- Resting ABI ≤0.9 p is diagnostic of PAD.
- Resting ABI >1.4 indicates the presence of noncompressible, calcified arteries in the lower extremities and is considered uninterpretable, so a toe-brachial index is indicated for diagnosis.
- Toe-brachial index <0.7 is diagnostic for PAD

An exercise ankle-brachial index is used if there is high clinical suspicion for PAD, but a normal able-brachial index.

### Further Management Plan

1. Stop smoking (provide both counseling and medication; varenicline [**most effective**] should be used in combination with short-acting nicotine replacement such as nicotine gum or lozenges)
2. Aspirin or other antiplatelet drugs such as clopidogrel
3. Graded exercise program (most effective in improving functional status)
4. BP goal < 130/80 mm Hg
5. Meticulous foot care (keep clean/dry and use well-fitting shoes)
6. Cilostazol (contraindicated in systolic dysfunction)
7. High intensity statin
8. Possible revascularization with angioplasty or surgery

**CLINICAL PEARL**

CCBs do not help peripheral vascular disease.

### Discussion

The patient should be advised to stop smoking and continue on a supervised exercise program. Most patients who stop smoking and maintain an exercise program will remain stable or improve their claudication, and will not require surgery. If the clinical situation deteriorates, however, to the point where the patient develops rest pain or becomes incapacitated (to the point of not being able to function), or sees no improvement with conservative changes above, then arteriography and consideration for surgical revascularization will be necessary.

Arteriography is not necessary for routine evaluation. It is useful only for planning surgical bypass or angioplasty by helping to determine the exact site of the lesion.

Cilostazol is an agent used in PAD that is both a vasodilator and an antiplatelet agent. It has shown significant effects in prolonging exercise tolerance and decreasing symptoms. It is clearly superior to pentoxifylline (there is no clear benefit of pentoxifylline). Cilostazol is contraindicated in systolic dysfunction.

In the past there has been concern about the use of beta blockers in those with PAD. Metoprolol and beta-1 specific agents do not worsen claudication. If a patient needs beta blockers for ischemia, arrhythmia, or CHF, they can be given safely.

Adding very low-dose rivaroxaban to aspirin reduces the occurrence of cardiovascular death, MI, or stroke by 2%, and increases the risk of bleeding by 1%.

### Follow-up Management and Prevention

- Checkups at 1-month intervals to confirm adherence to diet and exercise programs
- Smoking cessation counseling; varenicline or bupropion to help stop smoking
- ACE inhibitor (e.g., enalapril or lisinopril) for hypertension in PAD
- High intensity statin for all patients
- Combination of both aspirin and clopidogrel for severe disease
- Beta-blocker as needed for other indications when PAD is present (metoprolol is safe)
- Revascularization for persistent symptoms

### Final Diagnosis

Peripheral arterial disease (PAD)/claudication

# CASE 11

## Chief Complaint

"I can't breathe so well."

## History and Physical Examination

A 56-year-old man is in a motor vehicle accident and sustains chest wall trauma. He is brought to the emergency department an hour later with shortness of breath. He is generally healthy. He takes no medications and has no drug allergies.

He is afebrile. BP is 114/70 mm Hg, pulse 118/min, and respirations 26/min. Physical examination reveals chest contusions visible over the sternum and several tender ribs. Jugular venous distention is noted.

## Differential Diagnosis

1. Pneumothorax
2. Congestive failure
3. Tamponade

## Initial Management

**Setting:** emergency department

## Diagnostic/Therapeutic Plan

- Normal saline bolus
- Oxygen
- Chest x-ray
- Oximeter
- EKG
- Arterial blood gases

## Test Results

- Chest x-ray: rib fractures, no infiltrates
- Oximeter: 93% saturation on room air
- EKG: sinus tachycardia; QRS complexes vary in size from beat to beat
- Arterial blood gases: pH 7.53, $pCO_2$ 24 mm Hg, $pO_2$ 74 mm Hg

### Assessment

Tachycardia, hypotension, and distended neck veins are the signs of cardiac tamponade. The compression of the heart will cause decreased cardiac output and the backup of blood into the neck veins. BP will drop on inspiration normally; this drop in BP is exaggerated in cardiac tamponade.

A drop in BP on inhalation >10 mm Hg is called 'pulsus paradoxus.' It is a 'paradox' because when BP drops below 90 mm Hg, the radial pulse will disappear. This is the paradox: the pulse disappears but the patient is still alive.

Tamponade is associated with pulsus paradoxus. Constrictive pericarditis is associated with Kussmaul sign. Kussmaul sign is an increase in jugulovenous pressure on inhalation. Chest wall trauma can cause tamponade. Anything that causes pericarditis can cause tamponade if there is enough extravasation of fluid into the pericardial space to compress the heart.

The variation in the height of the QRS from beat to beat is called 'electrical alternans.' It is from the heart flopping backward and forward in the chest.

### Further Management Plan/Results

| | |
|---|---|
| Assess pulsus paradoxus | Systolic BP drops 20 mm on inhalation |
| Echocardiogram | Diastolic collapse of right atrium and right ventricle |

### Discussion

Cardiac tamponade is an emergency. Compression of the right side of the heart occurs first because the walls of these chambers are thinner than those on the left side of the heart. Death occurs from hypotension. Needle decompression of as little as 50–100 mL of fluid can be life-saving.

Diuretics should not be given because they decrease right ventricular filling pressure and can make the collapse of the right side of the heart even worse. Occasionally, a right-sided catheterization is performed. There is equalization of pressures in all 4 chambers of the heart in diastole.

### Follow-up Management and Prevention

- Continue IV normal saline
- Pericardiocentesis with a needle
- Possible placement of a pericardial window
- Surgical consultation
- Transfer to ICU

### Final Diagnosis

Cardiac tamponade

### CLINICAL PEARL

**Tamponade**

- Jugular venous distention, hypotension, tachycardia
- Pulsus paradoxus
- Electrical alternans on EKG
- Right atrial and ventricular diastolic collapse on echocardiogram

**Pneumothorax**

- Distended neck veins
- No pulsus paradoxus
- Visible on chest x-ray
- Needle or chest tube decompression

**Pericarditis**

- Chest pain that changes with respiration and position
- ST elevation everywhere on EKG
- PR segment depression
- Treat with NSAIDs; if no response, use steroids
- Use colchicine to prevent recurrences

# CASE 12

## Chief Complaint

"I passed out."

## History and Physical Examination

A 72-year-old man comes to the emergency department with an episode of syncope lasting <10 minutes, witnessed by his family. He was getting up from a seated position and started to play with his grandson when he suddenly lost consciousness. Within 5 minutes of hitting the floor, he fully regained consciousness. He denies a history of dyspnea and chest pain.

BP is 110/88 mm Hg, pulse 96/min, respirations 18/min. There is no fever. Chest is clear to auscultation. Cardiovascular exam reveals III/VI murmur at the second upper right intercostal space. The murmur radiates to the carotid arteries. The murmur is worse with leg raise and squatting and better with Valsalva. HEENT reveals a diminished carotid upstroke. On the exterior, no edema is found.

## Differential Diagnosis

- Vasovagal
- Orthostatic due to volume depletion or medications such as alfa-blockers
- Cardiogenic: sinus bradycardia, AV block
- Tachyarrhythmia, mechanical (AS, HOCM, PE)
- Seizure

## Initial Management

**Setting:** emergency department

## Diagnostic/Therapeutic Plan

- IV normal saline
- Oxygen
- Oximeter
- EKG
- Telemetry monitoring
- CK-MB and troponin

### Test Results

- Oximeter 97% room air saturation
- EKG: SV1 and RV5 >40 mm; no ST changes; T-wave inversions in lateral leads that are old
- Telemetry monitoring: unrevealing so far
- CK-MB and troponin: normal

### Assessment

The most important element of the evaluation of syncope is to exclude cardiac ischemia or arrhythmia as the cause. The majority of the mortality is associated with cardiac syncope; that is why an EKG, cardiac enzymes, and telemetry monitoring are done in almost all cases. Ventricular arrhythmia leads to syncope, and cardiac ischemia is the most common cause of arrhythmia.

It is important to determine the following 3 things.

1. **Did the loss of consciousness occur suddenly?**

   Sudden loss means a cardiac or neurologic abnormality
2. **Did the regaining of consciousness occur suddenly?**

   Sudden regaining means a cardiac problem
3. **Is there a murmur on exam?**

   An abnormal exam means aortic stenosis (AS), HOCM, or mitral stenosis

In this case, even before a single test is done, we know the origin of the loss of consciousness has to be cardiac. In addition, the murmur heard at the right second intercostal space has to be AS.

Also, with AS:

- There is an association with a decreased carotid upstroke and the signs of left ventricular hypertrophy on EKG (found here)
- Murmur decreases in intensity with Valsalva and standing position

### Further Management Plan/Results

| Transthoracic echocardiogram | Severe AS, valve diameter 0.8 $cm^2$ |
|---|---|

### Discussion

AS most commonly presents with chest pain because 50–70% of patients also have coronary disease, and the valvular damage limits the amount of blood flowing into the coronary blood vessels. The high frequency of coronary artery disease in these patients warrants excluding ischemia first. After chest pain, the next most common symptoms are syncope and dyspnea. Anyone with symptomatic AS needs treatment.

Transthoracic aortic valve repair (TAVR) is the first-line treatment. Surgical valve repair is optimal. If the patient is undergoing valve replacement and the chest is going to be opened, the

**CLINICAL PEARL**

Aortic stenosis should be distinguished from HOCM.

- Syncope, dyspnea, and chest pain
- Systolic murmur better with squatting and leg raise
- Diagnose with echocardiogram
- Treat with beta blocker or verapamil
- Catheter decompression with alcohol infusion or surgical myomectomy

patient should be evaluated for coronary artery disease. Use the opportunity for bypass surgery at the same time if needed.

### Follow-up Management and Prevention

- Cardiology evaluation
- Cardiothoracic surgery evaluation
- Valve replacement surgery

### Final Diagnosis

Syncope due to aortic stenosis

# CASE 13

## Chief Complaint

Follow-up of heart failure

## History and Physical Examination

A 67-year-old woman is evaluated during a follow-up visit for heart failure with reduced EF. She reports stable dyspnea with exertion when carrying groceries from her car or walking up a hill. She has no other symptoms. She has a history of COPD. Medications are lisinopril, furosemide, tiotropium, and albuterol.

On physical exam, BP is 138/82 mm Hg and pulse is 78/min. The lungs are clear and she has no edema. Laboratory studies reveal a creatinine of 1.3 mg/dL. Echocardiogram shows and left ventricular ejection fraction of 37%.

## Differential Diagnosis

None; follow-up of known diagnosis

## Initial Management

**Setting**: clinic

## Diagnostic/Therapeutic Plan

- Echocardiogram
- Chest x-ray
- TSH: normal
- Renal function: normal

## Test Results

- Echocardiogram: low EF
- Chest x-ray: normal
- TSH:
- Renal function:

## Assessment

Heart failure is a clinical syndrome characterized by fluid overload and decreased cardiac output. It can result from impairment in ejection of blood (systolic dysfunction) or ventricular filling (diastolic dysfunction), both of which lead to increased ventricular filling pressures and ultimately to classic signs and symptoms of heart failure (dyspnea orthopnea, peripheral edema, crackles).

In systolic dysfunction the LV ejection fraction is reduced (now called heart failure with reduced ejection fraction [HFrEF]) and is defined by EF <40%. Common causes are coronary artery disease (>50%), hypertension, diabetes, obesity, valvular heart disease.

In response to low cardiac output, the neurohormonal systems including renin-angiotensin-aldosterone system and sympathetic nervous systems are active; angiotensin II leads to vasoconstriction, increasing blood pressure, and increased afterload. Aldosterone leads to increased volume retention by increasing sodium retention, leading to increased preload.

Chronic activation of the neurohormonal systems in HFrEF causes not only hemodynamic alteration by increasing afterload and preload, but also structural and functional changes in individual myocytes, leading to worsening global LV function and dilations. Ischemic workup should be done in high-risk patients (diabetes, hypertension, smoking history, family history).

Diastolic dysfunction is characterized by a stiffened LV with abnormal relaxation, resulting in an increased in LV preload. EF >50% hypertension is the most common cause, but other causes include aging, obesity, DM, atrial fibrillation, and CAD.

Diastolic dysfunction can also be caused by amyloidosis, hemochromatosis, and sarcoidosis. These patients will have low voltage on EKG.

### Further Management Plan

There are several changes that should be made to this patient's care.

- Start metoprolol succinate, carvedilol, or bisoprolol.
- Change lisinopril to sacubitril-valsartan.
- Add spironolactone.
- DO NOT start digoxin.
- In 90 days, assess for cardiac device with another echocardiogram.
- Send to cardiac rehab.

### Discussion

This patient has a history of heart failure with low EF. She has stable symptoms. Examining her for volume overload is extremely important. If she were volume overloaded, the next step would be to increase the loop diuretic dose but not start a beta-blocker (not safe). However, because she is not volume overloaded, it is time to start thinking of medications that will reduce her mortality for HFrEF. There are many and it is very important to know them and when they should be started.

- Sacubitril/valsartan (**recommended over an ACE inhibitor or angiotensin receptor blocker**, as long as the BP can tolerate it)
  - Within a new class of drugs called angiotensin receptor neprilysin inhibitors (ARNI)
  - Significantly reduces heart failure hospitalization and mortality in patients with symptoms heart failure with reduced ejection fraction
  - Reduces mortality and heart failure hospitalization by 20%, as compared to enalapril (however, increases hypotension as compared to enalapril, so monitor as needed)
  - If patient is on an ACE-I, hold for 36 hours before starting sacubitril/valsartan to reduce risk of angioedema (neprilysin breaks down bradykinin).

#### CLINICAL PEARL

Sacubitril inhibits neprilysin, an enzyme that breaks down ANP and BNP (which both cause vasodilation and natriuresis/diuresis, reduce sympathetic tone, reduce cardiac fibrosis/hypertrophy, and reduce renin release). Neprilysin also breaks down bradykinin (hence the angioedema).

- Beta blocker
  - Initiate at a low dose and increase slowly (over weeks, not days) until HR <60/min if tolerated. Do not initiate if volume overloaded—only if euvolemic.
  - Beta-blockers are safe in stable pulmonary disease, but do not give if there is wheezing.
- Aldosterone antagonist (spironolactone, eplerenone) for all cases of symptomatic heart failure with reduced EF and normal kidney function (GFR >30) to improve survival; watch potassium closely (eplerenone is a more selective aldosterone blocker and will cause less gynecomastia)
- Ivabradine, an inhibitor of the funny current in the SA node (helpful only in sinus rhythm, not in atrial fibrillation)
  - Slows sinus heart rate
  - Add to regimen if HR >70/min while on maximum beta blocker dose (should not replace the beta blocker)
- Calcium channel blocker
  - Diltiazem and verapamil have negative inotropic properties and can worsen symptoms/mortality; never use in low EF.
  - If needed for additional BP control, amlodipine and felodipine are safe.
- Mechanical devices to further improve prognosis (can be considered only after patient has tried medical therapy for 40 days post-MI or 90 days all others):
  - Automatic implantable cardioverter/defibrillator (AICD), standard therapy for patients with EF <35%, which interrupts arrhythmia and lowers mortality in patients with systolic CHF; indications include ischemic or non-ischemic dilated cardiomyopathy with persistent ejection fraction <35% and NYHA class II–III or ejection fraction <30% and NYHA class I on medical therapy
  - Biventricular pacemaker, which "resynchronizes" the heart when there is dilated cardiomyopathy; the device also includes an automatic defibrillator (since patients are at risk for ventricular arrhythmia); indications include dilated cardiomyopathy with QRS wider than 120 msec (mortality benefit is greatest for LBBB with QRS >150 ms)
- Sodium-glucose cotransporter 2 (SGLT2) inhibitors (empagliflozin, canagliflozin, and dapagliflozin)
  - Proven to significantly reduce cardiovascular events and reduce risk for heart failure hospitalizations by 35%
  - Initiate in patients with HFrEF and NYHA class II-IV with or without type 2 DM, in addition to guideline-directed medical therapy to reduce worsening heart failure and death. GFR of at least 30 for dapagliflozin and 20 for empagliflozin is recommended.

The goal treatment regimen for mortality reduction in patients with HFrEF is an angiotensin receptor-neprilysin inhibitor, a beta-blocker at max-tolerated dose (with goal HR <60/min), an aldosterone antagonist, and SGLT2 inhibitor.

Loop diuretics play an important role in symptoms and maintaining euvolemia, but do not have an effect on mortality. If someone has volume overload on PE, increase the dose of loop diuretic. If the patient becomes hypotensive, decrease the dose or hold it.

### Final Diagnosis

Heart failure with reduced ejection fraction (HFrEF)

#### CLINICAL PEARL

All patients with HFrEF should be given **both a beta-blocker and an RAAS blocker** (sacubitril-valsartan preferred). Start both at a low dose and increase as the BP tolerates.

#### CLINICAL PEARL

Digoxin reduces the risk for heart failure hospitalization but does not reduce mortality. It is occasionally used in patients with HFrEF and atrial fibrillation when heart failure symptoms are refractory to other therapies, but it requires careful management due to significant toxicity. On the exam, digoxin is almost never the correct answer for heart failure questions.

#### NOTE

The key clinical pearls for HFpEF are cardiac rehab; controlled BP and heart rate if patient has atrial fibrillation; and loop diuretics as needed for volume overload.

A beta-blocker is not standard of care; use only if needed for rate control if there is atrial fibrillation.

# Pulmonology 4

## CASE 1

### Chief Complaint

Increasing shortness of breath with cough and wheezing

### History and Physical Examination

A 24-year-old woman comes to emergency department during wintertime with severe shortness of breath for 2 to 3 days. Her family states that she has a history of asthma and a chronic "nasal stuffiness." She has been maintained on bronchodilators and steroid inhaler. She recently developed an upper respiratory infection and began to mildly wheeze. She has been taking an over-the-counter cold medicine over the last day. This afternoon she developed acute worsening of her breathing and called 911.

She has low grade fevers (Tmax 100.4). Her BP is 180/100 mm Hg, pulse 120/min, and respirations 36/min. The patient appears agitated, restless, and is unable to speak in full sentences. She is using accessory muscles to breathe. Physical exam shows discharge from a nasal polyp. She has a paradoxical pulse with inspiration; no jugular venous distention is noted. Pulmonary exam shows minimal breath sounds, and faint expiratory wheezes are heard throughout with prolonged expiratory phase. The heart is tachycardic, S1 with prominent split S2, no S3, no murmurs. Examination of the abdomen is normal, and examination of extremities shows no thigh swelling or edema.

#### CCS NOTE

Only patients who are hypoxemic should receive supplemental oxygen and get a chest x-ray. Pulse oximetry is part of vital signs. ABG should not be done as a routine lab but should be ordered if the results will aid in diagnosis or change your clinical management.

### Differential Diagnosis

1. Asthma exacerbation
2. Secondary pneumothorax from underlying asthma
3. Pulmonary embolism from a lower extremity DVT above the knee
4. Congestive heart failure from a viral cardiomyopathy
5. Community-acquired pneumonia

**Setting**: emergency department

| Initial Diagnostic Plan | Test Results |
|---|---|
| • Arterial blood gas | pH 7.36; $PCO_2$ 44 mm Hg; $PO_2$ 60 mm Hg (results do not mean intubation is needed, but rather that patient is decompensating and requires immediate, more aggressive therapy, i.e., critical care evaluation for possible ICU admission) |
| • PA and lateral chest x-ray | Normal heart size; no acute cardiopulmonary process, no pneumothorax |
| • Peak flow (not usually performed during an exacerbation and mainly helpful if patient's baseline peak flow is known) | 100 L/min (baseline 400–500 L/min) |
| • Influenza nasal swab | Negative |
| • Sputum culture and Gram stain | Gram stain negative and no growth |

### Assessment

The patient has a history of asthma and a recent upper respiratory infection, and she now presents with wheezing, acute shortness of breath, and a markedly diminished peak flow. The presence of diffuse wheezing on examination with a peak expiratory flow significantly below the patient's baseline suggests a severe asthma attack. The history of rhinitis and nasal polyps with recent use of cold medication raises the question of an exacerbation associated with aspirin sensitivity.

In a young patient presenting with shortness of breath with an underlying pulmonary disease such as asthma, a secondary pneumothorax needs to be considered. The chest x-ray (especially an expiratory film) in this case would aid in the diagnosis.

### Further Treatment Plan

1. Repeated nebulizer or metered-dosed inhaler with a spacer, with short-acting beta-agonist-2 agonists (first-line bronchodilator); can add nebulized short acting anti-cholinergics
2. Supplemental oxygen if patient is hypoxemic
3. IV glucocorticoids (e.g., methylprednisolone)
4. IV magnesium sulfate
5. Intubation and mechanical ventilation if no response

### Diagnostic Plan

Look for a precipitating cause. Viral infection is the most common. Bacterial pneumonia is not likely here given the negative chest x-ray. If in doubt, consider getting sputum culture with Gram stain and blood cultures before starting antibiotics.

## Discussion

Asthma is a disease characterized by inflammatory hyperreactivity of the respiratory tree to various stimuli, resulting in reversible airway obstruction. The combination of mucosal inflammation, bronchial musculature constriction, and excessive secretion of viscous mucus-causing mucous plugs produces bronchial obstruction. The bronchial hyper reactivity occurs in an episodic pattern with interspersed normal airway tone.

Asthma can occur at any age but is usually seen in the young, 80% of whom "outgrow" the condition by adulthood. There are 2 types, and many patients have features of both.

- **Intrinsic (idiosyncratic) asthma** occurs in 50% of asthmatics who are nonallergic. A bronchial reaction occurs secondary to nonimmunologic stimuli, such as infection, irritating inhalant, cold air, exercise, and emotional upset. The attacks are severe, and prognosis is less favorable.
- **Extrinsic (allergic) asthma** (20% of cases) results from sensitization and is precipitated by allergens. Specific immunoglobulins (IgE class) are produced, and the total serum IgE concentration is elevated. There is a positive family history of allergic disease. Other symptoms include allergic rhinitis, urticaria, and eczema. Prognosis is good.

The stimuli causing asthma exacerbation are varied.

- Respiratory infection is the most common stimuli, including viruses (e.g., respiratory syncytial, corona, rhino, influenza, depending on patient age and time of year)
- Pharmacologic stimuli (aspirin, NSAIDs, coloring agents, and beta-antagonists the most common)
  - The typical aspirin sensitivity affecting adults (10%) is nasal polyposis syndrome, which usually starts with perennial vasomotor rhinitis; later, asthma appears that occurs with minimal ingestion of aspirin.
  - There is significant cross-reactivity between aspirin and other NSAIDs (ibuprofen, naproxen). Patients can be desensitized by daily administration of aspirin (cross-tolerance also develops to other NSAIDs).
  - The mechanism by which aspirin and similar drugs cause asthma seems to be chronic overexcretion of leukotrienes, which activate the mast cells; that is why leukotriene synthesis inhibitors and antagonists are considered to be effective.

In a mild asthma attack, slight tachypnea, tachycardia, prolonged expirations, and mild, diffuse wheezing is seen. In a severe attack, the use of accessory muscles of respiration, diminished breath sounds, loud wheezing, and intercostal retraction are seen.

Poor prognostic factors include fatigue, diaphoresis, pulsus paradoxus (>20 mm Hg), inaudible breath sounds, decreased wheezing, cyanosis, and bradycardia.

## Variants of Asthma

- Cough variant asthma
- Exercise-induced bronchoconstriction

**NOTE**

Use of LABAs without ICS is associated with increased mortality and should never be used.

In the **acute phase**, ABG abnormalities are as follows: decrease in $PaCO_2$, increase in pH, and normal/low $PaO_2$. In **severe asthma**/status asthmaticus, there is a decreased $PaO_2$, increased $PaCO_2$, and decreased pH (bicarbonate level usually is normal in acute phase but becomes elevated in chronic). A normal $PCO_2$ may indicate respiratory muscle fatigue in an acute asthmatic patient.

Chest x-ray findings are nonspecific in an asthmatic attack. Chest x-ray may help to rule out acute bacterial infection and pneumothorax.

Asthma is a clinical diagnosis based on the history and physical examination. PFTs in a poorly controlled asthmatic can show an obstructive pattern with a significant bronchodilator response defined as a 12% improvement in the $FEV_1$ or FVC and/or increase of 200 ml post-bronchodilator challenge. PFTs may also be normal in a well-controlled asthmatic. A provocative challenge may be performed with methacholine, cold air, or exercise, which typically shows a decrease in $FEV_1$ and /or FVC of at least 20%.

**CLINICAL PEARL**

**New Guidelines as of 2019**

- All patients diagnosed with asthma should be prescribed an inhaled corticosteroid at a minimum (as-needed albuterol, as monotherapy is discouraged).
- Recommendation is to start with a ICS-LABA for almost all patients, even those with mild asthma.
- For those with moderate or severe asthma, the ICS-LABA may be used as maintenance (daily) preventive treatment, and also as a rescue inhaler, with extra inhalations taken for breakthrough asthma symptoms as needed.

## Management

Essential components of asthma management are routine monitoring of symptoms and lung function, patient education, control of trigger factors, and pharmacology. The goals of treatment are to reduce impairment from symptoms, minimize hospitalizations and loss of lung function, and minimize adverse effects from asthma medications. Effective asthma management requires a preventative approach, with regularly scheduled visits during which symptoms are assessed, pulmonary function is monitored, medications are adjusted, and ongoing education is performed.

Patients with poor perception of increasing asthma symptoms may also benefit from assessment of their peak expiratory flow rate at home. A very common cause of poorly controlled asthma is the inappropriate use of inhalers (monitor at every visit). Pets, dust, and cockroaches are common triggers.

Pharmacologic therapy varies according to asthma severity and asthma control. Asthma control is based on the current level of symptoms, $FEV_1$ or PEFR values, and number of exacerbations requiring oral glucocorticoids per year.

A stepwise approach to therapy is recommended, in which the dose of medication, number of medications, and/or frequency of administration are increased as necessary and decreased when possible. At each return visit, the patient's asthma control is evaluated. If the asthma is not well-controlled, therapy should be "stepped up." If the asthma is well-controlled, therapy can be continued or possibly "stepped down" to minimize medication side effects.

- For **mild intermittent** asthma, recommend a short-acting inhaled beta-2-selective adrenergic agonist. Recommend use as-needed for relief of acute symptoms as well as for prevention of symptoms caused by exercise or trigger exposure, as opposed to regularly scheduled administration.
- For **mild persistent** asthma, recommend inhaled glucocorticoids as initial long-term controller therapy, along with short-acting inhaled beta-2 agonists as needed.
- For **moderate persistent** asthma, it is very reasonable to add a long acting beta-2 agonist to the inhaled glucocorticoid (preferred) or medium-dose ICS.
- For **severe persistent** asthma:
  - Monoclonal antibody to IgE (omalizumab) for moderate to severe persistent asthma that is inadequately controlled with ICS/LABA, when patient is allergic, or IgE 30–700

- Anti-IL-5 monoclonal antibody (mepolizumab, reslizumab) to reduce symptoms, exacerbations, and need for oral steroids in those with absolute eosinophil count >150 cells/uL and severe asthma not controlled with standard therapy.
- In poorly controlled asthma with marked eosinophilia, high IgE, and intermittent pulmonary infiltrates, think of allergic bronchopulmonary aspergillosis. Diagnose with positive skin test for *Aspergillus* and IgG and IgE antibodies to *Aspergillus*. Treatment is systemic steroids and antifungal agents.

For patients with dysphonia and throat tightness who do not respond to asthma treatment, perform laryngoscopy or flow-volume loop to look for vocal cord dysfunction (improves immediately after intubation).

### Basic Science Correlate

Physiology of airflow obstruction limitation in asthma is a result of a narrowing of the airway lumen, causing variable reductions in airflow is a pathognomonic feature of asthma. The mechanisms causing airflow limitation include contraction of airway smooth muscle, thickening of the airway wall due to inflammation and edema, and plugging of airways with mucus. The main component of the rapid changes in airflow limitation is the smooth muscle, and is the basis for beta-agonist therapy that directly relaxes smooth muscle. Bronchoconstriction may be due to direct effects of contractile agonists released from inflammatory cells such as leukotrienes and histamine, which are potent bronchoconstrictors released by mast cells and eosinophils.

Airway inflammation also plays a critical role in airflow obstruction; this inflammation occurs throughout the tracheobronchial tree with varying degrees of obstruction dependent upon the diameter of the airway. Usually obstruction in large airways leads to airflow limitation with decreased flow rates. Conversely, obstruction in small airways leads to airway closure, air trapping with an increase in residual volume seen on PFTs (increased TLC, RV and FRC), and in many cases dynamic hyperinflation. Clinically the patient complains of chest tightness, and the discomfort of an asthma attack may be due to air trapping and breathing at higher lung volumes to maintain airway patency and sustain adequate ventilation.

Bronchial hyperresponsiveness (BHR) is another defining feature of asthma and is a manifestation of reversible airflow obstruction due to smooth muscle contraction. BHR represents an exaggerated constrictor response to a variety of physical, chemical, or environmental stimuli. BHR can be quantitated by the dose response to pharmacologic agents such as methacholine or histamine, causing a 20% fall in FEV1 or FVC.

TH2 plays a major role in asthma. It secretes IL-5, which attracts eosinophils and differentiation of B-cells and leads to production of IgA. It secretes IL-4, which leads to class switching to IgE and IgG. IgE leads to histamine and leukotriene release from mast cells. Leukotrienes cause bronchoconstriction and histamine leads to mucus production and inflammation.

## Final Diagnosis

Asthma exacerbation

# CASE 2

## Chief Complaint

Chronic cough

## History and Physical Examination

A 28-year-old woman comes to the clinic for evaluation of intermittent cough over the last few months. She recently started running several times a week and has noticed that the cough is much worse after she returns. She has noted occasional wheezing as well, particularly on very cold days. She is a nonsmoker and is otherwise healthy.

She is in no acute distress. Her temperature is 36.7 C (98.1 F), BP 108/70 mm Hg, pulse 64/min, and respirations 18/min. Physical examination is unremarkable.

## Differential Diagnosis

1. Exercise-induced asthma/exercise-induced bronchoconstriction
2. Gastroesophageal reflux
3. Postnasal drip (upper airway cough)

## Initial Management

**Setting**: outpatient

| Initial Diagnostic Plan | Results |
|---|---|
| • Pulmonary function tests | FEV1 108% of predicted, FVC 111% of predicted, FEV1/FVC 93%. TLC and DLCO within normal limits; flow volume loop is normal |
| • Methacholine challenge test | Significant drop in both the FVC and FEV1 >20% with administration of methacholine |

Chronic cough is defined as cough >8 weeks. The most common cause is post-nasal drip. Management is as follows:

- Chest x-ray first (all patients)
- If patient is taking an ACE inhibitor, stop for 4 weeks before any additional evaluation is done. Look for frequent throat clearing, nasal discharge, cobblestone appearance in the oropharyngeal mucosa, or mucus dripping down the oropharynx.
- Treatment is a first-generation antihistamine or intranasal corticosteroid.
- If there are GERD symptoms, start a PPI (3 months may be required to take effect).

## Assessment

This clinical presentation of exercise-induced cough is a common variant of asthma. Symptoms are often worse after exercise is completed. The normal PFTs (performed at rest) do not rule out this diagnosis. A methacholine challenge test should be performed to confirm this diagnosis. However, the clinical scenario is probably adequate, and the patient may be empirically treated.

Other common noninfectious causes of cough include allergic rhinitis, postnasal drip, and gastroesophageal reflux disease. However, there is no evidence to support these other causes in this patient.

### Treatment Plan

1. Inhaled beta agonists before exercise, such as albuterol

### Discussion

The term "exercise-induced asthma" or "cough-variant asthma" is used to describe episodic bronchoconstriction following exercise or cold exposure in asthmatic patients. This terminology can be misleading since exercise is not an independent risk factor for asthma, but can be categorized as a bronchoconstriction in patients with underlying asthma. In the pulmonary literature there is some research which shows that decreased physical activity/exercise is a risk factor for the development of asthma and that exercise may prevent the onset of asthma especially in the pediatric population.

The term "exercise-induced bronchoconstriction (EIB)" is a more accurate reflection of the underlying pathophysiology and is generally preferred. EIB varies from 5–20% of the population in the United States. The proposed mechanism of action of EIB is mainly based on the concept of minute ventilation (MV) rising with exercise. EIB probably results from changes in airway physiology triggered by the large volume of relatively cool, dry air inhaled during exercise.

- In patients with well-documented asthma and typical asthma symptoms following exercise, formal exercise/provocative testing is not usually needed.
- In patients without documented asthma, an exercise challenge test is the most direct way to establish a diagnosis of EIB. This usually involves an ergometer or treadmill exercise, sufficient to raise the heart rate to 85% of the predicted maximum.

Alternatively, surrogate tests to assess bronchial hyperresponsiveness (example, cold air hyperventilation, methacholine, histamine, or mannitol inhalation challenge) may be performed in the pulmonary function lab, but do not always correlate with the presence of EIB.

Measurement of peak expiratory flow rates before and after exercise help with the diagnosis. Therapy of EIB varies somewhat with the clinical setting. All patients with asthma should have a rapid-acting beta agonist available when exercising for relief of symptoms.

- For patients with uncontrolled asthma, the first priority is to step up treatment to achieve control of asthma.
- For patients with well-controlled asthma but frequent asthma symptoms with exercise, use a prophylactic rapid-acting beta agonist 10 minutes prior to exercise. (When a prophylactic beta agonist is proven to be effective, it is better to add an inhaled glucocorticoid or leukotriene agent than to use a long-acting beta agonist). May take 6 weeks to respond.
- If a prophylactic beta-agonist causes side effects, use a cromoglycate 15–20 minutes prior to exercise.

### Final Diagnosis

Exercise-induced asthma

# CASE 3

## Chief Complaint

Dyspnea on exertion with generalized fatigue

## History and Physical Examination

A 25-year-old African American woman comes to the clinic complaining of dyspnea on exertion along with a cough on and off for 1 year. The cough is nonproductive, and it has worsened in the last 4 months. She feels tired, has occasional low-grade fever, mild dyspnea on exertion, and has lost 5 pounds in 1 month. The patient has no history of asthma or tobacco use. She has experienced intermittent pain in her shoulder and knees. She has also noticed that her vision has worsened in the last 2 weeks.

She is well nourished and is in no acute distress. Pulmonary examination reveals bilateral dry crackles. She has knee pain with motion. Painful red nodules are seen on the anterior aspect of the legs with tenderness on palpations of both Achilles tendons.

## Differential Diagnosis

1. Tuberculosis
2. Lymphoma, especially Hodgkin
3. Sarcoidosis with Löfgren's syndrome
4. Systemic lupus erythematosus

### CCS NOTE

If you are asked what type of chest x-ray to request, the most appropriate is a posteroanterior and lateral done in the radiology department.

- Lateral decubitus films are for effusions
- Portable films are for patients too ill to move or stand
- Lordotic films are no longer useful

Anytime you need additional details, order a chest CT scan.

## Initial Management

**Setting**: outpatient

| Initial Diagnostic Plan | Results |
|---|---|
| 1. Chest x-ray, then chest CT | CXR: symmetric bilateral hilar enlargement. CT chest: reticular nodular disease involving the bronchovascular bundle with paratracheal and bilateral hilar adenopathy |
| 2. CBC | Normal |
| 3. Purified protein derivative skin test & IGRA | < 5 mm, negative |
| 4. Acid-fast stain and sputum culture | Negative and no growth |
| 5. Antinuclear antibodies and C-ANCA | Both negative |

## Assessment

The patient presents with progressive cough and constitutional symptoms. There is also evidence of erythema nodosum, polyarthralgias, and enthesitis. The differential is broad and includes rheumatologic diseases, collagen vascular disease, sarcoidosis, malignancy, infection (including HIV disease).

A young woman with the symptoms of polyarthralgia, visual changes, erythema nodosum, and bilateral hilar adenopathy is likely to have sarcoidosis. Patients are PPD and gamma release assay negative ruling out latent TB. Elevation of angiotensin-converting enzyme is nonspecific and not part of the diagnostic criteria. An elevated 24-hour urine calcium is sometimes evident and due to increased conversion of vitamin D.

Lymphoid malignancy may present as a mediastinal mass, nodal involvement, or pulmonary involvement inducing chronic cough with associated constitutional symptoms. However, the symmetrical nature of the hilar involvement is atypical. Since lymphoma and sarcoidosis mimic each other, it is important to make a tissue diagnosis through transbronchial biopsy or endoscopic bronchial ultrasound fine needle aspiration to confirm a diagnosis.

Infectious etiologies include other granulomatous diseases such as fungus and tuberculosis. Infection would be higher on the differential diagnosis if there were a history of exposure or immune suppression.

Collagen vascular disease is not supported by the negative serologies. However, small vessel vasculitis such as granulomatosis with polyangiitis (Wegener's) can also present on biopsy with non-caseating granulomas. Also the occupational lung disease known as berylliosis, or chronic beryllium disease (CBD) can also present with non-caseating granulomas on biopsy. HIV disease may also present as fever, weight loss, interstitial pneumonia, and adenopathy (there should be a low threshold to screen for HIV).

| Further Diagnostic Plan | Results |
|---|---|
| 1. Bronchoscopy (commonly done with endobronchial ultrasound) with biopsy is the gold standard. It needs to be done especially in patients with symptoms of weight loss and other constitutional symptoms to exclude lymphoma and tuberculosis. | Noncaseating granulomas, AFB negative and culture negative |
| 2. PFTs with bronchodilator response | • Decreased FEV1 and FVC<br>• Normal to high ratio of FEV1/FVC<br>• Decreased TLC and mildly decreased DLCO with no significant bronchodilator response<br>Findings consistent with a restrictive intrinsic pattern; baseline PFT usually needed before initiating therapy, particularly for sarcoid patients with respiratory issues |

## Treatment Plan

1. Oral corticosteroids

## Discussion

Sarcoidosis is a multisystem disorder of unknown etiology that is characterized pathologically by the presence of noncaseating granulomas in involved organs. It typically affects young adults. In ~50% of cases, it is detected in asymptomatic individuals as a result of incidental radiographic abnormalities (e.g., bilateral hilar adenopathy, reticular opacities). Common presenting symptoms include cough, dyspnea, chest pain, eye lesions, and/or skin lesions. Perform a comprehensive evaluation on all those with suspected sarcoidosis, including history, physical exam, chest x-ray, PFTs, peripheral blood counts, serum chemistry, urinalysis, EKG, ophthalmologic exam, and an evaluation for latent TB (PPD or interferon gamma release assay). The purpose is to obtain additional data supporting the diagnosis of sarcoidosis and to assess disease severity, while eliminating alternative diagnoses.

Pulmonary imaging plays an essential role in the diagnosis of sarcoidosis, starting with a chest x-ray and often followed by high-resolution CT. The classic chest x-ray reveals bilateral hilar adenopathy. This finding, however, may be absent or, if present, may occur in combination with parenchymal opacities.

PFTs are obtained in all patients with suspected sarcoidosis to assess for respiratory impairment; they characteristically demonstrate a restrictive defect with reduced gas exchange and reduced functional status. The diagnosis of sarcoidosis requires compatible clinical and radiographic manifestations, exclusion of other diseases that may present similarly, and histopathologic detection of noncaseating granulomas. Patients who present with asymptomatic bilateral hilar adenopathy or a classical Löfgren syndrome of fever, erythema nodosum, arthralgias, and bilateral hilar lymphadenopathy or Heerfordt syndrome (uveitis, parotid gland enlargement, facial nerve palsy, and fever) do not require biopsy. If available, biopsy of accessible peripheral lesions (e.g., cutaneous lesions, palpable lymph nodes, conjunctival lesions) is preferred to an invasive procedure.

- If an accessible lesion cannot be identified, the choice of procedure depends on the pattern and location of lung parenchymal abnormalities, the presence and location of enlarged thoracic lymph nodes, and the available expertise and equipment.
- If U/S-guided endoscopy or flexible bronchoscopy cannot be performed or is nondiagnostic, the next step is usually surgical mediastinal lymph node biopsy, followed by surgical lung biopsy via thoracoscopy or thoracotomy.

Noncaseating granulomas are the characteristic histopathologic abnormality in sarcoidosis. The differential diagnosis of granulomatous lung diseases includes many conditions; it is particularly important to exclude infections and malignancy. Most patients with pulmonary sarcoidosis do not require treatment, as a high proportion have asymptomatic, nonprogressive disease or experience a spontaneous remission.

- For asymptomatic patients with no significant extrapulmonary involvement, do not initiate therapy with oral glucocorticoids; just monitor symptoms, chest radiograph, and pulmonary function.
- For patients with bothersome symptoms, worsening radiographic opacities, and increasing pulmonary function impairment, initiate oral glucocorticoids rather than continued observation.

## Final Diagnosis

Sarcoidosis

# CASE 4

## Chief Complaint

Purified protein derivative skin test results

## History and Physical Examination

A 39-year-old man comes to your office as part of a routine screening examination for a new job. He is without symptoms and feels generally well. He is HIV-positive and has had a purified protein derivative (PPD) skin test in the past. His CD4 cell count is 550, and he is on no medications. He comes today for a routine examination and for the results of his PPD test, which your nurse placed 2 days ago.

His temperature is 37 C (98.6 F), blood pressure 110/70 mm Hg, pulse 72/min, and respirations 12/min. Physical examination shows normal eyes, ears, nose, and throat. The chest is clear bilaterally, and cardiovascular exam is normal. Abdomen is normal. There is no lymphadenopathy present. His skin test shows 8 mm of induration.

## Differential Diagnosis

1. Active tuberculosis (TB)
2. Latent TB (prior infection)
3. Bacille Calmette-Guérin administration

## Initial Management

**Setting**: outpatient

| Initial Diagnostic Plan | Results |
| --- | --- |
| The initial diagnostic plan should always be to rule out active TB. | |
| • Chest x-ray | Normal |
| • Liver function tests | Normal |

### CLINICAL PEARL

Develop the habit of thinking about what vaccinations should be given in any office or clinical setting. Because of the HIV, this patient should receive both influenza and pneumococcal vaccines.

## Assessment

A PPD skin test is generally considered positive if the induration >10 mm, but in an HIV-positive patient that cutoff is lowered to >5 mm to be considered positive. (Other conditions which similarly lower the cutoff to 5 mm are steroid use, organ transplantation (recipients), close contact with those who have active TB, and chest x-ray findings consistent with old (nonactive) TB.) Generally, nontuberculous mycobacteria will not give >5 mm of induration.

A positive PPD test should never be considered as a result of the Bacille Calmette-Guérin administration. This patient is considered to have a positive PPD because of the size of the induration of the reaction.

The question then becomes, which type of TB does this patient have.

### Treatment Plan

1. Isoniazid and vitamin B6 for 9 months

### Discussion

TB is caused by *Mycobacterium tuberculosis*, which is spread from person to person through the air. It usually affects the lungs (primary or pulmonary TB), but can also affect other parts of the body, such as the brain, kidneys, and spine. Not everyone infected with TB bacteria becomes sick. As a result, 2 TB-related conditions exist: **latent TB** and **active TB**.

- **Latent TB** infection causes no symptoms and patients do not feel sick; they are infected with *M. tuberculosis* but do not have active TB disease.
  - The only sign of TB infection is a positive reaction to the tuberculin skin test or TB blood test.
  - Patients are not infectious and cannot spread TB infection to others.
  - Treatment is isoniazid with no hospitalization needed
- **Active TB** infection causes weight loss, fever, cough, sputum, and night sweats; chest x-ray shows evidence of an apical lesion consistent with reactivation. Treatment is mandated hospitalization and isolation, with a 4-drug regimen.

**The Mantoux test** consists of **intradermal** injection of 0.1 mL of PPD in the forearm. The injection site is evaluated in 48–72 hours after injection. The reading is based on the diameter of the induration/swollen area (**not the red area**). Measure **perpendicularly** to the long axis of the forearm.

- Current recommendations from the **CDC** as to what constitutes a positive reading take into account the degree of clinical suspicion of latent TB infection. Never place a PPD first in acutely symptomatic patients.
- What is the **booster effect**? Some patients, especially the older adult who were infected with TB in the distant past, may no longer react to a TB skin test ("amnestic"). The PPD may boost their immune system enough so that they react to subsequent skin tests. The "2-step testing" assesses the responses to skin-test antigens to which a cell-mediated, delayed-type hypersensitivity (DTH) response is expected.
- Two interferon-gamma release assays (IGRAs) are available in the United States:
  - QuantiFERON®–TB Gold In-Tube test (QFT-GIT): an alternative to skin testing, this test incubates the patient's blood for 16–24 hours with synthetic peptides representing 2 TB specific antigens; the antigens will stimulate interferon-gamma release from the patient's WBCs, which is then measured by ELISA. Results are reported as positive, negative, or indeterminate.
  - T-SPOT® TB test (T-Spot): a unique, single-visit blood test; it is the only blood test for latent TB that has demonstrated both sensitivity and specificity greater than 95%
- Advantages of IGRAs: patient does not need to return for a read, results are available within 24 hours, there is no booster phenomenon, and there is no reader bias. Also, the result is not affected by prior BCG vaccination and not affected by HIV status.

- In patients presumed to have latent TB, it is essential to rule out active TB. If latent TB treatment is given to someone with active TB, there is a serious risk of developing drug-resistant strains of TB.
- There are 4 (CDC 2014) treatment regimens:
  - 9 months of isoniazid (**gold standard**; 93% effective)
  - 6 months of isoniazid is also acceptable based on cost-effectiveness, patient compliance, and drug toxicity
  - 4 months of rifampin for those who are unable to take INH or had exposure to INH-resistant TB
  - 3 months (12 dose) regimen of weekly rifapentine and isoniazid
- In order to become infected with TB, you need consistent exposure to the contagious person for a long time. For that reason, you're more likely to catch TB from a relative than a stranger.
- Latent TB is assumed by most doctors today to be the normal or regular strain of TB. There are 3 other types of TB recognized in the world today:
  1. Multi-drug resistant TB (MDR TB)
  2. Extensively drug resistant TB (XDR TB)
  3. Totally drug resistant TB (TDR TB)

A positive PPD skin test indicates an exposure to TB, not necessarily an active infection. About 10% of healthy individuals who have a positive PPD test develop active TB in their lifetime. Most cases (>90%) occur within the first 2 years after a negative test converts to a positive test.

**PPD Conversion:**

| | |
|---|---|
| >5 mm | Close contacts of active TB, HIV-positive, steroid users |
| >10 mm | Patients from endemic areas; health care workers; and those living in shelters, long-term facilities, and jails. Also, patients with chronic diseases, e.g., silicosis, diabetes, alcoholics, renal failure, and cancer |
| >15 mm | Patients with no risk factors |

## Final Diagnosis

Positive PPD skin test; latent TB

# CASE 5

## Chief Complaint

Fever, chills, and productive cough for 3 months

## History and Physical Examination

A 39-year-old man who is homeless presents with a several-month history of a productive cough. He also reported nightly fevers to 39.5 C (103.1 F) associated with chills. During the past 6 months he has had a 20-lb weight loss. He is a nonsmoker, and his medical history is significant for a hospitalization for pneumonia 4 months ago. He was lost to follow-up after discharge.

His T is 38.4 C (101.1 F), BP 105/60 mm Hg, pulse 88/min, and respirations 20/min. He is thin and unkempt-appearing in no acute distress. He has bitemporal wasting, poor dentition, and multiple 1- to 2-cm mobile cervical lymph nodes. His cardiac and pulmonary examinations are normal. Examination of the abdomen is benign, and extremities are normal.

## Differential Diagnosis

1. Tuberculosis
2. Lung abscess
3. Bronchiectasis
4. Lung cancer
5. Pneumonia

## Initial Management

**Setting**: emergency department (patient may come to the clinic initially but should be transferred to the hospital setting promptly)

| Initial Diagnostic Plan | Results |
|---|---|
| • Chest x-ray | Cavitary lesion in right upper lobe |

| Further Diagnostic Plan | Results |
|---|---|
| • Respiratory isolation and sputum for acid-fast bacillus stain and culture | Rare acid-fast bacilli seen |

## Assessment

Given the chronicity of the patient's symptoms in association with fever, weight loss, and hemoptysis, tuberculosis must be highly considered in the differential diagnosis. Although a primary lung cancer may present similarly (with a cavitary lung lesion), this would be less likely given the patient's age and lack of smoking history.

### Treatment Plan

Begin antituberculous drug therapy with 4 agents: isoniazid (INH), rifampin, pyrazinamide, ethambutol, which are used with vitamin B6 for the first 2 months. After that, isoniazid and rifampin are continued for 4 months, making it a 6-month total.

### Further Results (Weeks Later)

Culture is positive for *M. tuberculosis.*

### Discussion

TB must be suspected in patients who present with the classic findings of cough, fever, and weight loss in association with an infiltrate on chest x-ray. When there is clinical suspicion for TB, respiratory isolation must be promptly instituted regardless of whether an initial sputum smear reveals acid-fast bacilli.

All cases of TB must be reported to the Department of Health as a measure of infection control. Given the recent emergence of multi-drug-resistant strains, the current recommendation is to begin therapy with 4 drugs until the specific drug sensitivities become available. Directly observed therapy programs (DOT), available in most inner cities, have improved the compliance rates with multiple drug regimens.

The purified protein derivative (PPD) skin test was not used in this case because it is used as a screen of asymptomatic patients. The PPD is not used to make a diagnosis of TB in acutely ill patients such as are described here.

For most patients, the duration of therapy is 6 months total.

### Epidemiology

TB is still a leading cause of death in the world. The World Health Organization (WHO) estimates that about 1/3 of the world's population is infected. The global incidence of active TB is increasing, mainly due to TB associated with HIV infection.

- **Sites of TB disease**
    - Lungs (80–85%)
    - Pleura
    - Central nervous system
    - Lymphatic system
    - Genitourinary system
    - Bones and joints
    - Peritoneum
- **Terminology for TB**
    - Ghon focus is a primary lesion usually subpleural caused by TB.
    - If the Ghon focus also involves infection of adjacent lymphatics and hilar lymph nodes, it is known as the Ghon's complex.
    - When a Ghon's complex undergoes fibrosis and calcification, it is called a Ranke complex.

- The lungs are the major site for *M. tuberculosis* infection. Clinical manifestations of pulmonary TB include:
    - Primary TB
    - Reactivation TB
    - Laryngeal TB
    - Endobronchial TB
- Pulmonary complications of TB include:
    - Hemoptysis
    - Pneumothorax
    - Bronchiectasis
    - Extensive pulmonary destruction
    - Lung cancer
    - Chronic pulmonary aspergillosis
- Manifestations of active TB:-
    - Fever
    - Night sweats
    - Weight loss
    - Chronic cough (>3 weeks)
    - Hemoptysis
    - Local signs/symptoms for extrapulmonary disease
- Suspect the diagnosis of active TB in:
    - High-risk group
    - Worrisome chest x-ray
    - Consistent symptoms
- Isolate early
    - Airborne precautions
    - Negative pressure ventilation room
    - Use an N-95 respirator
- Diagnosis for active TB
    - Chest x-ray / CT chest
    - Infiltrates typically upper lobe or superior segments of lower lobes
    - Sputum for AFB stain and culture × 3
    - Note: CXR can be normal in HIV (+) patients

- **Diagnosis of extrapulmonary TB**
    - Pleural
- Pleural fluid stain/culture
- Adenosine deaminase
- *Mycobacterium tuberculosis* PCR
- QuantiFERON Gold on the fluid
- Pleural biopsy (gold standard)
- Meningitis
    - CSF stain/culture
    - Meningeal biopsy
- The first successful treatments for TB were surgical. They were based on the observation that healed TB cavities were all closed. Surgical management was therefore directed at closing open cavities in order to encourage healing. These procedures were all used in the pre-antibiotic era.

  There also exists a misconception that the purpose was to deprive the organism of oxygen; however, it is well known that TB survives anaerobic conditions. **Plombage** involved inserting porcelain balls into the thoracic cavity to collapse the lung underneath and thus reduced the need for a disfiguring operation.

## Final Diagnosis

Active TB

# CASE 6

## Chief Complaint

Shortness of breath for several months

## History and Physical Examination

A 66-year-old retired construction worker comes to the office for evaluation of increasing shortness of breath over the past 5 months. He describes a dry, nonproductive cough that began about 1 month before the onset of his shortness of breath. He has been in excellent physical condition, walking 2 miles daily for many years. Recently, however, he has been unable to walk 3 blocks without stopping to rest. He is a former smoker of 2 packs per day for 20 years. He quit 3 months ago because of his difficulty breathing.

Upon examination the patient is fit, well-nourished, and in no acute distress. His T is 36.7 C (98.1 F), BP 140/85 mm Hg, pulse 86/min, and respirations 22/min. Physical examination shows bibasilar coarse crackles on chest auscultation but is otherwise clear. Examination of the extremities shows clubbing. The remainder of the physical examination is unremarkable.

## Differential Diagnosis

1. Interstitial lung disease
    - Occupational etiologies:
        - Organic source: hypersensitivity pneumonitis
        - Nonorganic source: asbestosis, silicosis, berylliosis, coal worker's pneumoconiosis
    - Non-occupational etiologies: idiopathic pulmonary fibrosis
2. Bronchogenic carcinoma (squamous cell carcinoma and small cell carcinoma)
3. COPD / emphysema
4. Congestive heart failure

### Initial Management

**Setting**: outpatient

| Initial Diagnostic Plan | Results |
|---|---|
| • Chest x-ray (PA & lateral) | Reticular marking predominantly in the mid to lower lung with calcified pleural plaques mainly on the diaphragm |
| • EKG | Right axis deviation; normal sinus rhythm; prominent P waves in lead II; no ST changes |
| • Pulmonary function tests | Low FEV1, low FVC, normal FEV1/FVC, decreased total lung capacity and residual volume with a decrease in DLCO |
| • Echocardiogram | Normal ejection fraction, elevated right ventricle systolic pressure with tricuspid regurgitation |

### Assessment

This is likely an interstitial lung disease for an inorganic occupational etiology or obstructive lung disease given the patient's extensive smoking history or a combination of both. The presence of a dry cough for many months in association with dyspnea on exertion and clubbing can suggest a pulmonary process as the etiology of this patient's problem; however, none of these physical findings are pathognomonic. The radiographic finding of calcified pleural plaques is classic for asbestos exposure.

#### CCS NOTE

Echocardiography should be ordered in cases with unexplained dyspnea to exclude ventricular dysfunction. It will also help in the evaluation of pulmonary hypertension secondary to hypoxia.

| Further Diagnostic Plan | Results |
|---|---|
| Bronchoscopy with bronchoalveolar lavage and transbronchial biopsy | Gram stain negative, culture negative, cell differential predominantly macrophages, biopsy of the right lower lobe shows diffuse inflammatory changes with areas of fibrosis; asbestos fibers were noted |

### Treatment Plan

1. Close observation and follow-up PFTs and chest imaging in the future; consider a 6 min walk test to evaluate for desaturations
2. No specific medication or treatment exists at this time; in smokers, encourage cessation

### Discussion

Asbestosis is a common environmental cause of interstitial lung disease. It is produced by mineral silicate fibers that lodge in the lung and are phagocytosed by pulmonary macrophages, which are damaged and release lysosomal enzymes. This results in an inflammatory process that eventually leads to fibrosis.

Construction workers are commonly exposed to large amounts of asbestos. Other industries associated with asbestos exposure include automobile repair, insulation, textiles, mining, milling, and shipbuilding.

The disease often develops many years after exposure. There may be a dose-response relationship between the amount of exposure and the biologic agent. In addition, the fitness of the exposed individual is important. Because poorly conditioned persons ventilate more, they are more likely to have a higher exposure and subsequent disease.

There is no definitive therapy for asbestosis. This disorder, characterized by progressive dyspnea and cough in association with interstitial fibrosis, is only one of many potential pulmonary complications of asbestos exposure. Radiographic abnormalities, including pleural plaques and rounded atelectasis, are attributed to asbestos exposure.

Patients can demonstrate clinical evidence of progressive pulmonary failure with associated right heart dysfunction.

- Chest x-ray reveals the formation of pleural plaques, which are not associated with pulmonary compromise.
- As the disease progresses, linear opacities may appear in the lower lung lobes.
- Patients may develop honeycomb lung consistent with severe compromise and end-stage disease.

High-resolution CT may aid in the diagnosis.

Patients with a history of asbestos exposure are also at increased risk for the development of bronchogenic carcinoma. This risk increases dramatically with concomitant asbestos exposure and cigarette smoking (to 70× when compared to the risk of the general population). Finally, there is a strong association between asbestos and mesothelioma, although the risk is less than that of developing bronchogenic carcinoma.

## Final Diagnosis

Interstitial lung disease due to asbestosis

# CASE 7

## Chief Complaint

"I'm breathing worse."

## History and Physical Examination

A 65-year-old white man comes to the office with worsening dyspnea on exertion over the last year. He was recently treated for an episode of infectious bronchitis characterized by fever and a productive cough. He now has a persistent mild nonproductive cough. He notes a 10-lb weight loss over the last year and has increasingly restricted his activities because of respiratory compromise. He has a history of smoking 2 packs per day for 50 years but denies alcohol intake.

His T is 37.0 C (98.6 F), BP 150/80 mm Hg, pulse 90/min, and respirations 28/min. He is thin and frail, using accessory muscles of respiration at rest. He is sitting in a tripod position. Examination shows no sinus tenderness, decreased breath sounds with scattered rhonchi, increased anteroposterior diameter, and hyper resonance to percussion. His cardiac impulse is visible in the subxiphoid area; there is a regular rhythm, distant heart sounds, and an increased S2. His abdomen is soft, non-tender, with no hepatosplenomegaly. Examination of the extremities shows no cyanosis and no edema.

## Differential Diagnosis

1. Emphysema
2. Asthma exacerbation
3. Congestive heart failure (CHF)
4. Coronary syndrome, angina
5. Post-obstructive pneumonia for a primary lung tumor
6. Interstitial lung disease

| Initial Diagnostic Plan | Results |
|---|---|
| • PFTs with bronchodilator response | Decreased FEV1, decreased FVC, decreased FEV1/FVC, decreased $FEF_{25-75\%}$; decreased DLCO, increased TLC, increased RV, and increased FRC<br>Flow volume loop shows an obstructive contour on the expiratory portion of the loop. There was minimal bronchodilator response. |
| • Chest x-ray: PA and lateral | Flat diaphragm, narrow cardiac silhouette, apical bullae; no infiltrates are noted |
| • ABG (not diagnostic but helpful in the acute setting, especially if baseline ABG is known) | 7.35/60/74/32/94% in room air (consistent with a chronic respiratory acidosis with renal compensation based on the normal pH with an elevated $PaCO_2$ and elevated $HCO_{3-}$) |

**CLINICAL PEARL**

In patients presenting with acute exacerbation of COPD, the PFT will be unreliable. The first test to do is chest x-ray.

In patients without a documented diagnosis of COPD and mild to moderate symptoms, the first test to do is the PFT, to confirm diagnosis and assess prognosis.

### Assessment

Emphysema should be considered first because of physical findings and CXR imaging, and most importantly the PFTs are consistent with obstructive lung disease. This is not a clinical picture consistent with asthma, even though poorly controlled asthma can result in an obstructive process; it is less likely given the age of the patient and significant smoking history.

CHF should also be considered in an older adult patient complaining of dyspnea, but there is no evidence of increased jugular venous pressure or pulmonary edema on the examination. If CHF is truly a concern, consider ordering a BNP level or transthoracic echocardiogram. Patients with COPD and significant hypoxemia can develop pulmonary hypertension and cor pulmonale.

Coronary syndrome would be a consideration if this patient had chest pain or discomfort and/or history of coronary risk factors. Post-obstructive pneumonia, secondary to a primary lung tumor, can be a strong consideration based upon the significant smoking history. Bronchogenic tumors such as squamous cell carcinoma and small cell carcinoma would be the most likely tumors seen in smokers, and both can invade the bronchus resulting in a post-obstructive pneumonia. However, given the absence of radiographic findings this would be less likely. Interstitial lung diseases associated with smoking may present with shortness of breath and involve the lung parenchyma, however the PFTs are not consistent with a restrictive intrinsic process.

### Chronic Treatment

1. Smoking cessation (cognitive behavioral therapy, nicotine replacement and medications)
2. Home $O_2$ if the patient has $PaO_2 \leq 55$ or saturation <88%, or patient has cor pulmonale and $PaO_2$ >55 to 59, consider 6 minute walk test to evaluate for desaturation on exertion.
3. Treatment guidelines are based upon severity of disease. Inhaled bronchodilators are the cornerstone therapy (both long and short acting). In severe COPD, studies have shown a role for inhaled corticosteroids.
4. Pulmonary rehabilitation
5. Lung volume reduction in specialized group of emphysema patients
6. Referral for lung transplant in some
7. Screening for lung cancer with low dose CT chest in high-risk patients (smokers)

**CCS NOTE**

Acutely ill patients in the office should be transferred to the emergency department. The first dose of medication can be given in the office (such as bronchodilator and steroid) *before* the transfer.

### Acute Treatment (Exacerbation/Inpatient)

1. Oxygen to maintain $O_2$ saturation at approximately 90%
2. Inhaled bronchodilators: anticholinergic agents (ipratropium bromide) and/or beta-agonists (e.g., albuterol)
3. Oral antibiotics if treating for a bacterial pneumonia or bronchitis (e.g., azithromycin and ceftriaxone or fluoroquinolones)
4. Sputum culture and Gram stain; send for *Legionella* urinary antigen if considering atypical bacteria
5. Corticosteroids
6. Strongly consider noninvasive positive pressure ventilation (BiPAP) for increased work of breathing and to hopefully prevent intubation and mechanical ventilation
7. Mechanical ventilation is a clinical decision, not based upon a lab value or radiographic imaging, and should be discussed with the patient and family if possible

The only treatments that have increased survival in chronic obstructive pulmonary disease are home $O_2$, smoking cessation, and lung transplant.

Pneumococcal vaccine should be given every 5 years and influenza vaccine yearly to all patients with chronic obstructive pulmonary disease.

## Discussion

Emphysema, a major category of COPD, is defined as irreversible dilatation of the distal air space with associated destruction of the alveolar septae. It is subdivided into pathologic patterns in which either the respiratory bronchioles alone (centroacinar) or more distal portions (panacinar) are involved. Cigarette smoking causes the following changes, all contributing to the generation of emphysematous changes.

- Abnormalities in ciliary movement
- Hyperplasia of mucous-secreting glands
- Inhibition of the alveolar macrophages
- Release of proteolytic enzymes from neutrophils
- Inhibition of antiproteolytic enzymes

Antitrypsin is an enzyme responsible for the inhibition of trypsinase and elastinase in the lung, and patients deficient in this enzyme experience severe panacinar emphysema. Always consider alpha-1 antitrypsin deficiency in patients with emphysema involving the base of the lung and liver abnormalities.

Emphysema is characterized by a loss of airway elastic recoil and caliber resulting in collapse during forced expiration (referred to as the loss of radial traction). This leads to a prolonged expiratory phase, an increase in residual capacity, and air trapping with increases in lung volumes. This also results in increased work of breathing because tidal breathing takes place on a less compliant part of the pressure/volume curve.

Mismatching of ventilation and pulmonary blood flow is a cause of hypoxia (emphysema is dead space physiology). Alveolar hypoxia eventually leads to pulmonary hypertension with cor pulmonale.

## Final Diagnosis

Emphysema

# CASE 8

## Chief Complaint

"I wake up in the middle of the night gasping for air."

## History and Physical Examination

A 50-year-old man is evaluated for a 9-month history of loud snoring and "gasping" during sleep. He also frequently falls asleep in a chair while reading during the day. His medical history is otherwise unremarkable. Patient denies symptoms of narcolepsy (cataplexy, sleep paralysis, and visual hallucinations upon transitioning into sleep) or restless leg syndrome.

On physical examination, his T is afebrile, BP 150/82 mm Hg, pulse 70–80/min, and respirations 12–14/min; BMI is 36. Neck circumference is 18 inches, with notable macroglossia, micrognathia, and a high-arched hard palate.

## Differential Diagnosis

1. Obstructive sleep apnea (OSA)
2. Primary snoring
3. Poor sleep hygiene with insufficient sleep syndrome
4. Hypersomnia of central etiology

## Initial Management

**Setting**: outpatient

## Diagnostic/Therapeutic Plan

- Split night nocturnal polysomnography with CPAP titration with apnea hypopnea index >15

## Test Results

- Apnea hypopnea index (AHI) of 65 events per hour during the first half of the study
- Patient successfully titrated with nasal CPAP mask to pressure 15 cm/$H_2O$, which alleviated all respiratory events and resulted in AHI 0.0

### Discussion

OSA is a common chronic disorder that often requires lifelong care. Cardinal features in adults include the following:

- Obstructive apneas, hypopneas, or respiratory effort related arousals
- Daytime symptoms attributable to disrupted sleep, such as sleepiness, fatigue, or poor concentration
- Signs of disturbed sleep, such as snoring and restlessness

OSA is an important disorder because patients are at increased risk for poor neurocognitive performance and adverse medical outcomes, due to repeated arousals and/or hypoxemia during sleep. The severity and duration of OSA necessary for development of these sequelae vary among individuals. In addition, moderate to severe untreated OSA has been associated with increased all-cause and cardiovascular mortality.

The prevalence of OSA in the general adult population is ~20–30% in men and 10–15% in women if it is defined as an apnea hypopnea index (AHI) >5 events per hour. When defined as AHI ≥5 events per hour **plus** at least 1 symptom/sign of OSA, the prevalence is ~15% in men and 5% in women.

Well-defined risk factors for OSA include older age, male gender, obesity, craniofacial abnormalities, and upper airway soft tissue abnormalities. Potential risk factors include smoking, nasal congestion, and family history. Snoring and daytime sleepiness are common manifestations of OSA. Additional symptoms and signs include restless sleep, periods of silence terminated by loud snorts or snoring, nocturnal angina, poor concentration, and awakening with a sensation of choking, gasping, or smothering. The physical exam can be normal, although obesity, elevated blood pressure, a narrow airway, and a large neck circumference are common.

Polysomnography is the preferred diagnostic study when OSA is suspected. There are several interventions that may benefit patients with OSA. These include behavior modifications, including weight loss, and OSA-specific therapies such as positive airway pressure, oral appliances, hypoglossal nerve stimulator, and surgery.

The most appropriate next step in treatment is CPAP. Obstructive sleep apnea (OSA) is defined by upper airway narrowing or collapse resulting in cessation (apnea) or reduction (hypopnea) in airflow despite ongoing efforts to breathe. Severity is commonly measured using the apnea-hypopnea index (AHI), the sum of apneas and hypopneas per hour of sleep.

- **AHI 5–15** indicates **mild OSA**
- **AHI 16–30** indicates **moderate sleep apnea**
- **AHI >30** indicates **severe OSA**

CPAP should be considered first-line therapy in any patient who has OSA and associated symptoms, particularly excessive daytime sleepiness. Optimal positive airway pressure therapy may have salutary effects on cardiovascular diseases that are associated with OSA. Suboptimal adherence to CPAP and bilevel positive airway pressure devices are common in clinical practice, and rates of discontinuation are high. Therefore, objective monitoring of use and periodic follow-up are important to ensure adherence.

- Nocturnal oxygen therapy alone is inadequate to prevent complications associated with OSA because it does not correct upper airway obstruction, which is the primary problem related to oxygen desaturation.
- Oral devices may be considered for patients who cannot tolerate or are unwilling to use positive airway pressure therapy but are usually reserved for patients with mild to moderate OSA.
- Surgery may be indicated for specific underlying surgically correctable craniofacial or upper airway abnormalities that contribute to OSA, including nasal polyps, nasal septal deviation, tonsillar enlargement, or retrognathia, although positive airway pressure therapy may be preferred for such patients.
- Upper airway surgery may also be considered in selected patients with OSA who desire surgery, reject other therapeutic modalities, and can undergo the procedure.

### Final Diagnosis

Obstructive sleep apnea

## CASE 9

### Chief Complaint

"I've been coughing and spitting up yellow stuff."

### History and Physical Examination

A 35-year-old woman is evaluated for a 1-week history of cough associated with yellow phlegm production. She has a 5-pack-year history of cigarette smoking but stopped smoking 15 years ago. She received albuterol and ipratropium earlier, but the cough did not improve. Chest x-ray today shows a right middle lobe nodule. There are no old images available for comparison. A mammogram and Pap smear earlier this year were normal.

On physical examination she is afebrile, BP is 120/80 mm Hg, pulse 80/min, and respirations 12-14/min. Heart and lung examination are unremarkable, no wheezing, rhonchi or rales. S1 and S2 are present with no murmurs, rubs, or gallop. No lymphadenopathy is noted. Laboratory studies, including CBC and basic metabolic panel, are normal.

### Differential Diagnosis

1. **Malignancy**
    - Bronchogenic carcinoma
    - Pulmonary metastases
    - Carcinoid tumors
2. **Benign disease**
    - Granulomas
    - Benign tumors (hamartomas)
    - Resolving infarction
    - Rheumatoid and vasculitic nodules
    - AV malformations
    - Trauma
    - Rounded atelectasis

### Initial Management

### Diagnostic/Therapeutic Plan

- CT chest with IV contrast

### Test Results

- Chest CT: dense, centrally calcified smooth contoured 2-cm nodular opacity in right middle lobe with no mediastinal adenopathy or other lung abnormality

## Further Evaluation

Recommendations in "low risk patients" (such as this patient) are to repeat imaging in 3–6 months and confirm there is no growth of the nodule.

## Discussion

The nodule described in the results of the CT chest is dense, centrally calcified and smoothly bordered, consistent with a granuloma. The likelihood that a nodule is malignant depends on such factors as its size, surface characteristics and the patient's age, smoking history, and history of previous malignancy. Nodules with smooth borders are usually benign; nodules with spiculated borders have a high likelihood of being malignant. Central and diffuse patterns of calcification are associated with benign disease (the calcifications are described as "popcorn," "onion skin," "bull's eye."

Although this patient is at risk for lung cancer secondary to her smoking history, this benign nodule needs no further evaluation.

Not all patterns of calcification are associated with benign disease. A nodule that has "eccentric" or "off-center calcification" may be either benign or malignant, and further evaluation or follow-up is advised. Bronchial carcinoid tumors are low-grade malignant neoplasms that consist of neuroendocrine cells and account for 1% to 2% of all tumors of the lung. Patients may present with hemoptysis, have evidence of bronchial obstruction, or be asymptomatic. Carcinoid tumors are often located within a bronchus, resulting in lobar atelectasis. A history of malignancy is another indicator of possible cancer. The lung is a common site of metastasis from various tumors, but this patient does not have a history of cancer, and metastases are usually multiple, peripheral, and not calcified.

Note: Patients age $\geq$45 with significant tobacco history should receive further work-up. This may include bronchoscopy with biopsy, open lung biopsy, or CT-guided biopsy.

## Final Diagnosis

Solitary pulmonary nodule; granuloma

# Emergency Medicine 5

## CASE 1

### Chief Complaint

"Leave me alone!"

### History and Physical Examination

A 64-year-old man with a history of chronic alcoholism is brought to the emergency department by the police, who found him agitated, combative, and shouting at imaginary monsters. Vital signs are T 39 C (102.2 F), BP 130/85 mm Hg, pulse 110/min, and respirations 24/min.

The patient appears disheveled and agitated and is sweating profusely. He is staring around. Examination of the head, eyes, ears, nose, and throat shows poor dentition, a supple neck, and intact cranial nerves. Cardiovascular exam shows tachycardia, with no rubs or gallops. Lungs are clear and the abdomen is benign. There is no clubbing, cyanosis, or edema of the extremities, although there is a resting tremor of the hands. Neurologic exam is nonfocal, and there is no evidence of external injury.

**CCS NOTE**

A patient with a high fever on the CCS should undergo blood cultures, chest x-ray, and urinalysis. This is a generic fever evaluation.

### Differential Diagnosis

1. Delirium tremens
2. Alcoholic hallucinosis
3. Acute intoxication
4. Acute schizophrenia
5. Bacterial meningitis
6. Subdural hematoma

**CCS NOTE**

The CCS will value an 'appropriate process' more than 'jumping straight to the diagnosis.' Hence, CT scan of the head is acceptable for a patient presenting with fever and change in mental status, even if the results are normal.

### Initial Management

**Setting:** emergency department

### Diagnostic/Therapeutic Plan

- Electrolytes
- Blood alcohol level
- Serum magnesium level
- Arterial blood gases
- CT scan of head
- Lumbar puncture
- Toxicology screen
- Blood cultures
- Urinalysis

### Test Results

- Sodium 146 mEq/L; chloride 108 mEq/L; BUN 30 mg/dL; creatinine 1.3 U/L
- Blood alcohol 0.00 mg/dL
- Serum magnesium 0.8 mg/dL (1.8–3.0 normal)
- pH 7.46; $pCO_2$ 32 mm Hg; $pO_2$ 84 mm Hg; $HCO_3$ 24 mm Hg; $O_2$ saturation 96%
- CT scan: no evidence of bleeding or trauma
- Lumbar puncture: normal WBC, protein normal, glucose normal
- Toxicology negative
- Blood cultures: no growth
- Urinalysis: no WBCs

### Assessment

The presentation of a patient with a history of alcohol abuse who is disoriented, agitated, hallucinating, and perspiring is classic of delirium tremens. Acute confusion and fever are suggestive of meningitis and this can be excluded with a lumbar puncture if the diagnosis is not certain. The acute change in mental status may also be due to a CNS bleed precipitated by falling. The more mild alcohol withdrawal syndrome is often referred to as "impending DTs." The symptoms can generally be managed with oral benzodiazepines. Alcoholic hallucinosis presents with visual hallucinations (as opposed to auditory hallucinations) and is generally distinguished from acute schizophrenia by the history of prolonged alcohol use followed by a period of cessation. The treatment is the same as for delirium tremens.

**CCS NOTE**

There is no specific test to diagnose alcohol withdrawal. It is a diagnosis of exclusion, along with a history of high-volume alcohol consumption.

| Further Management Plan | Results |
|---|---|
| 1. Chest x-ray | No infiltrates |
| 2. Vitamin B12 level | Normal |
| 3. Liver function tests | Normal |

### Treatment Plan

- IV chlordiazepoxide 50–100 mg every 4–6 hrs and as needed (could also choose other agents, e.g., diazepam, lorazepam, or phenobarbital)
- IV thiamine and folic acid
- Start IV fluids D5NS and adjust depending on patient's hemodynamic status
- Magnesium sulfate replacement
- Clonidine can also be helpful to suppress some of the cardiovascular hyperexcitability
- Atenolol can be used as an adjunct to the benzodiazepines for the tachycardia
- Admission to general floor if the withdrawal is mild or to the ICU if patient has severe symptoms (e.g., seizures)

### CCS NOTE

In patients with a clear presentation of alcohol withdrawal and delirium tremens, medical therapy such as lorazepam and chlordiazepoxide should be ordered before the results of the tests are known.

### Discussion

Abstinence or withdrawal syndrome refers to a constellation of symptoms that develop only after a period of relative or absolute abstinence from alcohol. The syndrome may develop in the periodic drinker, as well as the chronic drinker.

Delirium tremens is the most serious form of the syndrome and an acute medical emergency. It should not be confused with the more mild signs and symptoms of alcohol withdrawal such as tremulousness. Seizures may develop, which may be fatal, and if left untreated mortality rate is up to 15%.

It is characterized by:

- Delusions
- Generalized seizures
- Profound confusion
- Visual hallucinations
- Tremor
- Agitation
- Increased activity of ANS, e.g., dilated pupils, fever, tachycardia, perspiration

Symptoms generally develop 9–12 hrs after the last drink, peaking at 48–72 hrs. Laboratory hallmarks include hypomagnesemia, decreased arterial pH, and decreased $pO_2$. There are also derangements in the serum electrolytes that are most often related to dehydration.

The initial evaluation should be thorough, paying special attention to possible injuries the patient may have sustained while in an altered mental status. Falls are common, as is malnutrition.

Special attention should be given to the issue of glucose administration in the IV fluids. The alcoholic patient generally lives on a diet high in carbohydrates (alcohol) and low in thiamine and tends to have no vitamin B reserves. The administration of glucose will consume the patient's last stores of thiamine and may precipitate Wernicke's syndrome. There is no definitive proof, however, that giving the thiamine just before or after the dextrose really makes any difference because they are given so closely together.

The goal of therapy is to provide medication that (a) is cross-tolerant for alcohol and (b) will blunt the patient's state of agitation and thereby prevent exhaustion. This is best achieved with benzodiazepines or chlordiazepoxide; however, the specific agent used is not as important as using a sufficiently high amount of the medication.

- Phenytoin is not useful for withdrawal-related seizures.
- Haloperidol should be avoided because it can lower the seizure threshold.
- If the patient has liver failure, lorazepam and oxazepam are the only safe agents.
- If the patient is refractory to benzodiazepines, barbiturates or propofol can be effective.

### Basic Science Correlate

Benzodiazepines activate GABA receptors, which increase the chloride current in neurons of the CNS. This leads to hyperpolarization of neurons and inhibits firing of action potentials (inhibitory potentials).

Thiamine deficiency can lead to **Wernicke–Korsakoff** syndrome. Wernicke is the triad of confusion, ataxia, and **ophthalmoplegia** (weakness or paralysis [-plegia] of $\geq$1 extraocular muscles). It is reversible with thiamine treatment. Korsakoff is amnesia with confabulation. It is irreversible.

Thiamine deficiency may also lead to wet beriberi, which is high cardiac output failure. This, like other causes of high cardiac output failure (chronic anemia, arteriovenous fistula, Paget's disease of bone, hyperthyroidism), is due to intense vasodilation of the peripheral arterioles because of the loss of ability to vasoconstrict secondary to low ATP levels. This leads to increases in cardiac output because of the decrease in resistance (low afterload) and an increase in venous return. The chronically elevated venous return overworks the heart and leads to eccentric hypertrophy (dilated cardiomyopathy). The patient presents with edema and shortness of breath due to pulmonary edema.

### Basic Science Correlate

Patents with thiamine deficiency have decreased activity of 3 important enzymes:

- Pyruvate **dehydrogenase**
- α-**keto**glutarate **dehydrogenase**
- Trans**keto**lase

Thiamine is a cofactor for the enzymes above. All of these enzymes are necessary for normal production of ATP, and patients with thiamine deficiency have decreased utilization of glucose because they are not able to produce ATP.

Pyruvate dehydrogenase complex catalyzes the following reaction:

$$\text{Pyruvate} + \text{NAD} + \text{CoA} \rightarrow \text{acetyl-CoA} + CO_2 + \text{NADH}$$

The pyruvate dehydrogenase complex requires 5 cofactors:

1. Pyrophosphate (B1, thiamine, TPP)
2. FAD (B2, riboflavin)
3. NAD (B3, niacin)
4. CoA (B5, pantothenate)
5. Lipoic acid

The end product of the pyruvate dehydrogenase complex is acetyl-CoA, which then enters the citric acid cycle. Impairment of the complex can cause tissues (e.g., brain and heart) to be affected by low ATP.

### Final Diagnosis

Alcohol withdrawal with delirium tremens

# CASE 2

## Chief Complaint

"I can't walk right."

## History and Physical Examination

A 19-year-old man who was playing rugby 6 hrs ago comes to the emergency department complaining of a severe headache for the last 2 hrs. While playing, he sustained head trauma and had a brief period of loss of consciousness from which he awoke and was his normal self. He then started to complain of nausea, vomiting, and weakness of the right side, as well as an inability to walk. He has no other medical problems.

Vital signs are T 37.8 C (100 F), BP 120/80 mm Hg, pulse 88/min, and respirations 18/min. Neurologic examination shows a small laceration of the left temporal region. His right eye is normal, and his left eye is dilated. There is a right hemiplegia. The remainder of the physical examination is unremarkable.

**CCS NOTE**

All patients with head trauma and a loss of consciousness should undergo a head CT scan without contrast, no matter how brief the loss of consciousness.

## Differential Diagnosis

1. Subdural hematoma
2. Concussion
3. Epidural hematoma
4. Contusion
5. Subarachnoid hemorrhage

## Initial Management

| Initial Management Plan | Results |
|---|---|
| • CT scan of head, without contrast | Convex hyperdensity between the brain and skull, consistent with an acute epidural hematoma. A midline shift to the right is seen. |

**Setting:** emergency department

## Assessment

Rapidly evolving and often lethal, acute epidural hematomas are formed by laceration of a dural vessel, which produces a clot between the skull and the dura. Hemorrhage originates most often from a branch of the middle meningeal artery that has been lacerated by a fracture. In 90% of adult patients with an epidural hematoma, skull fracture is demonstrated by x-ray or at surgery or autopsy. The classic history is a brief loss of consciousness from which the patient awakens and is completely well; then the clot forms, compressing the brain surface and increasing the overall intracranial pressure. The increased pressure results in headache, vomiting, and weakness of contralateral limbs. The temporal lobe is displaced, compressing the brainstem and the adjacent ipsilateral oculomotor nerve.

**CCS NOTE**

Although not repeatedly mentioned in every one of these cases, every patient scheduled to have surgery should have a CBC to assess the platelet count and a prothrombin time to assess the risk of bleeding during the procedure.

### Treatment plan

1. Intubation and hyperventilation to a $pCO_2$ of 25–30 mm Hg
2. IV mannitol use
3. Neurosurgical evaluation for surgical evacuation of the hematoma
4. Maintain systolic BP greater than 100 mm Hg
5. Stress ulcer prophylaxis with proton pump inhibitors, $H_2$ blockers, or sucralfate
6. Admission to the intensive care unit

### Discussion

In acute epidural hematoma, careful observation of the level of consciousness and the neurologic status is imperative if an epidural hematoma is considered. Earliest possible evacuation of the hematoma before transtentorial herniation can occur is essential for a favorable outcome. Studies have shown that once signs of herniation are present, approximately 73% of patients who were decerebrate before surgery died. However, only 1% of patients died before surgery when they presented conscious, with no signs of herniation prior to surgery. The 2 essential components of a successful procedure are (a) removing the clot to relieve brain compression and (b) securing the source of bleeding to prevent recurrence. As the clot is removed, hemostasis is achieved by electrocoagulation and ligation of the main trunks of the middle meningeal vessels as they appear on the dura.

The acute management of increased intracranial pressure involves hyperventilation and mannitol injection. Hyperventilation lowers the $pCO_2$ of the arterial blood, and the cerebral vessels will therefore constrict. This will reduce intracranial pressure. Mannitol is an osmotic diuretic that also acutely decreases intravascular volume.

Steroids are of no benefit in intracranial bleeding. Their best indication is to decrease swelling around brain tumors, such as neoplasms and infection, which lead to increased intracranial pressure from edema.

### Final Diagnosis

Epidural hematoma, acute

#### CCS NOTE

Stress ulcer prophylaxis is given for any patient who has had head trauma, burns, or intubation.

#### CCS NOTE

For every CCS case, make sure to address location. Don't leave your patient in the ED after the initial management is complete. This patient will be transferred to the surgical ICU or directly to the OR.

## CASE 3

### Chief Complaint

Nausea and vomiting

### History and Physical Examination

A 21-year-old college student is brought to the emergency department with nausea and vomiting. Her roommate states that she has been depressed lately and is sleeping more than usual. Things got worse after she failed 2 final exams last week. Since the day before, she has not seemed herself. She started complaining of nausea this morning and has been vomiting for the past 6 hrs. She has no other medical problems and denies daily use of medicines. Her roommate is worried that she took some pills.

She is awake but appears somnolent and in mild respiratory distress. Vital signs are T 38.3° C (101° F), BP 110/60 mm Hg, pulse 130/min, and respirations 26/min. Cardiovascular exam shows a regular rhythm and hyperdynamic precordium. Lungs are clear and the abdomen has normal bowel sounds with slight tenderness. There is no evidence of edema in her extremities.

### Differential Diagnosis

1. Drug overdose, unspecified
2. Acetaminophen overdose
3. Salicylate (aspirin) overdose
4. Alcohol intoxication
5. Gastroenteritis

**CCS NOTE**

All patients with acute altered mental status of unclear etiology can receive naloxone, thiamine, and dextrose as part of their initial set of orders.

| Initial Management Plan | Results |
|---|---|
| • CBC | WBC 12,000/mm$^3$; platelets and hemoglobin WNL |
| • Serum electrolytes | Sodium 146 mEq/L, potassium 5 mEq/L, chloride 108 mEq/L, bicarbonate 17 mEq/L, glucose 110 mg/dL |
| • BUN, creatinine | BUN 28 mg/dL, creatinine 2.1 U/L |
| • Anion gap | 21 mEq/L |
| • ABG | pH 7.46 $pCO_2$ 23 mm Hg/$pO_2$ 90 mm Hg/$HCO_3$ 17 mm Hg |
| • Serum ethanol level | 0 mg/dL |

### Assessment

The presentation of an acute change in mental status in a depressed patient should lead you to suspect a possible drug overdose. A respiratory alkalosis and metabolic acidosis should prompt you to suspect salicylate intoxication. A blood alcohol level can help to rule out this ingestion. The management approach should take into account the patient's altered mental status. Other complications of aspirin overdose (not present in this patient) are tinnitus, pulmonary edema, and coma (resulting from edema).

Aspirin is a very complex metabolic poison. It causes an acute respiratory alkalosis at first by central brainstem stimulation. Later, there is predominant metabolic acidosis. The acidosis is actually a lactic acidosis because aspirin poisons the mitochondria, leading to anaerobic metabolism and the production of lactate. Aspirin is directly toxic to the kidney tubules and lung parenchyma and may give acute tubular necrosis and acute respiratory distress syndrome. The direct effect of aspirin on the brain leads to encephalopathy.

| Further Management Plan | Results |
|---|---|
| 1. Plasma salicylate level | Salicylate level 100 mg/dL (elevated) |
| 2. Urine or blood toxicology screen | Negative for all but salicylate |

#### CCS NOTE

For patients with potential overdose, it is acceptable to order activated charcoal before obtaining the results of specific diagnostic tests. Although charcoal may not help every overdose, it has no adverse effects.

### Treatment plan

1. Activated charcoal to block further absorption of the drug
2. IV fluids to help restore volume status
3. IV bicarbonate for urine alkalinization, which aids drug excretion
4. Psychiatric consultation when patient is stable

### Discussion

Salicylates (aspirin) have great potential for both accidental ingestion by children and as a suicide substance for adults. Acute ingestion of >100 mg/kg leads to an initial respiratory alkalosis and later may cause a mixed respiratory alkalosis and metabolic acidosis. Acute ingestion invariably presents with vomiting, and this often aids in distinguishing aspirin from acetaminophen overdose.

Winter's formula is helpful in evaluating acid-base disorders associated with metabolic acidosis. It tells you the expected (corrected) $pCO_2$ in a patient with a metabolic acidosis.

$$pCO_2 = 1.5(HCO_3) + 8\ (+/-2)$$

For example, if bicarbonate is 10 mm/L, the expected $pCO_2$ is 1.5(10) + 8 = 23 mm Hg.

If the $pCO_2$ is lower than this, the patient has an additional respiratory alkalosis. This is not respiratory compensation for a metabolic acidosis. Overcompensation is impossible.

**CCS NOTE**

Consultations should rarely, if ever, be ordered for single-best answer questions. However, you are expected to ask for them much more often on the CCS.

The initial management calls for the prevention of absorption. This is best accomplished at home by induced emesis (with an agent like ipecac syrup) and should be considered for all patients without altered mental status. Gastric lavage, used more often in the ED, is used when patients present within 1 hour of ingestion as another method to empty the gastric contents. Activated charcoal is administered to absorb the ingested toxin, thereby blocking further systemic absorption. Following these initial measures, alkalinization of the urine should be performed to promote ionization of the salicylate and to thus reduce further reabsorption. For this purpose, IV bicarbonate is given. Effectiveness is monitored by measuring the pH of the urine, not serum.

Lastly, hemodialysis would be indicated for:

1. Persistent acidosis with pH <7.1
2. Initial salicylate levels >160 mg/dL or >130 mg/dL after 6 hrs
3. Coma/seizures
4. Renal failure
5. Congestive heart failure

### Final Diagnosis

Salicylate intoxication

# CASE 4

## Chief Complaint

"I have blood in my stool."

## History and Physical Examination

A 76-year-old man comes to the emergency department after passing stool surrounded by a large volume of blood. The patient states he had 2 similar episodes 7 months ago but did not seek medical attention. He denies abdominal pain, fever, and diarrhea. He has a history of a myocardial infarction and valvular disease. He takes no medications.

Vital signs are T 37.0 C (98.6 F), BP 90/70 mm Hg, pulse 100/min, and respirations 16/min. There are orthostatic changes. The abdomen is soft and nontender. Rectal exam shows no hemorrhoids or stool, but there is bright red blood in rectum. Cardiovascular exam shows a 3/6 systolic ejection murmur radiating to carotids.

### CCS NOTE

On the CCS in GI bleed, the most important initial consideration is hemodynamic stability. If the patient is hypotensive or tachycardic, a bolus of IV normal saline or Ringer's lactate should be ordered with the first set of orders.

## Differential Diagnosis

1. Hemorrhoids
2. Angiodysplasia
3. Colonic polyps
4. Ulcerative colitis
5. Crohn's disease
6. Diverticulosis with diverticular bleeding
7. Rectal ulcer

### CCS NOTE

Specific endoscopy is not as important as fluid resuscitation and correction of coagulopathy. Order fluids, CBC, type and cross first, then do endoscopy or other procedures later.

| Initial Management Plan | Results |
|---|---|
| • CBC | Hematocrit 29% (normal 39–49%) |
| • BUN | 32 mg/dL (normal 8–18 mg/dL) |
| • Creatinine | 0.9 mg/dL (0.6–1.3 mg/dL) |
| • PT/PTT | Normal |
| • EKG | Normal |

**Setting:** emergency department

**CLINICAL PEARL**

If a patient with hematochezia has hypotension and elevated BUN, do an upper endoscopy before a colonoscopy. The reason is that 10% of patients presenting with hematochezia will have an upper GI bleed, and if the patient is unstable it is more likely to be an upper bleed (which needs to be addressed immediately).

### Assessment

Large volume bleeding from the colon in adults is usually caused by diverticular disease, angiodysplasia, or ulcerative colitis. Benign or malignant neoplasms and ischemic colitis rarely cause massive bleeding. The site of bleeding in the colon can be identified in 70–80% of patients. Massive bleeding originates in the right as often as in the left colon. Diverticulosis is most often left-sided. Bleeding diverticula and angiodysplasia are common in the right colon. When active hemorrhage is occurring, radionuclide scintigraphy or angiography can be performed to identify the site of hemorrhage.

Colonoscopy will show lesions in the colon also, but they are harder to see during large-volume bleeding. Colonoscopy is the primary method of identifying angiodysplasia. Nasogastric tube placement is occasionally useful because 10% of cases of hematochezia originate from the upper GI tract. BUN characteristically rises because of absorption of nitrogenous breakdown products of blood from the GI tract.

| Further Management Plan | Results |
|---|---|
| 1. Colonoscopy | Spider angioma-like lesions in right colon |
| 2. Radionuclide scintigraphy (RBC scan), if bleeding is too rapid to make colonoscopy effective | Negative |
| 3. Nasogastric tube placement (if uncertain whether upper or lower GI source of bleed) | Negative |

**CCS NOTE**

Nasogastric tube placement is one of the least useful tasks in GI bleeding. Lavaging the stomach with saline or ice has no efficacy in stopping the bleeding. The nasogastric tube is useful in guiding the site of the initial endoscopy.

### Treatment plan

1. Normal saline infusion until blood is available for transfusion
2. Endoscopic electrocoagulation
3. Blood transfusion if patient symptomatic from anemia or if active ongoing bleed
4. Surgical consult for possible colonic resection if bleeding is persistent and massive (>4–6 units of blood in <24 hrs)

### Discussion

Angiodysplasia is sometimes associated with aortic stenosis. It is characterized by painless bleeding, from mild to massive; signs of bleeding can range from brisk hematochezia to occult blood loss leading to iron-deficiency anemia. Many patients are older adult with a history of cardiac disease, especially aortic stenosis. "Hematochezia" refers to the passage of gross blood per rectum. Recent transfusion guidelines are more liberal and recommend giving packed RBC transfusions at hemoglobin <7 and hemoglobin <8–9 in those with cardiac disease.

Brisk colonic hemorrhage due to angiodysplasia responds to endoscopic electrocoagulation. In high-risk patients unable to be controlled by endoscopy, selective arterial catheterization should be performed for deliberate embolization. Vasopressin is rarely necessary and should be avoided in a patient with cardiac disease because it causes vasospasm. Most cases of GI bleeding stop spontaneously. If massive bleeding continues, subtotal colectomy, laser therapy, or electrocoagulation is indicated. Fresh frozen plasma is used with coagulopathy.

Aortic stenosis with bleeding from angiodysplasia has been called Heyde's syndrome. A possible mechanism by which aortic stenosis may lead to the development of angiodysplasia is through the development of an acquired form of von Willebrand disease (vWD). Acquired vWD is thought to result from mechanical disruption of von Willebrand multimers during turbulent passage through the narrowed valve and from a von Willebrand factor interaction with platelets that triggers platelet clearance.

In patients with recurrent bleeding due to AVM and aortic stenosis, an aortic valve replacement should be done to prevent recurrent bleeding.

### Final Diagnosis

Lower GI bleed

# CASE 5

## Chief Complaint

Confusion and irritability

## History and Physical Examination

A 73-year-old woman with insulin-requiring diabetes mellitus is brought to the emergency department by her family for a flu-like illness earlier in the week and because she has not been eating well. Over the past 24 hrs she has "not been herself," with marked irritability and confusion. This morning she was difficult to awaken. There is no history of fever, neck stiffness, or focal neurologic deficits. She is on no other medications. She is currently lying on a stretcher and is difficult to arouse.

Vital signs are T 37.8 C (100.0 F), BP 105/72 mm Hg, pulse 110/min, and respirations 16/min. Her pupils are equal, round, and reactive to light and accommodation. She has normal heart sounds and tachycardia. Her lungs are clear and examination of the abdomen is benign. Changes consistent with venous stasis are evident in the extremities. Neurologic exam is nonfocal; there are no gross deficits; however, she is unable to follow commands.

## Differential Diagnosis

1. Hypoglycemia
2. Acute delirium
3. Drug overdose
4. Cerebrovascular accident
5. Sepsis syndrome

## Initial Management

**Setting:** emergency department

## Diagnostic/Therapeutic Plan

- Measurement of blood glucose by finger stick
- Serum electrolytes
- CBC

## Test Results

- Blood glucose 35 mg/dL
- Serum electrolytes: normal
- CBC: normal

### Assessment

Hypoglycemia is a relatively common complication of therapy with insulin and oral hypoglycemic agents. It should be thought of first when seeing a diabetic patient with change in mental status. Other common symptoms include irritability, tremulousness, diaphoresis, seizure, stupor, and coma. Meningitis is unlikely in the absence of fever and neck stiffness. Stroke usually presents with a focal deficit rather than a generalized delirium, as seen in this patient.

### Further Management Plan/Results

1. Treatment with IV dextrose (50 mL of 50% dextrose should be given initially). Avoid oral administration in patients who are not alert.
2. If patient does not recover after the administration of glucose, consider thyroid function tests, vitamin B12 level, lumbar puncture, toxicology screen, and CT scan of the head.
3. Blood cultures: no growth
4. Urine cultures: no growth

### Discussion

In diabetic patients, the most common causes of hypoglycemia are as follows:

- Change in dietary habits without an appropriate change in medication
- Increase in metabolic demands (e.g., increase in physical activity)
- Medication overdose
- New onset renal failure

Diagnosis is easy to establish and the condition must be corrected promptly.

In non diabetic patients, there are several possible causes:

- Insulinoma
- Severe liver disease
- Alcohol intoxication
- Adrenal insufficiency
- Myxedema
- Severe malnutrition
- Factitious disorder with abuse of insulin or sulfonylureas

### Final Diagnosis

Hypoglycemia

#### CCS NOTE

Treating an unstable patient is always more important on the CCS than doing a specific diagnostic test. Giving glucose to a disoriented person is more important than waiting for specific diagnostics.

#### CLINICAL PEARL

- If a patient presents with the triad of hypoglycemia, elevated insulin, and low c-peptide levels, suspect factitious use of insulin.
- If a patient presents with hypoglycemia with elevated insulin and c-peptide levels, check sulfonylurea levels for overdose of sulfonylurea hypoglycemic drugs.

Insulinoma also causes elevated insulin levels and elevated c-peptide, but is rare. Reactive hypoglycemia occurs following a meal, usually 2–4 hrs after eating. It is due to an excess of insulin released after glucose stimulation often after gastric resection. When the diagnosis is in question, an insulin level can be obtained.

## CASE 6

### Chief Complaint

"I'm wheezing, and my lips are swollen."

### History and Physical Examination

A 27-year-old woman comes to the emergency department complaining of wheezing and swelling of the lips. The symptoms began acutely just after eating a chicken-and-nut dish at a nearby Chinese restaurant. She also complains of tightness in her chest and mild difficulty breathing. She has no significant past medical history and is not taking any medications. She had a similar episode a year ago after she had eaten some cookies at a friend's house.

Vital signs are T 36.8 C (98.2 F), BP 110/50 mm Hg, pulse 110/min, and respirations 24/min. The patient appears anxious and in mild respiratory distress. She has diffuse facial erythema and swelling of the lips and tongue. There is no stridor. Her heart has a regular rhythm and is tachycardic. There is diffuse bilateral wheezing on auscultation. The remainder of the physical examination is unremarkable.

### Differential Diagnosis

1. Acute anaphylaxis
2. Foreign body aspiration
3. Asthma

### Initial Management

**Setting:** emergency department

### Diagnostic/Therapeutic Plan

- Pulse oximetry

### Test Results

- Oxygen saturation 92%

### Assessment

The onset of wheezing, shortness of breath, facial erythema, and swelling of the tongue are common manifestations of anaphylaxis. The diagnosis is made easier by the development of these symptoms occurring shortly after exposure to the causative agent—in this case, nuts. There are no tests that will determine the specific agent. The most important factor in a case of acute allergic reaction is evidence of instability, such as dyspnea, hypotension, or signs of airway obstruction, such as stridor. An allergic reaction characterized only by a rash is much less dangerous. The presence of wheezing in this case is very worrisome.

### Further Management Plan

- Epinephrine 1:1,000 subcutaneously every 15 minutes until improvement
- Supplemental oxygen
- Establish IV access and start normal saline
- Diphenhydramine intramuscularly or intravenously every 4–6 hrs
- IV corticosteroids every 6 hrs
- Endotracheal intubation if there is severe airway obstruction secondary to laryngeal edema that does not rapidly improve with epinephrine
- Albuterol inhalers in patients who are wheezing

### Discussion

Anaphylaxis is an acute systemic reaction resulting from the interaction of a foreign antigen with surface immunoglobulin E located on mast cells and basophils in a previously sensitized person. This results in the release of histamine, leukotrienes, and other factors that lead to smooth-muscle contraction causing bronchoconstriction and smooth-muscle relaxation leading to vasodilation. Anaphylactic reactions can present with a spectrum of symptoms and, in the majority of cases, will develop within one hour of exposure to the offending agent.

Vasodilation results in the leakage of plasma into the extravascular space, which may result in urticaria and angioedema, hypovolemia and shock, pulmonary edema, obstruction of the upper airway, and cardiac arrhythmias. The most critical issue in anaphylaxis is whether or not the person's airway is obstructed and if their BP is low. IV fluids must be given with epinephrine at the beginning if BP is low.

The systems most frequently affected are the skin, lungs, GI tract, and cardiovascular system. The diagnosis is generally easily made if the symptoms occur shortly after exposure to the causative agent. If not, the diagnosis may be more difficult and can be confused with such diagnoses as a vasovagal episode, foreign body aspiration, and cold urticaria.

Countless substances can cause anaphylactic reactions, but the most common offenders are drugs, insect stings, and food substances, such as peanuts and fish. Because anaphylaxis may be rapidly fatal, the most important step in management involves a rapid assessment of the patient's airway, breathing, and cardiovascular status.

#### Basic Science Correlate

Anaphylaxis is a classic type I hypersensitivity reaction, but know the other hypersensitivity reactions and their associated clinical conditions and mechanisms.

### CCS NOTE

An oximeter alone is sufficient when one is not investigating $CO_2$ retention and when a specific A-a gradient is not important. An ABG is important in COPD or *Pneumocystis* pneumonia.

### CCS NOTE

Oxygen should be administered at the same time as ordering the oximeter in a patient with shortness of breath. When a test and a treatment are ordered at the same time, the test reflects the pretreatment state.

### CLINICAL PEARL

Diphenhydramine is the superior antihistamine in case of anaphylaxis. It is more effective than the others.

Following an initial assessment, epinephrine should be administered as the first-line agent. Then, antihistamines (such as diphenhydramine or hydroxyzine), H2 blockers, and steroids may be added. All patients with an episode of severe anaphylaxis should be observed for at least 6 to 8 hrs, due to the possibility of a late second reaction.

Beta-blockers are contraindicated in those at risk for anaphylaxis because they can make it worse. Also, because epinephrine is used as one of the main treatments for anaphylaxis, beta-blockers will interfere with the ability of the epinephrine to be effective.

**Type I hypersensitivity**

- Anaphylactic and atopic
- Free antigen cross-links IgE on mast cells and basophils and triggers immediate release of histamine and bradykinin, which act on postcapillary venules; this leads to edema formation, vasodilation, and bronchoconstriction.
- Delayed response follows, due to production of leukotrienes from arachidonic acid.
- Examples:
  - Allergic and atopic (rhinitis, asthma, hay fever, hives, eczema)
  - Patients with IgA-deficiency can have severe anaphylactic reaction to blood products (dyspnea, bronchospasm, hypotension, respiratory failure, shock); administer washed RBCs.

**Type II hypersensitivity**

- Cytotoxic (antibody mediated) IgM, IgG bind to fixed antigen on cell leading to cellular destruction
  - Opsonization leading to phagocytosis
  - Complement-mediated lysis
  - Antibody-dependent cell-mediated cytotoxicity usually due to NK cells or macrophages
- Examples:
  - Autoimmune hemolytic anemia
  - Pernicious anemia
  - Rheumatic fever
  - Goodpasture's syndrome
  - Bullous pemphigoid
  - Idiopathic thrombocytopenic purpura

**Type III hypersensitivity**

- Immune complex mediated
- Complexes activate complement, which attracts neutrophils; neutrophils release lysosomal enzymes
- Examples:
  - SLE
  - Polyarteritis nodosa
  - Post-streptococcal glomerulonephritis
  - Serum sickness
  - Arthus reaction (e.g., swelling and inflammation following a vaccination)

**Type IV hypersensitivity**

- Delayed (T-cell mediated)
- Sensitized T lymphocytes encounter antigen and then release lymphokines, leading to macrophage activation
- Only hypersensitivity type that does not involve antibodies
- Examples:
  - Multiple sclerosis
  - Guillain-Barré syndrome
  - Graft-vs-host disease
  - PPD
  - Contact dermatitis

## Final Diagnosis

Anaphylaxis, secondary to nuts

# CASE 7

## Chief Complaint

Extensive body burns

## History and Physical Examination

A man is trapped in a house fire for 20 minutes. When he is finally rescued, he is noted to be alert and breathing. He suffers extensive burns on his right arm and anterior chest and is brought by ambulance to the emergency department.

He is currently awake and alert with a patent airway and moving air without difficulty. There is some soot around his mouth, and he is not hoarse. Vital signs are stable. There are extensive second- and third-degree burns along the entire right arm and anterior torso, with some scattered first-degree burns over both lower extremities and back. He weighs 220 lb. Heart and lung examinations are normal except for tachycardia; there is no wheezing. His abdomen is soft and nontender.

## Differential Diagnosis

1. Skin burns
2. Airway burn
3. Carbon monoxide poisoning

## Initial Management

**Setting:** emergency department

## Diagnostic/Therapeutic Plan

- Carboxyhemoglobin level
- Chest x-ray
- CBC
- Electrolytes (chemistry)

## Test Results

- Carboxyhemoglobin elevated at 23%
- Chest x-ray: normal
- Hemoglobin 14 g/dL
- Electrolytes: normal

**CLINICAL PEARL**

The most common cause of death in burns is carbon monoxide poisoning. That makes 100% oxygen administration the most important initial therapy for burns.

### Assessment

Diagnosing skin burns in this case is not difficult; the challenge is to determine the exact extent of the burns. Burn depths are graded as first-, second-, and third-degree.

- **First-degree burns** are erythematous, and only the superficial layer of skin is affected.
- **Second-degree burns** are often associated with blistering and a white or fibrinous exudate.
- **Third-degree burns** may appear blackened, charred, or leathery. Patients often lack sensation in these areas because of loss of both epidermal and dermal elements, including hair follicles and pain receptors.
- The most common causes of death in the initial period following second- and third-degree burns are hypovolemic shock, infection, and airway injury.
  - Airway injury is a variable problem, depending on the nature of the burn. Even without a direct burn of the airway, inhalation injury can lead to serious illness because of the elevation of carboxyhemoglobin levels. Carboxyhemoglobin does not deliver oxygen to tissues, and functionally, it is the same as being anemic.

Evidence of respiratory tract injury includes tachypnea, soot in the mouth, erythema of the palate, stridor, laryngospasm, and other evidence of respiratory distress. Laryngeal edema and respiratory failure can develop 6–24 hrs after the injury. The airway and lung may appear normal at first, but life-threatening abnormalities may appear later.

**CCS NOTE**

Order a bolus of fluids with the initial set of labs in serious burns; you can only specify "bolus" or "continuous," not the specific amounts.

**Further Management Plan/Results**

- Immediate bronchoscopy: reveals no significant airway injury

### Further Management Plan

1. 100% oxygen
2. Fluid resuscitation 4 mL/kg% BSA burned (Ringer's lactate)
3. Prevention of infection with topical antibiotics
4. Endotracheal intubation if there is evidence of significant respiratory injury

**CCS NOTE**

In burn cases with evidence of respiratory burn (e.g., hoarseness, wheezing, stridor, burns in the mouth), perform endotracheal intubation with the first set of orders.

### Discussion

Care in the acute period should focus on maintaining adequate ventilation and oxygenation, replacing acute volume loss, correcting metabolic abnormalities, and preventing infectious complications. The decision to use intubation is based on the degree of airway inflammation and level of oxygenation. The patient should be started on 100% supplemental oxygen, as oxygen therapy decreases the half-life of the carboxyhemoglobin. The full extent of an inhalation injury may not be apparent for 12–24 hrs.

Hypovolemic shock often results from second- or third-degree burns encompassing >25% of the BSA.

- Fluid is infused at 2–4 mL per kg per %.
- Fluids are given in first 24 hrs; normal saline or Ringer's lactate is acceptable.
- Patients may require replacement of plasma and albumin as well.
- Emphasis should be placed on maintaining adequate urine output to avoid renal failure.
- Hypovolemia can result in metabolic acidosis.

**CCS NOTE**

The CCS asks route of administration, not dose. Hence, in burns, topical antibiotics, not systemic or IV antibiotics, are used prophylactically.

If the patient is not tolerating PO intake, control the pain with IV morphine drip or PCA pump; if the patient is tolerating it, use extended-release morphine or methadone.

Calculations for BSA are as follows:

- Head 9%
- Arms 9% each
- Legs 18% each
- Chest 18%
- Back 18%
- Perineum 1%

Silver sulfadiazine is administered topically to all burned areas, and the wounds should be debrided and dressings changed 2x daily. Operative debridement of deep partial-thickness burns and skin grafting should be done as soon as feasible. This helps to avoid subeschar infection and improves wound closure. Streptococcal and staphylococcal infection often complicate the initial course.

Excision of burn eschar may be done to improve healing or if evidence of arterial compression is present. Patients may require skin grafting.

### Final Diagnosis

Burns

# CASE 8

## Chief Complaint

"I have a weird feeling in my chest."

## History and Physical Examination

A 66-year-old man comes to the emergency department complaining of a several-day history of an intermittent sensation of fluttering in his chest. He feels weak when the episodes occur, but denies chest pain or shortness of breath. He presents today because the symptoms are now constant. He has had hypertension for 20 years, which is well-controlled with enalapril, and he takes albuterol for asthma. He denies any alcohol use.

Vital signs are temperature 36.8° C (98.2° F), blood pressure 140/80 mm Hg, pulse 140/min, and respirations 12/min. Physical examination shows a supple neck and no jugular venous distention or thyromegaly. Cardiovascular exam shows an irregularly irregular rhythm with no rubs or gallops. The chest is clear, the abdomen is benign, and there is no edema in his extremities.

## Differential Diagnosis

1. Atrial fibrillation
2. Multifocal atrial tachycardia
3. Supraventricular tachycardia
4. Cardiomyopathy
5. Pulmonary embolism
6. Thyrotoxicosis
7. Sinus tachycardia with ectopy
8. Hypoglycemia

### CCS NOTE

Fluttering or palpitations do not necessarily signify hemodynamic instability, but they do mean that an EKG should be ordered.

## Initial Management

**Setting:** emergency room

## Diagnostic/Therapeutic Plan

- EKG

## Test Results

- EKG: irregular tachycardia with absent P waves; ventricular response 140/min; pulse irregularly irregular

#### CCS NOTE

If the EKG does not reveal the etiology of the palpitations, order telemetry monitoring or ambulatory Holter monitoring.

### Assessment

The presentation of palpitations and a rapid pulse is suggestive of a cardiac arrhythmia. Sinus tachycardia is due to underlying medical disorders such as fever, pain, anxiety, dyspnea, and many other causes.

The irregularly irregular pulse should make you suspect atrial fibrillation. Prompt evaluation of the patient's hemodynamic status is crucial. An EKG will confirm the diagnosis.

By itself, the sensation of "fluttering in his chest" or palpitations is extremely nonspecific. Many patients with palpitations are never found to have a cardiac problem of any kind. Any form of arrhythmia may cause palpitations. Atrial flutter and supraventricular tachycardia will generally not give an irregularly irregular heart rhythm.

The tests described below represent a systematic evaluation to determine the etiology of atrial fibrillation.

#### CCS Note

The cases in this course give groups of diagnostic tests because each case is meant to cover a whole area of medicine. You might not have to order all these tests if the diagnosis on the CCS case is obvious.

| Further Management Plan | Results |
|---|---|
| 1. Thyroid function tests | Normal |
| 2. Cardiac enzymes | Normal |
| 3. Echocardiogram | Normal ejection fraction; left atrial enlargement; no pericardial disease |
| 4. Arterial blood gases | Normal |

### Treatment Plan

- IV diltiazem
- Admit to telemetry unit

#### CCS NOTE

On the CCS, you must order drugs by a specific name, not just by class.

### Discussion

Atrial fibrillation ("a-fib") is most commonly due to hypertension. Chronic hypertension leads to increased afterload, and as a result the heart has to increase contractility to maintain the stroke volume. This increase in contractility places the heart under a high pressure state, which leads to concentric hypertrophy. Concentric hypertrophy causes a stiff, non compliant left ventricle. This causes left atrial dilatation.

Mitral stenosis and mitral regurgitation may also cause atrial fibrillation. A-fib may also occur in the setting of any underlying heart disease, lung disease, or hyperthyroidism. The differential diagnosis includes multifocal atrial tachycardia, which most often can be distinguished by the presence of 3 distinct P-wave morphologies on the EKG. Paroxysmal supraventricular tachyarrhythmias have a regular rhythm and more commonly must be distinguished from atrial flutter. Precipitating conditions such as thyrotoxicosis, pulmonary embolus, pericarditis, alcohol intoxication, the use of catecholamine-like drugs, and myocardial infarction should be excluded.

There are 3 things to consider with a-fib:

- Rate control
- Anticoagulation
- Rhythm control

Treatment is directed at restoring normal sinus rhythm and preventing the paroxysms and slowing conduction through the atrioventricular node (with agents like digoxin, beta-adrenergic blocking agents, and CCBs). When a patient presents with a-fib and rapid ventricular response, the first step is to determine stability. Emergency cardioversion is indicated for patients with hemodynamic instability or angina. For patients who are stable, rate control should be achieved with an AV nodal blocking agent (i.e., a beta-blocker such as metoprolol or esmolol, or a non-dihydropyridine CCB such as diltiazem or verapamil). Digoxin is a good option for a patient with decompensated systolic heart failure, but not good for a normal cardiac patient who is ambulatory. It will only control the resting HR.

Rate control is usually preferred. Rhythm control is used when patients cannot tolerate the symptoms of atrial fibrillation (shortness of breath or palpations) or cannot be rate-controlled. For rhythm control, elective DC cardioversion is preferred. Chemical cardioversion may also be used. Amiodarone, sotalol, dofetilide, ibutilide, propafenone, and flecainide may all be used. In most case these agents will have to be continued for maintenance. Once rate control is achieved, the next step is to decide whether to continue with rate control or to proceed with rhythm control.

Long-term success of maintaining sinus rhythm is less likely if the arrhythmia has been present for a long period of time or if the left atrial size >45 mm. Anticoagulation should be given for 3 wks before elective cardioversion if the arrhythmia has been present for several days or if the patient is at increased risk for stroke (cardiomyopathy, rheumatic mitral valve disease, prosthetic valves, left atrial enlargement, or a previous stroke). Another option before elective cardioversion is to perform a transesophageal echocardiogram to exclude the presence of a thrombus.

Routine cardioversion of atrial fibrillation is not indicated. The vast majority of those who develop atrial fibrillation will not be successfully converted to sinus rhythm because they will slip back into atrial fibrillation. Therefore, rate control and anticoagulation with warfarin is the standard of care.

For a patient with non-valvular a-fib, we use the CHADS2 score to determine if an anticoagulant is needed.

**C** is for CHF

**H** is for HTN

**A** is for age >75

**D** is for DM

**S** is for stroke or TIA

Each condition gets 1 point, except for stroke/TIA, which gets 2 points.

| Score of 0 in lone a-fib | Give aspirin |
|---|---|
| **Score of 1** | Give aspirin or anticoagulant |
| **Score of 2+** | Give anticoagulant |

There are a few options for anticoagulation:

- Warfarin with goal INR 2–3
- Dabigatran is an oral direct thrombin inhibitor
- Rivaroxaban and apixaban are oral factor Xa inhibitors

These new agents have been clinically compared to warfarin. Results have shown that they are non-inferior or superior for stroke prevention, with less intracranial hemorrhaging (though more GI bleeding).

Long-term rate control with anticoagulation is equal in efficacy to elective cardioversion with either medication or electrical shock. Digoxin is preferable for rate control in patients with poor ventricular function. Diltiazem is just as rapid as verapamil with fewer adverse effects. Verapamil produces a rapid effect but because of its profoundly negative inotropic/dromotropic activity, it must not be used when there is evidence of ventricular dysfunction or conduction block. Beta-blockers such as metoprolol and propranolol are options as well to control rate; similar to calcium blockers, they are relatively contraindicated with atrioventricular block.

Most patients will go back into atrial fibrillation and will require anti arrhythmic agents for maintenance, and anticoagulation indefinitely. Amiodarone is superior for maintaining the patient in sinus rhythm after conversion when there is systolic dysfunction. The only 2 agents that are safe for rhythm control in systolic dysfunction are amiodarone and dofetilide.

**CCS NOTE**

Patients with atrial rhythm disorders do not have to go to the intensive care unit if the rate has been controlled to $<$100/min. They can go to the ward with telemetry monitoring.

Ablation is the answer for patients who cannot tolerate anti arrhythmic agents and have symptoms while in atrial fibrillation. If they have a high CHADS2 score, they will require anticoagulation after ablation indefinitely.

### Final Diagnosis

Atrial fibrillation with a rapid ventricular response

## Basic Science Correlate

Let's understand the drugs used to target the different phases of the action potential and their mechanisms of action. Antiarrhythmic drugs are useful not only for treatment of atrial fibrillation but also for the other cardiac arrhythmias. The 4 main classes of antiarrhythmic drugs are detailed below:

| | |
|---|---|
| **Class I: $Na^+$ channel blockers** | Class 1A<br>• Increase action potential duration (APD) and effective refractory period (ERP)<br>• Also blocks $K^+$ channels (prolongs repolarization)<br>• e.g., quinidine, procainamide<br>• Cautions and contraindications:<br>  • Prolongation of QRS and increased QT interval<br>Class 1B<br>• Block inactivated channels—increase threshold for excitation<br>• Decrease APD due to block of slow $Na^+$ currents<br>• e.g., lidocaine, mexiletine<br>• Lidocaine is safe in ischemic tissue<br>• Class 1C<br>• No effect on APD<br>• No ANS effects<br>• e.g., flecainide<br>• Cautions and contraindications:<br>  • Limited use due to proarrhythmogenic effects |
| **Class II: beta-blockers** | • Prevent β-receptor activation<br>• Decrease SA and AV nodal activity<br>• Decrease slope of phase 4 of AP in pacemaker cells<br>• e.g., propranolol (nonselective), acebutolol, and esmolol (cardioselective) |
| **Class III: $K^+$ channel blockers** | • Slows phase 3 (repolarization) of AP<br>• Increase APD and ERP<br>• e.g., amiodarone, sotalol<br>• Cautions and contraindications:<br>  • Long QT syndrome |
| **Class IV: $Ca2^+$ channel blockers** | • Decrease phase 0 and phase 4<br>• Decrease SA and AV nodal activity<br>• e.g., verapamil, diltiazem<br>• Cautions and contraindications:<br>  • Additive AV block with β-blockers and digoxin<br>• Verapamil displaces digoxin from tissue binding sites |

### CLINICAL PEARL

Class IA and III antiarrhythmic drugs block $K^+$ channels, prolonging repolarization and increasing the QT interval on EKG. **QT prolongation** leads to torsades de pointes. Hypokalemia, hypomagnesemia, and hypocalcemia may also inhibit the opening of the delayed rectifying potassium channels and prolong the refractory period, leading to QT prolongation. Other drugs such as macrolides, fluoroquinolones, and antipsychotics such as haloperidol have the same effect.

# CASE 9

## Chief Complaint

"I'm having palpitations."

## History and Physical Examination

A 65-year-old man, recently discharged from the hospital after being treated for an anterior-wall myocardial infarction, is brought to the emergency room by his family because of palpitations. As you are examining him, he becomes unresponsive and loses his pulse.

## Differential Diagnosis

1. Ventricular fibrillation
2. Ventricular tachycardia
3. Acute myocardial infarction
4. Asystole
5. Electromechanical dissociation
6. Pulmonary embolus

## Initial Management

**Setting:** emergency department

### CCS NOTE

Unsynchronized cardioversion is always the first thing to do if ventricular fibrillation is found. It's more important than any specific diagnostic test.

## Diagnostic/Therapeutic Plan

- EKG

## Test Results

- EKG: ventricular fibrillation

## Assessment

Ventricular fibrillation causes loss of cardiac output, and death occurs within a few minutes. It is not a realistic diagnostic consideration in the conscious patient. There is irregularly irregular undulation of the baseline at variable rates without any organized QRS activity.

Immediate direct-current defibrillation should be administered to all patients with ventricular fibrillation. Once the heart is successfully defibrillated, immediate attention must be given to correct underlying causes and to institute prophylactic antiarrhythmics. The absolute priority in any attempt to resuscitate from ventricular fibrillation is electrical defibrillation. Without an EKG, it is not possible to tell if the cause of a patient's loss of pulse is asystole, ventricular fibrillation, ventricular tachycardia, or electrical-mechanical dissociation.

Ventricular arrhythmia is a known complication after anterior-wall myocardial infarction.

| Further Management Plan | Results |
| --- | --- |
| Arterial blood gases | pH 7.12; $pCO_2$ 42 mm Hg; $pO_2$ 90 mm Hg; bicarbonate 14 mEq/L |

## Treatment Plan

1. Cardiopulmonary resuscitation until the defibrillator arrives
2. Defibrillate at 360 J, perform several cycles of CPR after defibrillation
3. Repeat defibrillation at 360 J
4. IV access
5. Intubate
6. Epinephrine intravenously or vasopressin once every 5 minutes
7. Repeat defibrillation at 360 J
8. Amiodarone or lidocaine; if both are answer choices, choose amiodarone
9. Consider bicarbonate
10. Repeat defibrillation at 360 J

## Discussion

In a case of ventricular fibrillation, immediate defibrillation is the critical intervention. Defibrillation is an unsynchronized shock. (When one delivers a synchronized shock, it is synchronized to the ventricular contraction, but in ventricular fibrillation there is no ventricular contraction.) There are 3 conditions where defibrillation should be delivered: ventricular fibrillation, pulseless ventricular tachycardia, torsades de pointes.

Precordial thumping is indicated only when the arrest is witnessed and no defibrillator is available. Cardiopulmonary resuscitation should not be interrupted except while defibrillation is being administered.

- First, administer 360 J of direct-current countershock with one paddle at the apex and the other at the aortic position.
- Proceed with 5 cycles of CPR immediately after the shock.
- Evaluate cardiac rhythm after the 5 cycles of CPR. Failure of ventricular fibrillation to revert to normal sinus rhythm after direct-current countershock may be due to severe acidosis, hypoxia, myocardial failure, or a combination of all 3.
- Continue CPR, correct abnormalities, and continue advanced cardiac life support protocol according to treatment guidelines.

### CCS NOTE

Patients with ventricular rhythm disturbances should be placed in the ICU.

Although medications such as amiodarone, lidocaine, and procainamide are used, their efficacy is considerably less than that of electrical defibrillation. Hence, the order is shock-drug-shock-drug-shock, etc.

- Vasopressin has been added as an alternative to epinephrine.
- Amiodarone has been added as an alternative to lidocaine.
- Bretylium should not be used.
- Magnesium can be used in any serious ventricular arrhythmia; its greatest efficacy is in patients with Torsade de pointes.

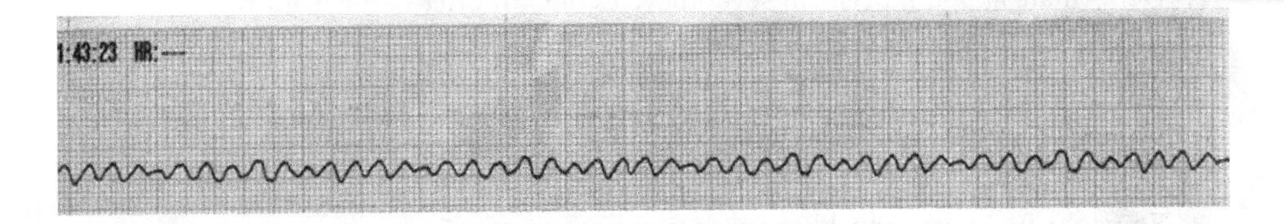


Ventricular Fibrillation

### CCS NOTE

Never order intracardiac administration of medications on the CCS.

## Final Diagnosis

Ventricular fibrillation

# CASE 10

## Chief Complaint

"I'm nauseous and can't stop vomiting."

## History and Physical Examination

A 44-year-old business executive comes to the emergency department with complaints of severe nausea and vomiting over the past 12 hours. He has been under a great deal of pressure recently and has been taking numerous over-the-counter cold preparations and acetaminophen around the clock for a severe upper respiratory tract infection. He has had several emergency department visits for alcohol intoxication, including one episode of alcohol withdrawal. He is a chain smoker, and has several glasses of wine with dinner each evening.

Vital signs are T 37.9 C (100.2 F), BP 110/75 mm Hg, pulse 100/min, and respirations 20/min. Physical examination is unremarkable, except for mild right upper quadrant tenderness without rebound or guarding.

## Differential Diagnosis

1. Acetaminophen overdose
2. Appendicitis
3. Acute gastroenteritis
4. Acute cholecystitis
5. Acute pancreatitis
6. Hepatitis

## Initial Management

**Setting:** emergency department or office

## Diagnostic/Therapeutic Plan

- CBC
- Electrolytes
- LFTs
- Prothrombin time
- Amylase level
- Abdominal U/S

### Test Results

- WBC count 12,800/mm$^3$, hemoglobin 13.0 g/dL, platelets 210,000/mm$^3$
- Electrolytes: normal
- AST (SGOT) 74 U/L, ALT (SGPT) 92 U/L, total bilirubin 1.6 mg/dL
- Prothrombin time: 12.2 sec
- Amylase: normal
- U/S: normal

**CCS NOTE**

Sometimes you cannot identify the diagnosis on the initial history in the CCS. Do not worry. Order tests around the history, and the specific diagnosis will be revealed later. Just don't count on consultants to help you.

### Assessment

The differential diagnosis in a 44-year-old patient presenting with nausea and vomiting is quite broad. It is important to recognize that many over-the-counter cold preparations contain acetaminophen. In addition, the patient has been taking large doses of supplemental acetaminophen.

Patients with significant alcohol ingestion are at increased risk for developing clinical acetaminophen toxicity, as they may have some level of baseline hepatic injury. The absence of significant associated fever and a normal WBC count speak against appendicitis, pancreatitis, and cholecystitis, though those are all considerations here.

### Further Diagnostic Plan/Results

- Serum acetaminophen level: 150 μg/mL
- Aspirin level: 0 mg/dL

**CCS NOTE**

Normal values are routinely provided with the test results on the CCS. Do not worry about memorizing uncommon test results, such as acetaminophen levels.

### Treatment Plan

1. Gastric lavage or induced emesis with ipecac if patient not already vomiting; most useful within 1 hour of ingestion. There is a non significant effect after 2 hrs.
2. Acetylcysteine (beneficial up to 24 hours after ingestion)
3. Charcoal administration in between the doses of acetylcysteine (administer 1 hr apart)

### Discussion

Early clinical manifestations of acetaminophen overdose include anorexia, nausea, vomiting, diaphoresis, and malaise. Hepatotoxicity is the major concern, with peak injury occurring 72–96 hrs after ingestion.

To determine if the patient is at risk for the sequelae of acetaminophen overdose, the serum acetaminophen level is plotted against time after ingestion. The level is more accurate after 4 hrs; prior to that, absorption is still occurring and the level may still be rising.

**CLINICAL PEARL**

Ipecac is rarely used in the ED, as it delays the administration of antidotes orally. It is most useful for those with an accidental ingestion at home.

### Further Management

The initial management of acetaminophen overdose focuses on minimizing absorption of the drug with gastric lavage or induced emesis.

- Ipecac is rarely, if ever, used in the ED; it is primarily for home management of overdose in those who have not yet arrived at the hospital.
- Charcoal may interfere with absorption of acetylcysteine (the antidote) if given at the exact same time, so the doses should be interspersed.
- Acetylcysteine should be administered as quickly as possible for up to 24 hrs after ingestion of acetaminophen.
- Acetylcysteine repletes glutathione stores.

Patients with hepatic injury due to acetaminophen toxicity may require liver transplant. One very important value to monitor is **prothrombin time**. If this rapidly increases along with signs of hepatic encephalopathy, the patient has fulminant hepatic failure and needs a liver transplant.

A single dose of 10–15 grams is sufficient to result in evidence of hepatic injury. Fatalities can occur with >15-gram ingestion; however, in chronic alcoholics, toxicity may begin with as little as 4 grams. In the first 4–12 hrs, the early symptoms are nausea, vomiting, diarrhea, and abdominal pain, which often resolve; 24–48 hrs later, evidence of hepatic injury begins. The injury is not directly caused by the acetaminophen but rather by a toxic metabolite formed by the hepatic cytochrome p450 system.

A common question seen on the USMLE is acetaminophen overdose in alcoholics. Chronic alcohol depletes the glutathione stores and can predispose to acetaminophen toxicity at lower levels than in non-alcoholics. One important point is that alcoholic hepatitis can never lead to AST >500. Thus, if a patient has AST and ALT in the thousands, it is very likely the patient has acetaminophen toxicity and needs to be treated with acetylcysteine.

### Final Diagnosis

Acetaminophen overdose

#### CCS NOTE

Order acetaminophen and aspirin levels with any overdose case on the CCS. Co-ingestion is frequent. You won't lose points, even if the aspirin level is normal (as seen here). On the CCS, missing an occult aspirin or acetaminophen overdose is more dangerous than finding an additional normal level.

#### CLINICAL PEARL

Acetaminophen toxicity causes hepatic injury, which elevates transaminase (ALT, AST) levels >1,000. When hepatic injury occurs in acetaminophen toxicity, **acetylcysteine is not** effective since this occurs typically 2 days after the ingestion.

# CASE 11

## Chief Complaint

"I've had shortness of breath for 5 hours."

## History and Physical Examination

A 25-year-old man with no significant past medical history comes to the emergency department with shortness of breath for the past 5 hours. He was reportedly doing well until this afternoon when he had difficulty going up a flight of stairs after getting home from the gym. He has never experienced this in the past. He reports having mild chest pain, especially when taking a deep breath. He denies fever/chills, cough, recent travel, and sick contacts. Additionally, he denies using tobacco products and believes there is no family history of hypercoagulability.

His temperature is T 37.2 C (99.0 F), blood pressure 118/65 mm Hg, pulse 105/min, and respirations 24/min. Height is 6 ft (1.8 m) and weight 179 lb (81 kg). He appears to be in mild distress. Examination of the head and neck shows no abnormalities. No carotid bruits are noted and the thyroid is not enlarged. Cardiac examination shows tachycardia without murmurs, gallops, or rubs. The PMI is not displaced. Lung examination shows few bibasilar rales. Abdominal examination is unremarkable. The extremities show no cyanosis, clubbing, or edema. There is no calf tenderness or palpable cords.

## Differential Diagnosis

1. Pneumothorax
2. Pulmonary embolism (PE)
3. Pneumonia
4. Arrhythmia
5. Acute coronary syndrome

## Initial Management

**Setting:** emergency department or office

## Diagnostic/Therapeutic Plan

- Pulse oximeter
- Chest x-ray
- EKG
- ProBNP
- Serum troponin
- Lactate
- ABG
- Serum electrolytes, BUN, creatinine, glucose
- D-dimer
- PT/PTT/INR

### CCS NOTE

Most of these tests will be completed simultaneously. While the results of the basic chemistry panel, lactate, troponin, and proBNP are pending, the chest x-ray, EKG, and ABG are being done. Results of these tests will be delivered within a short time frame.

### Test Results

- Pulse oximeter: 91% room air
- Chest x-ray: bilateral atelectasis and bilateral small pleural effusions, no pneumothorax seen
- EKG: sinus tachycardia at 105/min, no ST/T wave changes
- ProBNP: 800 pg/mL
- Serum troponin: <0.01 ng/L
- Lactate: 1.3 mg/dL
- ABG: pH 7.46, $PaO_2$ 85 mm Hg, $PaCO_2$ 30, $HCO_3$ 25, oxygen saturation 92%
- Serum electrolytes, BUN, creatinine, glucose: sodium 136 mEq/L, potassium 3.8 mEq/L, chloride 103 mEq/L, bicarb 23 mEq/L, BUN 10, creatinine 0.7, glucose 89 mg/dL
- D-dimer: 2,000 mg/L
- PT/PTT/INR: normal

### Assessment

At this point, the patient is hypoxic, tachycardic, and has an elevated A-a gradient. The patient is hemodynamically stable so the next step is CT angiogram of the chest ("gold standard"). A V/Q scan can also be completed if the patient has renal failure or allergy to contrast dye.

### Further Management Plan/Results

1. Supplemental oxygen
2. CT angiogram: right-sided PE
3. Echocardiogram: normal RV size, no tricuspid regurgitation, EF 55–60%
4. Admit patient to telemetry floor

### Treatment Plan

Since it has been determined that the patient has a PE, start anticoagulation therapy with IV unfractionated heparin (UFH), fondaparinux, or low-molecular weight heparin (LMWH), with the goal of simultaneous warfarin administration. LMWH has largely replaced UFH in the treatment of acute VTE because it has more reliable pharmacokinetics and facilitates outpatient management.

Warfarin therapy may be initiated on day 1 or 2 of heparin therapy. Because factor II and X levels require at least 5 days to decline, parenteral anticoagulation should overlap with warfarin for at least 5 days and until an INR $\geq$2 is achieved.

Rivaroxaban is approved by the FDA for the long-term prevention of recurrent PE; however, due to the paucity of long-term experience with it, warfarin or LMWH is preferred.

In patients with advanced cancer, the duration of therapy is indefinite or as long as the cancer is active or being treated.

Placement of a vena cava filter is the appropriate treatment of acute deep venous thrombosis or PE only in cases with contraindications to anticoagulation.

Persistent hypotension or shock (i.e., systolic BP <90 mm Hg or a decrease in systolic BP by ≥40 mm Hg from baseline) due to acute PE is the only widely accepted indication for thrombolysis. Systemic thrombolytic therapy with tPA should be considered only after acute PE has been confirmed because its adverse effects can be severe.

Additional workup for this young man with acute PE is warranted: lower extremity U/S Doppler, genetic testing for a hypercoagulable state, and occult malignancy.

### Follow-up Management

Currently, there are no guidelines for hypercoagulable workup for thromboembolic disease. However, it is very important to consider age-appropriate malignancy workup. In the older adult, for example, a full malignancy workup (mammogram, colonoscopy, CT chest, abdomen and pelvis, etc.) should be done. In this patient, a testicular exam would be appropriate.

Antiphospholipid antibodies should be considered because the antiphospholipid syndrome should be anticoagulated for life. These patients are at risk for both arterial and venous thromboemboli. They are also at increased risk for MI and cardiovascular mortality.

In women, it is important to test for factor V Leiden. Patients with factor V Leiden must not take oral contraceptive pills because the risk of VTE is very high with this combination. Those patients must also be anticoagulated with LMWH during pregnancy.

Lower extremity Doppler should be done to find the source. Most PEs originate as lower extremity DVTs.

### Discussion

The patient is presenting with acute PE. Patients with idiopathic (unprovoked) VTE are at high risk for recurrence, with approximately 50% experiencing a recurrence within 10 years.

Guidelines recommend the following:

- Patients with a first episode of acute unprovoked PE (i.e., acute PE that is NOT due to a temporary or reversible risk factor) should receive anticoagulant therapy for 6 months and possibly longer.
- Patients with recurrent acute PE should receive anticoagulant therapy indefinitely if they have a low or intermediate risk of bleeding.

**CLINICAL PEARL**

OPC and pregnancy can lead to a hypercoagulable state because estrogen causes an increase in liver production of clotting factors.

### Final Diagnosis

Pulmonary embolism

## Basic Science Correlate

The 3 pathways which make up the classical blood coagulation pathway are as follows:

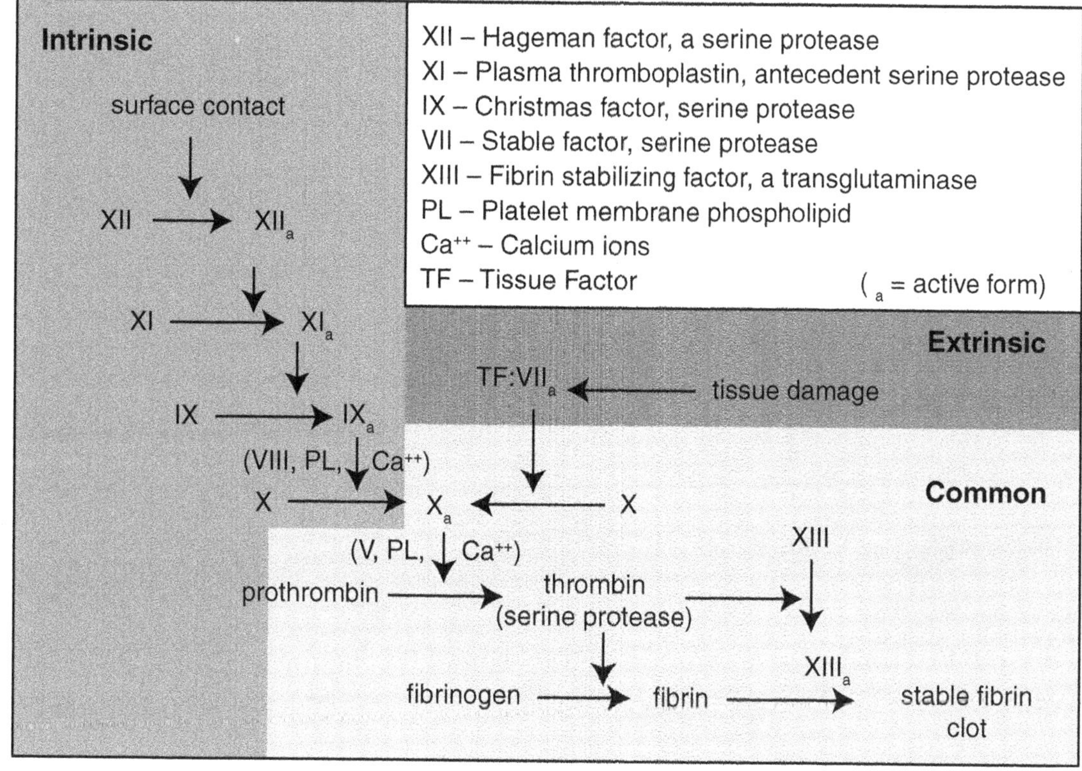


Source: Wikimedia

### Thrombus Formation

Thrombi can appear grossly (and microscopically) as laminations called **lines of Zahn;** these represent pale platelet and fibrin layers alternating with darker red cell–rich layers. Such lines are significant in that they are only found in thrombi that form in flowing blood; their presence can usually distinguish antemortem thrombosis from the bland nonlaminated clots that form in the postmortem state. Factors which play a role in thrombus formation are:

- Stasis or turbulent flow: immobility (e.g., surgery), aneurysm, atrial fibrillation, cardiomyopathy
- Endothelial damage
- Hypercoagulable states
  - **Common states**: factor V Leiden (a mutation of factor V, which makes it unable to be cleaved and inactivated); prothrombin mutation (G20210A variant); increased levels of factor VII, IX, XI, or fibrinogen
  - **Rare states**: antithrombin III deficiency, protein C and protein S deficiencies

**CLINICAL PEARL**

**Warfarin necrosis**

Vitamin K dependent factors are VII, II, IX, X, protein C, and protein S. Warfarin necrosis occurs in patients with protein C or S deficiency. When given warfarin, protein C and S levels decrease before the other factors because they have a shorter half-life and that leads to clot formation and necrosis of the fingers and toes. Prevent this by anticoagulation with heparin first

# Hematology 6

## CASE 1

### Chief Complaint

Fatigue, jaundice, back pain, dark urine, fever

### History and Physical Examination

A 30-year-old man of Greek origin presents to the emergency department with complaints of acute onset fatigue, back pain, and lightheadedness. He also notes the onset of jaundice and dark urine over the past several hours. He recently ate in a Middle Eastern restaurant but has no nausea or vomiting. He denies any bright-red blood per rectum and melena. He denies fever and chills. He states that in the past, a physician told him he has mild anemia. He had a recent cholecystectomy for recurrent gallstones and takes no medications.

He appears pale, icteric, and restless. Vitals signs are T 38.3 C (101.0 F), blood pressure 100/80 mm Hg, and pulse 120/min. Physical examination shows scleral icterus, tachycardia with regular rhythm, no hepatosplenomegaly, and no fecal occult blood.

### Differential Diagnosis

1. Acute hepatitis
2. Acute hemolysis
    - Autoimmune IgG hemolytic anemia
3. Cold agglutinin IgM disease
    - Glucose-6-phosphate dehydrogenase (G6PD) deficiency
    - Hereditary red cell membrane deficiency with associated infection
4. Paroxysmal nocturnal hemoglobinuria (PNH)
5. Cholangitis secondary to retained stone in common bile duct

### Initial Management

**Setting:** emergency department

### Diagnostic/Therapeutic Plan

- CBC
- Peripheral smear
- PT and PTT
- LFTs
- Urinalysis
- U/S of abdomen

### Test Results

- WBC: 5,000/mm$^3$ (normal 4,500–11,000/mm$^3$), hemoglobin 6 g/dL (normal 13–17 g/dL), platelets 180,000/mm$^3$ (normal 150,000–350,000/mm$^3$)
- Peripheral smear: bite cells present
- PT and PTT: normal
- Bilirubin: 10 mg/dL (normal 0.2–1.2 mg/dL) 90% unconjugated; AST and ALT normal
- No urobilinogen; hemoglobin-positive; no RBC or WBC
- U/S of abdomen: normal

#### CCS NOTE

The case simulations are liberal in accepting extra ordered diagnostic tests. Patients with fatigue should have a CBC. Jaundiced patients should have all LFTs.

### Assessment

The patient presents with an acute onset of jaundice and severe anemia, suggestive of hemolysis or liver dysfunction with associated bleeding. There is no clinical evidence of bleeding, coagulopathy, or hepatomegaly suggestive of a primary hepatic process.

The presence of markedly elevated serum indirect bilirubin and hemoglobin-positive urine in the absence of RBC is consistent with acute hemolysis with spillage of hemoglobin into the urine. Hemolytic anemia results from the premature destruction of circulating RBCs and is characterized by elevation of the reticulocyte count, lactate dehydrogenase, and unconjugated bilirubin and a decrease in haptoglobin.

Hemolysis may occur in the extravascular or intravascular space. The former generally presents in a subacute manner and results from premature destruction of RBC in the spleen and liver. This may occur in the setting of splenomegaly as a result of liver disease, infection, or hematologic malignancy. Extravascular hemolysis may be caused by autoantibodies directed against RBCs and is seen in the setting of autoimmune disease, lymphoproliferative disease, or drugs such as penicillin or alpha-methyldopa. The presence of autoantibodies bound to RBC membranes results in a positive direct Coombs test, whereas excess antibody in the serum leads to a positive indirect test. Extravascular hemolysis may also be caused by membrane abnormalities, such as hereditary spherocytosis, which renders RBCs more susceptible to splenic destruction.

The acute onset of symptoms in this patient with a dramatic drop in hematocrit is more suggestive of intravascular hemolysis. It is characterized by the presence of hemoglobinemia, which results in hemoglobinuria, hemosiderinuria, and a marked decrease in serum haptoglobin. Intravascular hemolysis may be caused by microangiopathic processes such as thrombotic thrombocytopenic purpura, hemolytic uremic syndrome, disseminated intravascular coagulation, and malignant hypertension, which are characterized by the presence of schistocytes on peripheral smear. Other potential causes include complement-mediated lysis, toxin-mediated lysis (*Clostridium perfringens* sepsis), and oxidant-mediated lysis (G6PD deficiency). The latter may be precipitated by exposure to oxidant stresses, such as fava beans, that the patient likely ingested. The most common type of oxidant stress causing hemolysis in G6PD deficiency is infection.

### Basic Science Correlate

Mechanism of Heinz bodies and bite cells:

- Oxidized Hg precipitates in RBC membrane as Heinz bodies
- Spleen "bites" out a piece of the membrane as bite cell

Mechanism of cold agglutinin disease:

- IgM destroys RBCs in Kupffer cells of liver
- This is why neither steroids nor splenectomy is an effective treatment

Mechanism of PNH:

- Genetic defect leads to loss of PIG-A, which is where complement-removing factor anchors to prevent cell destruction by C5
- Measure this as decreased CD55/59 by flow cytometry
- Acidosis increases complement activation at night in PNH

Why are there no fragmented cells on smear in G6PD hemolysis?

- Because the cells "melt" like ice in hot water from oxidant stress from infection
- They are not "broken" into fragments as in TTP, HUS, or DIC

## Further Management Plan/Results

| | |
|---|---|
| • Urine for hemosiderin and hemoglobin | Positive |
| • Haptoglobin | Low/absent |
| • Coombs test | Negative |
| • Supravital stain (crystal violet or methylene blue) of peripheral smear | Heinz bodies |
| • Hydration to prevent renal failure from hemoglobinuria | |

## Discussion

Glucose-6-phosphate dehydrogenase (G6PD) is the most common enzyme abnormality of RBCs and is thought to affect hundreds of millions of people worldwide. It is an X-linked disorder and therefore clinical disease is more prevalent in men. G6PD is an important enzyme in the hexose monophosphate shunt. This pathway is important in generating reduced glutathione in response to oxidant stresses, thus protecting hemoglobin from having sulfhydryl groups activated and causing precipitation. G6PD activity normally declines as the cell ages. This process is accelerated in patients with the deficiency and there are many degrees of severity.

**CCS NOTE**

Test results appear automatically as you advance the clock in the exam.

The A-variant of this deficiency is found commonly in central Africans and in 15% of African Americans. In general, these patients have a mildly decreased red-blood-cell survival time but are not anemic. However, when an exposure to an oxidant stress occurs (such as infection, sulfa drugs, diabetic ketoacidosis, antimalarials, or accidental ingestion of mothballs) acute hemolysis can occur. Other medications that can cause hemolysis are dapsone, primaquine, and nitrofurantoin.

Another population with a high incidence of G6PD deficiency is that of the Mediterranean basin. These patients tend to have a more severe form with lower enzyme levels and greater sensitivity to oxidants. Some of these individuals display a marked sensitivity to fava beans.

Clinically, patients present with signs of acute hemolysis, including indirect hyperbilirubinemia without the presence of bilirubin in the urine because unconjugated bilirubin is tightly bound to albumin. Haptoglobin binds free hemoglobin, but when this is overwhelmed, free hemoglobin is filtered by the glomeruli and is converted to hemosiderin in tubular cells. When this system is overwhelmed, free hemoglobin is put out in the urine, leading to a reddish-brown color.

The above patient is Greek and recently ate in a restaurant that might have served fava beans. Confirmation of the diagnosis is difficult in the acute situation because of the hemolysis of older RBC and the presence of only circulating young RBC and reticulocytes. These cells may have normal G6PD activity because it is a biased young population. The diagnosis may require repeating the test once the acute hemolytic period is over.

## Follow-up Management and Prevention

- Consider transfusional support if necessary
- Avoid offending drugs or foods in future
- Move clock forward 2 months and check G6PD level

### Basic Science Correlate

Why do you have to wait 2 months to check a G6PD level?

- Levels of G6PD are normal just after an episode of acute hemolysis
- The older cells with lower levels have already been destroyed, and all there is to test are younger cells with higher level

Mechanism of hemolysis in G6PD deficiency:

- Infection is most common oxidant stress
- Infection uses up small amount of G6PD in the cell and then it is destroyed prematurely

## Final Diagnosis

Acute hemolysis due to glucose-6-phosphate dehydrogenase (G6PD) deficiency

# CASE 2

## Chief Complaint

Nose bleed

## History and Physical Examination

A 25-year-old previously healthy woman comes to the local emergency department with epistaxis for several hours that has finally responded to pressure and elevation. The patient is bleeding from both nostrils. She denies fever, chills, and recent upper respiratory symptoms. She had noted multiple "spots" on both ankles, and she has gingival bleeding. A CBC is drawn which reveals platelet count 10,000/mm$^3$ (normal 150,000–400,000/mm$^3$). The patient takes no medications and has no significant past medical history.

Her blood pressure is 110/86 mm Hg and pulse 88/min. She is afebrile. Physical examination shows no focal lesion in the nasal mucosa. The oropharynx is not infected. Multiple petechiae are seen on both ankles. The remainder of the examination is unremarkable.

## Differential Diagnosis

1. Immune thrombocytopenic purpura (ITP)
2. Acute leukemia
3. Disseminated intravascular coagulation (DIC)
4. Drug-related thrombocytopenia
5. Aplastic anemia
6. von Willebrand disease (vWD)
7. Marrow infiltration (malignancy)
8. Systemic lupus erythematosus

## Initial Management

**Setting:** emergency department

## Diagnostic/Therapeutic Plan

- CBC, differential, peripheral smear
- PT/PTT
- Fibrinogen

## Test Results

- WBC 5,000/mm$^3$, hemoglobin 13 mg/dL, 67% granulocytes, 23% lymphocytes, 10% monocytes, no abnormal cells seen; large platelets (10,000/mm$^3$) noted
- PT 11 seconds (normal)/PTT 33 seconds (normal)
- Fibrinogen normal

## Assessment

The patient has the acute onset of thrombocytopenia without systemic symptoms. Thrombocytopenia results from a failure of platelet production or premature destruction. This distinction may be made by performing a bone-marrow examination in which the presence of increased numbers of megakaryocytes suggests peripheral consumption of platelets. The former is associated with marrow suppressive states and pancytopenia. Potential etiologies include drugs such as sulfa antibiotics, marrow failure due to aplastic anemia, vitamin B12 and folate deficiency, and marrow infiltrative disorders, such as hematologic malignancy, metastatic solid tumors, and disseminated mycobacterial or fungal infection. Because the patient is not acutely ill, is not on medications, and has no abnormalities on peripheral smear, these causes are unlikely.

Increased platelet destruction may be due to microangiopathic processes, such as disseminated intravascular coagulation, thrombotic thrombocytopenic purpura, or hypersplenism. However, isolated thrombocytopenia is more likely to be platelet autoantibodies. This may be seen in the setting of systemic lupus erythematosus, HIV, or lymphoproliferative diseases such as chronic lymphocytic leukemia (CLL). Infections such as Cytomegalovirus, herpes, and hepatitis can also cause antibody-mediated thrombocytopenia. In addition, drugs such as heparin, penicillin, or quinidine may stimulate antibodies that are cross-reactive with platelets or may bind as antigen/antibody complexes to the platelet surface (innocent bystander effect). If no clear underlying condition can be identified, it is most likely antibody-mediated thrombocytopenia, also known as ITP (diagnosis of exclusion).

### CLINICAL PEARL

Patients with a bleeding problem should have their PT checked and a CBC. Do not worry if the test results are normal. What matters is that the tests could have been abnormal.

## Further Management Plan/Results

| | |
|---|---|
| • Prednisone orally | |
| • HIV test | Negative |
| • Repeat CBC | Platelet count 12,000, increased mean platelet volume |
| • Hematology consult | No specific recommendations are made |
| • Bone marrow biopsy | Normocellular, normal erythroid and myeloid maturation; normal M:E ratio; markedly increased numbers of megakaryocytes with some immature megakaryocytes |
| • ANA | Negative |
| • Abdominal U/S | Normal-sized spleen |

## Discussion

Antibody-mediated thrombocytopenia (ITP) is characterized by immune destruction of circulating platelets by autoantibodies. In adults, it is seen more commonly in women. Immune-related thrombocytopenia may be triggered by medications, or it could be associated with collagen-vascular disease or lymphoproliferative diseases. Diagnosis of antibody-mediated thrombocytopenia is suggested by severe thrombocytopenia in the presence of increased megakaryocytes in the bone marrow. The presence of antiplatelet antibodies in the serum is not diagnostic because these are often found nonspecifically in nonimmune-related thrombocytopenia. Bone marrow biopsy shows increased megakaryocytes and excludes production problems.

The presentation usually consists of platelet-type bleeding such as petechiae, purpura, gingival bleeding, and epistaxis. The patient's platelets are young and effective, and patients can tolerate low counts without bleeding. Spontaneous bleeding with platelets $>30,000/mm^3$ suggests a separate problem of platelet dysfunction. Bleeding is occasionally seen in the GI or GU tracts. CNS bleeds are rare but can be fatal.

### CCS NOTE

If a patient has a serious problem, always initiate therapy and do not wait for specific test results. In this otherwise healthy patient with isolated thrombocytopenia and a normal spleen, initiating prednisone is more effective than waiting for specific tests.

In children, antibody-mediated thrombocytopenia often follows an antecedent viral illness. The disease is usually transient, resolving in 2 to 8 weeks, and therapy is needed only to help temporarily. In adults, the disease often becomes chronic or relapsing.

Prednisone is the initial therapy and is given for 4–6 wks and then tapered. IV immunoglobulin results in the more rapid improvement in the platelet count through the blockage of the RES system. Its effect is transient, and because it is quite expensive, its use is limited to patients who require an acute increase due to profoundly low counts or severe, life-threatening bleeding. Thrombopoietin-stimulating agents such as eltrombopag can also be used. Anti-RhD therapy is a less expensive alternative for Rh-positive patients. Adult patients typically relapse during steroid tapering, and second-line therapy is splenectomy. This is particularly effective in patients with an initial response to steroids. Adults have a lower risk of postsplenectomy sepsis than do children. Those patients with platelets >20,000/mm$^3$ and those without clinical symptoms may sometimes be followed without therapy. Splenectomy failures are treated with rituximab, romiplostim, or eltrombopag. Less effective agents are danazol or cytotoxic agents, such as vincristine or cyclophosphamide.

### Follow-up Management and Prevention

- One day after the start of steroids, repeat CBC
- Continue prednisone or dexamethasone until platelet count >50,000
- IV gammaglobulin (IgG) if acute increase in platelet counts are required with severe bleeding such as CNS or melena
- Splenectomy if thrombocytopenia continues to recur
- Treat recurrences after splenectomy with rituximab or thrombopoietin-stimulating agents such as romiplostim or eltrombopag
- Platelet transfusion is rarely effective since platelets are consumed as soon as they are infused. This should be considered only in life-threatening bleeding.

### Final Diagnosis

Immune (idiopathic) thrombocytopenic purpura

# CASE 3

## Chief Complaint

Shortness of breath with joint and back pain

## History and Physical Examination

A 25-year-old man with a history of sickle-cell anemia comes to the emergency department with acute onset of severe knee and back pain, typical of his vaso-occlusive crises in the past. In addition, over the last few hours, he has had the acute onset of pleuritic pain, severe shortness of breath, and fever. He typically suffers from a crisis every 3 months.

He appears to be in acute distress. Vital signs are temperature 38.3 C (101.0 F), blood pressure 180/100 mm Hg, pulse 120/min, and respirations 30/min. Physical examination shows tachycardia with I/VI systolic murmur at the left lower sternal border. There is no costovertebral-angle tenderness. The remainder of the physical examination is unremarkable.

## Differential Diagnosis

1. Vaso-occlusive crisis of sickle-cell disease
2. Pulmonary infarction (acute chest syndrome)
3. Pulmonary infection

## Initial Management Plan

**Setting:** emergency department

## Diagnostic/Therapeutic Plan

- Oxygen, IV normal saline
- Morphine or hydromorphone
- Ceftriaxone IV (or moxifloxacin or levofloxacin)
- Blood cultures
- CBC
- Bilirubin
- Urinalysis
- Chest x-ray
- ABG
- Smear

### Test Results

- Blood cultures negative
- WBC 14,500/$mm^3$ (normal 4,000–11,000/$mm^3$), hematocrit 25% (normal 37–44%), platelets 480,000/$mm^3$ (normal 150,000–400,000/$mm^3$), reticulocytes 15% (normal 1–2%)
- Bilirubin 2.3 mg/dL (normal 0.2–1.0 mg/dL), 85% unconjugated
- Urinalysis: hematuria, no WBC
- Chest x-ray: focal infiltrate peripherally on the right
- ABG: pH 7.5, $PCO_2$ 32 mm Hg, $PO_2$ 70 mm Hg
- Smear: sickle cells present

### Assessment

The cause of the patient's back and knee pain is most likely vaso-occlusive crisis, particularly given the history of recurrent crises of a similar nature in the past. Other potential etiologies for abdominal pain include cholecystitis and pancreatitis because patients often have gallstones due to chronic hemolysis.

Vaso-occlusive crisis is often precipitated by dehydration, hypoxia, or infection. Patients are particularly susceptible to dehydration because of an inability to concentrate their urine due to ischemic damage to the renal medulla. Hematuria is usually the result of renal tubular damage or papillary necrosis, but infection must be ruled out. The presence of dyspnea with exertion may be due to severe anemia precipitated by worsening hemolysis or aplastic crisis, as seen in parvovirus infection. However, the presentation above is suggestive of a primary pulmonary process, most likely infection or the acute chest syndrome.

Patients with sickle-cell disease are at increased risk for infection, particularly with encapsulated organisms such as *Pneumococcus, Haemophilus influenzae, Klebsiella pneumoniae*, and *Neisseria meningitidis*. The presence of fever or WBC higher than usual is an indication for antibiotics. Pleuritic pain, fever, and shortness of breath are characteristic of the acute chest syndrome. This is caused by sickling and vaso-occlusion of the capillaries of the pulmonary bed with resultant infarction. Meperidine is NOT the right pain medication to use. Repeated doses of meperidine can cause seizures.

**CCS NOTE**

All patients with an unexplained fever should have a chest x-ray, urinalysis, and blood culture.

**CLINICAL PEARL**

With sickle crisis, give antibiotics for fever or WBC higher than usual.

### Further Management Plan/Results

| | |
|---|---|
| • Repeated doses of morphine or hydromorphone | |
| • Continued IV saline and oxygen | |
| • Continued ceftriaxone | |
| • Reticulocyte count | 16% |
| • Hemoglobin electrophoresis | HgS 86%, HgF 12%, HgA 0%, HgA2 2% |

**CCS NOTE**

Sickle-cell disease is a perfect example where therapy should be initiated prior to obtaining the results of specific tests. If the patient has a fever, add a 3rd or 4th generation cephalosporine (cefotaxime, ceftriaxone, cefepime) to the initial set of orders even if the chest x-ray and urinalysis give normal results.

### Discussion

The cause of pulmonary symptoms may be infection and/or an infarction. In adults with negative sputum, the latter is more common. Empiric antibiotics may be given during the acute period. If the patient's oxygenation does not improve with supplemental oxygen, exchange transfusion should be considered.

Sickle-cell anemia is the result of a mutation in the beta-globin gene. Patients with sickle trait are heterozygous for this mutation, whereas those with sickle-cell anemia are homozygous. Eight percent of African Americans are heterozygous for HbS. In homozygous SS disease, RBC with the abnormal hemoglobin become sickled upon deoxygenation due to the formation of abnormal polymers of beta-globin strands within the cells. The sickled cells are nondeformable and block capillary flow. This leads to tissue hypoxia and lowered oxygen tension, further exacerbating the sickling process. The additional sickled cells are rapidly destroyed, leading to hemolysis and reticulocytosis. Acidosis increases sickling, whereas fetal hemoglobin helps prevent cells from sickling. Hemoglobin electrophoresis is used to make the diagnosis. Patients typically have:

- Hemoglobin F: 2–20%
- Hemoglobin A2: 2–4%
- Remainder hemoglobin S: remainder

Vaso-occlusive crisis is a common presentation. It is associated with an increased population of sickle cells and is probably due to tissue ischemia as a result of small-vessel obstruction. It is often precipitated by a viral or bacterial infection or dehydration.

Patients rarely present with focal complications of tissue ischemia, such as bowel infarction or central nervous system symptoms such as seizure or stroke. Acute chest syndrome is a common presentation and may be precipitated by hypoxia due to infection. Hematuria is often seen and is most commonly caused by renal tubular damage. Papillary necrosis of the kidneys sometimes occurs. Infection is common because patients are functionally asplenic and are susceptible to encapsulated organisms.

Hematocrit does not routinely drop with a sickle-cell crisis. A sudden drop in hematocrit >3–4 points should make you think of either parvovirus B19 or folic-acid deficiency. Parvovirus can be detected with an immunoglobulin M level or PCR for parvovirus DNA level. Parvovirus is treated acutely with IV immunoglobulin infusion.

Chronic organ damage includes decreased pulmonary function, probably due to chronic hypoxia and shunting. Bilirubin gallstones may occur owing to chronic hemolysis. Concentrating ability is impaired in the kidney, causing the patient to be prone to dehydration. Aseptic necrosis of the head of the femur and chronic skin ulcers are also seen.

Patients with a history of SS homozygous disease should be maintained on folate to support the increased RBC. Infections should be treated promptly. Care of vaso-occlusive crises is supportive with emphasis on pain management and hydration. Supplemental oxygen is used for respiratory symptoms. Exchange transfusions can be used to mitigate symptoms and are used particularly for severe hypoxemia, pulmonary infarction or acute chest syndrome, stroke, visual disturbance, and priapism. Long-term therapy concentrates on increasing the proportion of hemoglobin F with agents such as hydroxyurea. Increased hemoglobin F levels prevent sickling and decrease the frequency of crises.

**CLINICAL PEARL**

Parvovirus B19 causes a sudden drop in both hematocrit and reticulocyte count.

- PCR for parvovirus DNA is more accurate than IgM or IgG for parvovirus
- Marrow shows giant pro-normoblasts
- Treat with IV immunoglobulin

## Follow-up Management and Prevention

- Exchange transfusion if the hypoxia does not correct with supportive measures (to treat possible acute chest syndrome)
- Hydroxyurea to decrease frequency of crisis in future
- Pneumococcal vaccine if not previously given
- Folate supplementation chronically
- If reticulocyte drops test for parvovirus

## Final Diagnosis

Sickle-cell anemia with vaso-occlusive crisis

# CASE 4

## Chief Complaint

Bleeding

## History and Physical Examination

A 70-year-old woman was hospitalized last week for pneumonia and was treated with ceftriaxone and azithromycin. She was initially lethargic but has slowly improved. This morning she had an episode of coffee-ground emesis which appeared to be self-limiting. The patient has a history of peptic ulcer disease for which she takes pantoprazole. CBC shows WBC 5,000/mm$^3$ (normal 4,500–11,000/mm$^3$), hemoglobin 12 g/dL (normal 12–16 g/dL), platelets 250,000/mm$^3$ (normal 50,000–400,000/mm$^3$), and coagulation studies: PT 22 sec (normal <14 sec) and PTT 45 sec (normal <35 sec).

Her temperature is 37.0 C (98.6 F), BP is 120/80 mm Hg, and pulse is 90/min. In general, she is anicteric and appears somewhat debilitated. Physical examination shows that the eyes, ears, nose, and throat are normal, lungs are clear, and abdomen is soft with no hepatosplenomegaly. Rectal examination shows brown, guaiac-positive stool.

## Differential Diagnosis

1. Vitamin K deficiency
2. Factor deficiency
3. Factor inhibitor
4. Disseminated intravascular coagulation (DIC)
5. Liver disease

## Initial Management

**Setting:** inpatient hospital

## Diagnostic/Therapeutic Plan

- Fibrinogen level
- AST (SGOT)
- ALT (SGPT)
- Lactate dehydrogenase
- Alkaline phosphatase
- Bilirubin

## Test Results

- Fibrinogen 500 mg/dL (normal 200–400 mg/dL)
- AST 25 U/L (normal 10–30 U/L)
- ALT 22 U/L (normal 10–40 U/L)

- Lactate dehydrogenase 100 U/L (normal)
- Alkaline phosphatase 88 U/L (normal)
- Bilirubin 1.0 mg/dL (normal 0.2–1.0 mg/dL)

**CCS NOTE**

In the case simulations, any patient admitted to the hospital can have a CBC, chemistries, chest x-ray, and urinalysis. If the patient is age >40, EKG is acceptable as a routine screening admission test. You do not lose points if the tests show normal results.

### Assessment

Abnormalities of the coagulation profile are due to factor(s) deficiency or, rarely, an inhibitor. The intrinsic cascade is reflected in the PTT, whereas prolongation of the PT suggests a lesion affecting the extrinsic cascade. Deficiencies arise because of congenital abnormalities (hemophilia), consumption (DIC), or more commonly by inability to synthesize factors (liver disease or vitamin K deficiency). Factor inhibitors are seen in patients with autoimmune disease or in hemophiliacs who receive repeated infusions of concentrated products. This patient has an elevated PT and PTT, with some evidence of bleeding.

DIC is unlikely because the patient is clinically improving, with no signs of sepsis, and the platelet and fibrinogen levels are still normal. LFTs are normal; thus, liver failure is unlikely.

In hospitalized patients on antibiotics, the most likely etiology is a vitamin K deficiency. If the patient does not respond to a trial of vitamin K, a mixing study can be performed. In the presence of an inhibitor, the addition of normal plasma to the patient will not correct the abnormality. All factor deficiencies must correct the PT and PTT to normal when mixed with normal plasma.

### Further Management Plan

- Trial of subcutaneous vitamin K
- Repeat PT and aPTT

**CCS NOTE**

When PT and PTT are elevated, replacing vitamin K and checking for improvement is a faster method of obtaining a diagnosis than obtaining specific factor levels.

### Discussion

Vitamin K is a fat-soluble vitamin that is essential for the production of factors II, VII, IX, X, and proteins C and S. It is essential for the gamma-carboxylation of these factors and is necessary for their membrane-based activity. Warfarin inhibits this process and produces a coagulation defect identical to vitamin K deficiency. Vitamin K is absorbed by the small intestine and stored in the liver. It is also produced endogenously in the GI tract by the native bacterial flora. Deficiency occurs in 3 settings: poor intake, malabsorption, and loss of storage sites due to liver disease.

Acutely ill patients often become deficient due to poor oral intake and sterilization of the gut due to broad-spectrum antibiotics. It is also commonly seen in severe liver disease. Initially only the PT is elevated because factor VII has the shortest half-life in the cascade.

The INR is used to monitor therapy with warfarin. The INR is not necessary when initially assessing clotting factor levels and function. Vitamin K supplementation can be done parenterally but anaphylaxis can be seen. Fresh frozen plasma can be given when severe bleeding occurs.

### Follow-up management and prevention

- Continue vitamin K for 3 days
- Pneumococcal vaccine

### Final Diagnosis

Coagulation defect due to vitamin K deficiency

# CASE 5

## Chief Complaint

Fatigue, recurrent upper respiratory infections, and frequent bruising

## History and Physical Examination

A 25-year-old woman comes to the clinic because of progressive fatigue over the last 6 months. She has also noticed frequent colds and several sinus infections, which she never experienced in the past. Over the last 2 months she notes multiple bruises on her arms and legs without a history of obvious trauma. Her periods have also been particularly heavy, lasting 7 days. She denies recurrent fever and weight loss. Her appetite is intact, and she has no abdominal pain or fullness. The patient currently is unemployed but had worked as a painter for several years. She takes no medications.

Upon physical examination her temperature is 38 C (100.4 F), blood pressure 100/70 mm Hg, and pulse 100/min. CBC shows WBC 1,200/$mm^3$ (normal 4,000–11,000/$m^3$), hemoglobin 7.8 g/dL (normal 12–16 g/dL), platelets 30,000 $mm^3$ (normal 150,000–400,000/$mm^3$). She appears pale. With the exception of multiple bruises seen on her extremities, the remainder of the physical examination is normal.

### CCS NOTE

Most of the case simulations will not give you laboratory test results in the history. You need to order the tests.

## Differential Diagnosis

1. Aplastic anemia
2. Acute leukemia
3. Vitamin B12 or folate deficiency
4. Paroxysmal nocturnal hemoglobinuria
5. Drug- or toxin-induced marrow failure
6. Myelofibrosis
7. HIV
8. Systemic lupus erythematosus

## Initial Management

**Setting:** emergency department

## Diagnostic/Therapeutic Plan

- Peripheral smear
- Absolute neutrophil count
- HIV test
- Chest x-ray, urinalysis, blood cultures
- ANA
- B12 and folate

### Test Results

- Peripheral smear: no immature forms seen, no increase in reticulocytes, mean corpuscular volume 100 fL (normal 800–100 fL)
- Absolute neutrophil count: 500/mm$^3$ (low)
- HIV: negative
- Chest x-ray, urinalysis, blood cultures normal
- ANA negative
- B12 and folate normal

### Assessment

The differential diagnosis for pancytopenia is extensive and includes premature destruction of cells due to hypersplenism or autoimmune disease, marrow suppression secondary to nutritional deficiency (vitamin B12, folate), infection (tuberculosis, HIV), drugs (trimethoprim-sulfamethoxazole, chloramphenicol), or malignant infiltration. Drug-induced pancytopenia is usually dose-dependent and reversible. A rare idiosyncratic reaction to chloramphenicol is associated with irreversible marrow failure. Nucleated RBC on the peripheral smear are suggestive of marrow fibrosis or infiltration. There are no abnormal white blood cell forms on peripheral smear. The most likely cause is aplastic anemia, which may be related to her exposure to paints.

**CCS NOTE**

All patients with anemia should have a peripheral smear. A smear is most useful in macrocytic anemia and hemolysis.

Paroxysmal nocturnal hemoglobinuria may also present with a hypocellular marrow, although it is more commonly associated with hyperplasia of red blood cell precursor populations. Myelodysplasia may also yield a hypocellular biopsy but is usually associated with a hypercellular specimen with abnormal features of maturation and characteristic findings (deletion of chromosomes 5 or 7). Other potential etiologies for a dry aspirate include hairy cell leukemia, myelofibrosis, and M7 (megakaryocyte) acute myeloblastic leukemia (AML). Hairy cell leukemia is associated with characteristic abnormalities on immunophenotyping. Tartrate-resistant acid phosphatase (TRAP) staining is no longer considered accurate enough and diagnosis should be made based on morphology.

### Further Management Plan/Results

| | |
|---|---|
| • Bone marrow biopsy | • Unable to aspirate; biopsy profoundly hypocellular with fat replacing most hematopoietic elements<br>• No increase in reticulin fibers seen<br>• Bone marrow for AFB stain and fungal forms negative |

**CCS NOTE**

A consultant will arrive within 15 minutes if a consult is ordered "stat." A consultant will never tell you which specific tests or treatments to order.

### Discussion

Aplastic anemia is characterized by pancytopenia, thought to be due to stem cell injury. This can be acquired or congenital. In the acquired form, a known insult (such as one of the above toxins), drug, or infection is found in about 50% of cases.

Several drugs are associated with aplasia, such as indomethacin, gold, phenylbutazone, sulfonamides, phenytoin, nifedipine, and quinacrine. Chloramphenicol is associated with a dose-related pancytopenia and with an idiosyncratic, rare, profound, pancytopenia not related to dose.

Other causes of marrow aplasia include:

- Toxins such as benzene, arsenic, toluene found in glue, insecticides, paint thinners, and lacquers
- Infections such as hepatitis C and infectious mononucleosis
- Radiation and chemotherapeutic agents
- Occasionally, HIV and parvovirus (usually cause red cell aplasia but occasionally can cause aplastic anemia)

A careful history of prior toxin exposure is crucial because removal of the offending agent may reverse the disease.

In some cases, aplastic anemia is thought to arise from immune-mediated injury of stem cells. This is supported by the finding that some patients have been shown to respond to immunosuppressants such as antithymocyte globulin (ATG) and cyclosporine. Bone marrow transplant is often only successful when preceded by high-dose chemotherapy to eradicate the existing host immunity prior to transplant. Bone marrow transplant is also curative and is the best therapy in patients age <70 in good health and with an HLA-matched donor.

The clinical presentation includes bleeding, anemia, and recurrent infections. The latter is of particular concern in patients with neutrophil count $<500/mm^3$, who are at risk for nadir sepsis. The first principle in treatment is removal of the offending toxin or agent. Those patients who are fit and have HLA-matched siblings should undergo bone marrow transplantation. If possible, patients should not be transfused prior to transplant to avoid sensitization and rejection of the future graft. Those patients who are older adult or have no donor are given trials of immunosuppressive agents.

## Follow-up Management

- Removal of offending toxin if one is present
- Hematology consult to consider bone marrow transplantation in those age <50 with a matched donor
- Trial of immunosuppressive therapy with anti-thymocyte globulin and cyclosporine if transplant is not an option
- Alternate immunosuppressive medications are mycophenolate or cyclophosphamide

## Final Diagnosis

Pancytopenia, aplastic anemia

# CASE 6

## Chief Complaint

Fatigue, depression, and ataxia

## History and Physical Examination

A 75-year-old man is brought to the office by his son, who states that his father has been increasingly lethargic over the last few months. His father's mood has been erratic and volatile, and he drinks quite a lot of alcohol. The patient complains of increasing generalized weakness and fatigue. Over the last few weeks he has experienced worsening ataxia. He denies fever, chills, or difficulty with thyroid regulation. His appetite is unchanged and he maintains a balanced diet.

Vital signs are T 37.5 C (99.5 F), BP 140/85 mm Hg, and pulse 86/min. In general, the patient appears mildly confused but is oriented to person, place, and time. Examination shows a supple neck without adenopathy, a normal thyroid, and a clear chest. He has a regular heart rate and rhythm with an S1 and S2. Skin tone appears normal, and his abdomen is soft, nontender, with no hepatosplenomegaly. Neurologic examination shows muscle strength that is somewhat diminished throughout: a decreased sensation in the lower limbs with loss of position and vibratory sense, hyperreflexia in the lower extremities, and an ataxic gait.

## Differential Diagnosis

1. Vitamin B12 deficiency
2. Tertiary syphilis
3. Central nervous system vascular disease (multiple strokes)
4. Chronic alcoholism
5. Thyroid disease
6. Depression

## Initial Management

**Setting:** outpatient or emergency department if symptoms severe

## Diagnostic/Therapeutic Plan

- CBC
- Thyroid function studies (T4, TSH)
- BUN, creatinine
- Head CT
- VDRL or RPR

### Test Results

- WBC 4,000/mm$^3$ (normal 4,500–11,000/mm$^3$), hemoglobin 9.1 g/dL (normal 13.75–17.5 g/dL), platelets 190,000/mm$^3$ (normal 150,000–400,000/mm$^3$), MCV 110 $\mu m^3$ (normal 80–100 $\mu m^3$), differential: 60% granulocytes
- Hypersegmented neutrophils seen on smear
- T4, TSH normal
- BUN, creatinine normal
- Head CT: mild diffuse atrophy
- VDRL or RPR non reactive

### Assessment

The patient's primary manifestations are neurologic: motor deficits, sensory deficits, and ataxia. This makes primary motor neuron or muscle disease unlikely. The diffuse distribution makes stroke less likely. Fatigue, motor weakness, and confusion can be seen with both hypo-and hyperthyroidism in older adult patients, but no other signs of thyroid disease are present. The neurologic findings could be consistent with both vitamin B12 deficiency and syphilis. Macrocytic anemia can be caused by vitamin B12 deficiency, folate deficiency, alcoholism, or liver disease.

Given the neurologic symptoms in this patient, combined with macrocytic anemia and hypersegmented neutrophils, vitamin B12 deficiency or alcoholism is the most likely cause. Homocysteine levels are elevated in both folate and vitamin B12 deficiency, whereas methylmalonic acid levels are increased only in vitamin B12 deficiency. Folate will partially improve vitamin B12-induced anemia but do nothing for the neurological symptoms.

#### Basic Science Correlate

Why does B12 cause neurological symptoms and folate does not?

- B12 is needed to form myelin
- Any neurologic problem is possible but peripheral neuropathy is the most common (dementia is least common)

Why is the marrow hypercellular if there is a pancytopenia?

- B12 deficiency gives ineffective erythropoiesis
- Cells are made in increased number, but they rapidly self-destruct as they leave the marrow
- Cell destruction increases indirect bilirubin and LDH but keeps the reticulocyte count low

What is the mechanism of B12 deficiency?

- Pernicious anemia is an auto immune disorder
- Antibodies are made to intrinsic factor and parietal cells

### Further Management Plan/Results

| | |
|---|---|
| • B12 level | Borderline low |
| • Anti-intrinsic factor antibody | Present |
| • Methylmalonic acid level | High |

### Discussion

The Schilling test is rarely, if ever, necessary. It is performed to determine the etiology of the vitamin B12 deficiency when antiparietal-cell and anti-intrinsic factor antibody levels are normal.

Vitamin B12 is found in abundance in fish, meat, and dairy products. It is protein-bound in food, and in the acidic environment of the stomach, pepsin cleaves it to free product, which is then bound by intrinsic factor in the proximal ileum and is absorbed in the distal ileum. People usually have vast stores of the vitamin. Strict vegetarians over years may develop a deficiency. Vitamin B12 deficiency can also be seen with small-bowel bacterial overgrowth, Crohn's disease, celiac sprue, and ileal or gastric resections, resulting in malabsorption.

The most common cause is pernicious anemia, and its incidence increases with advanced age. It is found in 5–10% of patients age >65. It is an autoimmune process, which is characterized by autoantibodies against gastric parietal cells and intrinsic factor. Patients first develop achlorhydria, which is associated with gastritis that spares the antrum. The patients subsequently develop vitamin B12 malabsorption. Deficiency develops slowly over time (usually 3–6 yrs) if absorption stops abruptly.

**CCS NOTE**

CT scan of the head is always a good diagnostic test for unexplained change in mental status or memory.

The disease is characterized by macrocytic anemia with associated hypersegmented neutrophils. It may also present with pancytopenia. In addition, there are neuropsychiatric symptoms such as fatigue, weakness, paresthesia of the extremities, loss of vibratory and position sense, ataxia, dementia, and psychosis. Neurologic symptoms may precede hematologic ones. Patients with vitamin B12 deficiency and neuropsychiatric symptoms don't necessarily have macrocytosis or anemia. When vitamin B12 deficiency occurs with iron deficiency, it can result in a mixed microcytic/macrocytic population of red cells yielding an MCV that is normal. Serum gastrin levels are often high because the antrum is spared by the gastritis, and gastrin-producing cells do not have normal feedback inhibition from acid secretion.

**CCS NOTE**

Office-based cases require the clock to be moved forward by several days to weeks in "simulated" time.

Deficiency is suggested by low serum levels, although the condition may exist with low normal levels. In this circumstance, an elevation of the methylmalonic acid level suggests a vitamin B12 deficiency.

Another reason for an alteration in the Schilling test in the presence of vitamin B12 deficiency is if intrinsic factor is present but vitamin B12 is not absorbed because the vitamin that is bound to food cannot be released from the food due to achlorhydria. In this situation, both steps of the Schilling test will show absorption because free vitamin B12 is used. Anti-intrinsic factor antibodies are found in patients with pernicious anemia. Antiparietal cell antibodies are less specific. Pernicious anemia often coexists with other autoimmune diseases such as thyroiditis, vitiligo, MGUS, and Addison's disease.

### Basic Science Correlate

Vitamin B12 and folate are both necessary for the conversion of homocysteine to methionine, whereas the conversion of methylmalonyl CoA to succinyl CoA is dependent on vitamin B12 alone. The latter is thought to result in accumulation of nonphysiologic fatty acids, potentially leading to neurologic changes.

Vitamin B12 is an essential cofactor in folate metabolism necessary for DNA synthesis. Its absence results in megaloblastic changes in the bone marrow, characterized by asynchrony between nuclear and cytoplasmic maturation.

Why does treatment of B12 deficiency lead to low potassium levels?

- As cells are made in the marrow at a very rapid rate, all available potassium is used up.

## Follow-up Management and Prevention

- Methylmalonic acid levels if the B12 level is normal or borderline
- Injection of B12 as replacement
- Potassium levels with B12 replacement

## Final Diagnosis

Pernicious anemia/vitamin B12 deficiency

## CASE 7

### Chief Complaint

Fatigue

### History and Physical Examination

A 25-year-old woman comes to the office for a physical examination before starting a new job. She states that she has been feeling fatigued, particularly at the end of the day. She also notes palpitations with increasing frequency. Her menstrual cycle is regular and lasts 7–8 days. She does not drink alcohol or smoke cigarettes and is a vegetarian. Three weeks ago she completed a course of trimethoprim/sulfamethoxazole for a UTI.

Laboratory studies reveal hemoglobin 9.6 g/dL. Blood pressure is 110/70 mm Hg and pulse 100/min. She appears slightly pale. The heart has a regular rate and rhythm with occasional irregular beats, and normal S1 and S2. Rectal examination shows guaiac-negative stool. The remainder of the physical examination is unremarkable.

### Differential Diagnosis

1. Iron deficiency anemia
2. Folate deficiency
3. Vitamin B12 deficiency
4. Thalassemia
5. Sulfa-induced bone marrow suppression
6. Hemolytic anemia due to drugs or systemic lupus erythematosus
7. Myelodysplasia

**CCS NOTE**

In the initial visit of an office-based case, perform a complete physical examination. In a hospital-based case with an acutely ill patient, perform an examination focusing on the area of the body that is the center of the chief complaint.

### Initial Management

**Setting:** outpatient

### Diagnostic/Therapeutic Plan

- CBC
- MCV
- Peripheral smear
- Reticulocyte count

### Test Results

- WBC 4,800/mm$^3$ (normal 4,500–11,000/mm$^3$), hemoglobin 9.6 g/dL (normal 12–16 g/dL), platelets 500,000/mm$^3$ (normal 150,000–400,000/mm$^3$)
- MCV: 70 $\mu m^3$ (normal 80–100 $\mu m^3$)
- Peripheral smear: RBC appear hypochromic and microcytic
- Reticulocyte count: 1.0% (normal 1–2%)

## Assessment

The first issue to resolve in the evaluation of a patient with anemia is whether it is due to blood loss, increased peripheral destruction of RBCs, or a failure of marrow production. There is no clinical evidence of bleeding in the patient, and the lack of an elevated reticulocyte count in response to anemia suggests a primary problem with marrow production of RBCs.

Folate deficiency is seen in patients with poor diets, particularly alcoholics. Folate is found in leafy vegetables. Vitamin B12 deficiency can be seen in strict vegetarians but develops over years. It is often seen in the setting of pernicious anemia, which is unusual in this age group. Both folate and vitamin B12 deficiency produce macrocytic, not microcytic, anemia. Trimethoprim/sulfa can have a suppressive effect on the marrow but often suppresses white-blood-cell and platelet production as well. Sulfa drugs would be an unusual cause of an isolated decrease in red-blood-cell production. Myelodysplasia is a stem cell disorder of the marrow that affects all marrow cells. Anemia and dyserythropoiesis are seen.

The most likely cause of a microcytic anemia in an otherwise healthy young woman is iron deficiency. Other potential etiologies include thalassemia, anemia of chronic disease, or sideroblastic anemia. Iron deficiency results in an early elevation of the red cell distribution width (RDW) and is often associated with an elevated platelet count.

Thalassemia presents with a normal RDW, a disproportionately low MCV, and the presence of target cells on a peripheral smear. The diagnosis of iron deficiency is confirmed by examination of the iron studies. Serum iron is low, and total iron binding capacity (TIBC; a measure of iron binding sites available on circulating transferrin molecules) is high. This is in contrast to chronic inflammatory disease, where serum iron is low but so is the TIBC because of a defect in iron mobilization. Ferritin is the storage form of iron, and its level in the circulation reflects the level of iron stores. A low ferritin confirms iron deficiency. Ferritin is an acute-phase reactant, and a low-normal value can occur in an iron-deficient patient with an active inflammatory state. This means that you can have iron deficiency anemia with a normal ferritin level. In this situation, a bone marrow aspirate with direct examination of the iron stores may be necessary.

## Further Management Plan/Results

| | |
|---|---|
| 1. Ferritin | 5 ng/mL (low) |
| 2. Iron | Low |
| 3. TIBC | High |
| 4. RDW | High |

## Discussion

Iron deficiency is the most common nutritional deficiency in the world. It is believed that as many as 30% of the world's population may be anemic, and approximately 50% are believed to be iron deficient. In the United States, 20% of women of childbearing age are iron deficient. Daily iron losses from the skin and GI tract are approximately 1 mg for men and 1.5 to 2 mg for women. Daily iron intake is 10–20 mg a day in the United States, but it is poorly absorbed.

### CLINICAL PEARL

Iron studies must always be ordered before a transfusion is given. However, you do not have to wait for their results to give the transfusion.

Iron is primarily absorbed in the duodenum and proximal jejunum. Heme iron (meat) is better absorbed than non-heme iron. The latter requires the presence of stomach acidity and may be compromised in achlorhydria. Iron absorption is decreased by antacids and increased by ascorbic and citric acid. Iron absorption is also regulated by iron stores and increases during pregnancy and hemorrhage. Iron binds to transferrin in the circulation, which serves as a carrier molecule. It binds to apoferritin and is stored primarily in bone marrow and in the reticuloendothelial system as ferritin. Hemosiderin is a degraded form of ferritin that accumulates in iron overload.

Women are particularly at risk for iron deficiency due to increased losses secondary to menstrual bleeding, particularly if there is no iron supplementation in the diet. Pregnancy adds further risk in that the fetus takes approximately 750 mg of iron from the mother during gestation such that without supplementation, women will uniformly deplete their iron stores and become deficient by time of delivery. Infants are also susceptible, particularly if they are breast-fed and have no exogenous source of iron. Adolescents are susceptible because of increased iron requirements. Another cause, particularly in older patients, is occult GI bleeding. Iron deficiency due to malabsorption is less common and is seen in processes that diffusely affect the proximal small bowel, such as celiac and tropical sprue, giardiasis, or bacterial overgrowth.

Iron deficiency develops gradually. First iron stores are depleted. Then erythropoiesis is blunted, and anemia finally develops. Patients with longstanding anemia can occasionally develop glossitis and stomatitis due to dysfunction of iron-dependent enzyme systems that maintain epithelial cell integrity. Brittle fingernails and classic spooning of the nails can be seen. Patients can develop esophageal webs, resulting in dysphagia. This is known as the Plummer Vinson syndrome and may be a premalignant lesion. Pagophagia (craving for eating ice) is quite specific for iron deficiency.

**CLINICAL PEARL**

Serum iron can be normal in early iron deficiency. Anemia of chronic disease typically has low serum iron but the ferritin is elevated or normal (not low).

Oral ferrous sulfate is the most common form of repletion. Reticulocytosis is the first indication of response and peaks usually after 10 days of therapy. If the patient has severe malabsorption and cannot be repleted orally, parenteral iron dextran can be given intramuscularly or intravenously.

### Follow-up Management and Prevention

- Ferrous sulfate orally (325 mg 3x/day) until hemoglobin level recovers
- Repeat reticulocyte count in 2 wks
- Repeat CBC in one month
- Add oral vitamin C to increase iron absorption if cells are not being produced

**CLINICAL PEARL**

With unexplained iron-deficiency anemia in adults, always refer for colonoscopy to exclude colon cancer.

### Final Diagnosis

Iron-deficiency anemia

# CASE 8

## Chief Complaint

"I have been bleeding for 2 days after cutting myself."

## History and Physical Examination

A 22-year-old man comes to the clinic for evaluation of abnormal bleeding after shaving. This has been going on intermittently for years, but after he took aspirin this week (the first time in a long time) it became very severe. He has not had surgery in the past so he cannot tell if there is increased bleeding.

## Differential Diagnosis

1. Hemophilia A and B
2. Von Willebrand disease (vWD)
3. Immune thrombocytopenic purpura (ITP)
4. Factor XI deficiency

## Initial Management

**Setting:** outpatient

## Diagnostic/Therapeutic Plan

- CBC
- PT
- aPTT
- LFTs
- Discontinue aspirin
- Type and cross

## Test Results

- CBC normal, including normal platelet count
- PT normal
- aPTT prolonged at 55 seconds
- LFTs normal

## Assessment

Bleeding disorders should first be evaluated for whether they are from platelet or clotting factor disorders. Platelet disorder-type bleeding is superficial, such as from the gums, gingiva, epistaxis, or the skin. Vaginal bleeding is also from platelet disorders. The type of bleeding cannot determine if there is a platelet defect in function or just a decrease in the number of platelets.

Factor-type bleeding such as that from hemophilia is deep. Deep bleeding means into the joints or into the muscles. Bleeding of the GI tract, urine or into the brain can be from either etiology. All bleeding problems should always be evaluated with PT, aPTT, and CBC first.

The aPTT is elevated in vWD in about half of cases. This is because factor VIII antigen, which is the von Willebrand factor, travels bound to factor VIII coagulant, which is the hemophilia factor. It is very common that vWD presents with mild bleeding that is made worse after the use of aspirin.

A type and cross is useful in almost any form of severe bleeding. You want to be sure you have the ability to transfuse the patient, but you also want to show that you are thinking ahead. If this were a single best answer question, a type and cross would not be the most important thing to do.

You will never get into trouble on a CCS case by showing you are thinking ahead to the possibility of more severe bleeding. LFTs show that you know that clotting factors are made in the liver.

**CCS NOTE**

On a CCS case, doing a type and cross shows that you understand what is needed in advance for all potentially serious bleeding. On a type and cross, antibody testing is also done, which shows you are looking at the possibility of antibody inhibitors.

### Further Management Plan/Results

| | |
|---|---|
| • VWF or antigen level | Decrease in VWF level |
| • VWF activity (ristocetin cofactor assay) | Abnormal |
| • Repeat CBC | No significant change |

### Discussion

All clotting factors are made in the liver with the exception of factor VIII and VWF. These factors are made and stored underneath endothelial cells lining the vessel.

DDAVP causes the release of subendothelial stores of VWF and factor VIII. This is a safe way to rapidly increase blood levels of VWF without the risk of transfusion. This will rapidly increase the 'stickiness' of platelets. If DDAVP is not sufficient to stop bleeding, then factor VIII replacement contains both VWF and factor VIII. This is also why you can use DDAVP for mild hemophilia. Factor VIII antigen (the VWF) and factor VIII coagulant (the hemophilia factor) travel bound to each other.

**CLINICAL PEARL**

Always do a repeat CBC in any person with bleeding. It shows that you know the first CBC will not show the ultimate blood count.

The bleeding time is of equivocal value. When you cut a person and there is a prolongation of the bleeding time, this implies a defect in platelet function. It is not clear what the value is of this test if you can do VWF antigen and activity.

### Follow-up Management Plan

- Desmopressin (DDAVP)
- Factor VIII replacement if this is not effective (rarely)
- Avoid aspirin in the future

### Final Diagnosis

Von Willebrand disease

# CASE 9

## Chief Complaint

"How long do I have to stay in the hospital for my blood clot, doc?"

## History and Physical Examination

A 57-year-old man is admitted for shortness of breath after developing a pulmonary embolus. He has been administered IV unfractionated heparin for the last several days. On hospital day 3, his platelet count has dropped from 185,000 $mm^3$ to 62,000 $mm^3$ but he is otherwise improving. Warfarin was started 2 days ago.

Physical examination reveals chest is clear to auscultation, cardiovascular exam is normal with no murmurs or gallops. His extremities are normal.

## Differential Diagnosis

1. Heparin-induced thrombocytopenia (HIT)
2. Immune thrombocytopenia (ITP)
3. Thrombotic thrombocytopenic purpura (TTP)
4. Hemolytic uremic syndrome (HUS)

## Initial Management

**Setting:** inpatient hospital

## Diagnostic/Therapeutic Plan

- Discontinue all heparin
- Start argatroban or bivalirudin or fondaparinux
- Stop warfarin
- Repeat CBC
- PT, aPTT, INR

## Test Results

- Platelet count 54,000/$mm^3$
- PT, aPTT, INR: normal

## Assessment

Heparin-induced thrombocytopenia (HIT) is defined as >50% drop in the platelet count after several days of heparin use. HUS and TTP would also be associated with hemolytic anemia and an elevated BUN or creatinine. ITP does not develop in response to the use of heparin; however, ITP and HIT are both isolated decreases in the platelet count. ITP, however, causes bleeding from a low platelet count, while HIT results in thrombosis from the 'clumping' of platelets. HIT gives venous thromboses more often than arterial thromboses.

The diagnosis of HIT is **very dependent** on the temporal relationship of the start of heparin with the timing of the drop in platelet count.

### Further Management

- Serotonin release assay
- Platelet factor 4 assay
- Argatroban if renal failure present
- Fondaparinux if liver failure present

**CLINICAL PEARL**

HIT causes >50% drop in platelets with heparin.

- Causes clotting as a clinical manifestation; venous is 3x more common than arterial clotting
- Confirm with platelet factor 4 antibodies and serotonin release assay
- Remove **all heparins;** do **not** switch to low molecular weight
- Use argatroban or bivalirudin or fondaparinux as alternate therapy

**CLINICAL PEARL**

Lepirudin and danaparoid are not available in the United States.

### Discussion

HIT is increasingly recognized because of the increasing frequency of heparin use. If there is a drop in platelet count >50%, then stop all heparin and switch to a direct-acting thrombin inhibitor until there is no longer an indication for heparin.

You must **not** switch unfractionated heparin to low molecular weight heparin if HIT has developed. Although HIT is less common with low molecular weight heparin, once the patient develops HIT, **all** heparin products must be stopped.

When stimulated with serotonin, the platelets in a person with HIT will release labeled carbon. This helps confirm the diagnosis of HIT.

### Follow-up Management and Prevention

- Serotonin release assay is abnormal and platelet factor 4 antibodies are positive
- Continue argatroban or fondaparinux or bivalirudin for 5 days
- Oral anticoagulation for 6 months
- Do not start warfarin until argatroban or fondaparinux or bivalirudin are started
- Warfarin with INR 2–3 or rivaroxaban

### Final Diagnosis

Heparin-induced thrombocytopenia

# CASE 10

## Chief Complaint

"I fecl very weak and my urine is dark."

## History and Physical Examination

A 30-year-old woman is brought to the emergency department by her family because of the development of profound weakness over a few days. She also has dark urine. She went to see her family practice doctor who found blood on dipstick, but no red cells or white cells were seen on microscopic examination. She is brought now to the hospital because she developed left-sided weakness.

Upon examination blood pressure is 132/94 mm Hg, pulse 118/min, respirations 18 min, and temperature 100.8 F. Neurologic exam reveals left-hand weakness, though it is improved as compared to several hours ago. Cardiovascular exam reveals no murmurs. Skin has a yellow discoloration. In HEENT, scleral icterus is found. The abdomen is soft. Liver and spleen are normal.

## Differential Diagnosis

1. Hemolysis
2. Acute hepatitis
3. Thrombotic thrombocytopenic purpura (TTP)
4. Obstructive jaundice
5. Stroke
6. Paroxysmal nocturnal hemoglobinuria

## Initial Management

**Setting:** emergency department

## Diagnostic/Therapeutic Plan

- CBC
- LFTs
- Urinalysis
- Head CT
- Chemistry 7

## Test Results

- CBC: hematocrit 31%, platelets 42,000, WBC 7,500
- LFTs: total bilirubin 5.2 mg/dL, direct 0.8 mg/dL, alk phos normal AST, ALT normal
- Urinalysis: dip positive for blood, no cells seen; no bilirubin
- Head CT: normal
- Chemistry 7: BUN 34, creatinine 2.2 mg/dL

### Assessment

Dark urine can be either hemoglobin or bilirubin. This patient has hemoglobin in the urine turning it dark. The elevated total bilirubin with low direct means this is indirect or unconjugated bilirubin. Unconjugated bilirubin is not water soluble and cannot go into the urine. Unconjugated bilirubin is attached to albumin and does not filter.

This is not obstruction of the biliary system because obstruction gives an elevation of direct bilirubin. Obstruction would also increase the alkaline phosphatase and GGT. Acute hepatitis elevates the ALT>AST. Drug-induced hepatitis such as from alcohol increases the AST>ALT, and the bilirubin is direct or water soluble from conjugation to diglucuronide.

This patient has hemolysis. In addition there is a low platelet count, renal dysfunction and neurologic deficit. This is all consistent with thrombotic thrombocytopenic purpura (TTP). Although there is no identifiable cause for TTP or HUS in the history, it does not matter. Nearly half of cases have no identified cause. TTP is a pentad of intravascular hemolysis, low platelets, renal insufficiency, fever and neurologic problems. The absence of fever is not especially relevant since it is rare for all 5 criteria to be present at the same time.

### Further Management

- CBC
- Chemistry 7
- LDH
- Reticulocyte count
- Peripheral smear
- Normal saline
- Plasmapheresis

### Test Results

- CBC: hematocrit 27%, platelets 34,000, WBC 7,700
- Chemistry 7: BUN 36, creatinine 2.4 mg/dL
- LDH: elevated
- Reticulocyte count: 7%
- Peripheral smear: schistocytes and fragmented RBCs

### Discussion

There is no single diagnostic test for TTP. TTP is diagnosed with a combination of the findings such as we have here, which is evidence of intravascular hemolysis, low platelets, and renal dysfunction. The single most characteristic feature is fragmented cells on the smear. Schistocytes, helmet cells, and broken cells visible on routine blood smear are the main confirmatory features. This leads to intravascular microangiopathic hemolytic anemia and can cause stroke-like neurologic changes and acute glomerular renal injury.

The most common mistake in TTP is to give platelets when the level goes low. Giving platelets only makes TTP and HUS worse. The disorder is a deficiency of antibodies to a metalloproteinase (ADAMTS13) that breaks up VWF multimers. The multimers accumulate on the endothelium and lead to physical shearing of RBCs and depletion of platelets. If you give platelets they will only clog up the brain and kidney even more and worsen the hemolysis.

The best treatment for TTP is plasma exchange and replacement with donor plasma (plasmapheresis). They will remove anti-ADAMTS13 antibodies and replete ADAMTS13 levels.

### Follow-up Management and Prevention

- Repeat CBC and kidney function every 1–2 hours at the beginning
- Hematology consult
- IV saline
- Plasmapheresis (**treatment of choice**)
- Do not transfuse RBCs or platelets

### Final Diagnosis

Thrombotic thrombocytopenic purpura (TTP)

### CLINICAL PEARL

TTP results in intravascular hemolysis with fragmented cells on smear.

- Increasing BUN and creatinine
- Low platelets
- Neurologic problems
- Fever
- Treat with plasmapheresis to replace ADAMTS 13

# Oncology 7

## CASE 1

### Chief Complaint

"My right side is weak."

### History and Physical Examination

A 45-year-old woman comes to the emergency department because of a change in mental status and hemiparesis of the right side. She was well until 2 weeks earlier when she developed intermittent fevers and sore throat. She has suffered from several nosebleeds and gum bleeding over the last week. Her local internist evaluated her earlier this morning.

CBC shows WBC 1,500/mm$^3$, hemoglobin 7.0 mg/dL, and platelets 17,000/mm$^3$. She is lethargic and is not moving her right side. Her T is 38.3 C (101.0 F) and BP is 160/100mm Hg. Examination of her eyes, ears, nose, and throat is normal. Her neck is supple with no adenopathy. Her chest is clear, and her heart has a RRR with normal S1 and S2. There is no hepatosplenomegaly or peripheral edema noted. Neurologic examination shows that she is confused, oriented x1, has right hemiparesis, and upgoing toes on the right. She is uncooperative with sensory examination, but withdraws to painful stimuli on the left.

### Differential Diagnosis

1. Acute leukemia: myeloblastic or lymphoblastic
2. Aplastic anemia
3. Metastatic cancer
4. Bone-marrow invasion by infection
5. Myelodysplastic syndrome

### Initial Management

**Setting:** emergency department

### Diagnostic/Therapeutic Plan

- Peripheral smear
- Blood cultures, UA, chest x-ray
- Differential/absolute neutrophil count (ANC)
- PT, aPTT, D-dimers, fibrin split products, fibrinogen
- Head CT
- Platelet transfusion
- Meropenem, cefepime, or piperacillin/tazobactam IV

### Test Results

- Smear: multiple immature myeloid cells (blasts) seen with atypical folding pattern; Auer rods seen
- Blood cultures: pending for 1–2 days
- UA, chest x-ray normal
- Differential/ANC: 20% of 1,500 WBC or ANC 300
- PT, aPTT: 18 seconds, 78 seconds (elevated)
- D-dimers, fibrin split products: increased
- Fibrinogen decreased
- Head CT: left intraparenchymal hemorrhage in parietal lobe

### Assessment

The initial presentation of the patient is consistent with stroke syndrome. Given her platelet count and recent history of bleeding, a hemorrhagic stroke appears more likely.

Pancytopenia occurs with any primary cancer of the marrow, such as leukemia or any metastatic cancer that invades the marrow. Infections such as tuberculosis can also rarely cause a pancytopenia if they invade the marrow as well. Vitamin B12 and folate deficiency also rarely cause a pancytopenia, but they are not associated with disseminated intravascular coagulation, such as this patient has. The same is true of splenic sequestration and systemic lupus erythematosus. None of the causes of pancytopenia gives blasts on the peripheral smear, except for acute leukemia. The leukemia most commonly associated with disseminated intravascular coagulation is M3, or promyelocytic leukemia.

The most dangerous thing to this patient now is bleeding from the low platelet count and infection. Anyone with temp 38 and ANC <500 needs antibiotics within 60 minutes of it being found. Pseudomonal coverage is very important, so the initial choice can be a carbapenem (meropenem or imipenem), a synthetic penicillin such as piperacillin/tazobactam, or an anti-pseudomonal cephalosporin such as cefepime.

- Mechanism of AML: defect occurs shortly after the commitment of the stem cell to the myeloid line
- Stem cells are CD34+
- Definitive diagnosis is by flow cytometry: "CD" means "cluster of differentiation"

### Basic Science Correlate

Mechanism of DIC in M3 promyelocytic leukemia: release of azurophilic granules from promyelocytes that activate the clotting cascade

**CCS NOTE**

Once the clock is moved forward, nothing can be done to move it back. You can only go forward in time, even "simulated" time.

## Further Management Plan/Results

| | |
|---|---|
| 1. Bone marrow biopsy | Diffuse infiltration with monomorphic population of abnormal promyelocytes. Decreased megakaryocytes. |
| 2. Cytogenetic studies; FISH test for 5q deletion, 15:17 translocation | 15:17 translocation is present |
| 3. Add vancomycin, linezolid or daptomycin if still febrile after 48–72 hours | |

## Discussion

Acute myeloid leukemia is the most common acute leukemia of adults. Its incidence increases with age and is associated with previous radiation exposure, exposure to alkylating agents, benzene, and prior history of myelodysplasia. It is divided into seven morphologic types, including undifferentiated (M0), promyelocytic (M3), monocytic (M5), erythroleukemia (M6), and megakaryoblastic (M7). Undifferentiated forms may be difficult to discern from acute lymphocytic leukemia, but surface markers suggest myeloid origin. The presence of Auer rods or myeloperoxidase indicates myeloid origin of the cells.

Patients may present with high WBC. If WBC >150,000/mm$^3$, patients may experience complications of leukostasis, which include diffuse CNS changes caused by sludging or hemorrhage, blurry vision, and respiratory decompensation. Leukostasis can be treated with leukapheresis or cytoreduction with urgent hydroxyurea or chemotherapy administration. Patients may also present with low WBC counts. Monocytic disease may present with CNS, gum, or skin infiltration. Megakaryoblastic disease is characterized by marked marrow fibrosis.

Acute promyelocytic leukemia is a distinct form of acute myeloid leukemia and has the best prognosis among AML subtypes. It is caused by a translocation between the retinoic acid receptor and the PML gene (translocation 15:17). Acute promyelocytic leukemia cells contain procoagulant material that, when it gains access to the circulation, may initiate disseminated intravascular coagulation. Patients often present with complications of acute bleeding.

Treatment of acute promyelocytic leukemia has consisted of an induction regimen of an anthracycline such as daunorubicin or idarubicin, plus cytosine arabinoside. Many early deaths were a result of disseminated intravascular coagulation-related problems and were often exacerbated by cell lysis in the setting of treatment. Another form of therapy is all-trans retinoic acid; when exposed to this agent, it seems that acute promyelocytic leukemia cells undergo maturation. This may help to avoid problems seen with cell lysis during initiation of treatment.

The prognosis of acute promyelocytic leukemia is slightly better than it is with other forms of acute myeloid leukemia. In general, long-term survival with acute myeloid leukemia is approximately 40% without transplant.

**CLINICAL PEARL**

Acute myeloblastic leukemia

- Clinically: usually bleeding diathesis, infections, and anemia
- WBC may be increased, normal, or low
- Blasts $\geq$20% in marrow or peripheral blood
- Blasts: high cytoplasm-to-nucleus ratio, azurophilic granules, Auer rods
- Cytogenetics and cell markers consistent with myeloblasts

### Basic Science Correlate

The most important prognostic indicator is cytogenetic abnormalities on flow cytometry or bone marrow biopsy (PML/RARA—15;17).

**Why doesn't combining beta lactam antibiotics increase efficacy?** Penicillins, carbapenems, aztreonam, and cephalosporins all inhibit the cell wall. One mechanism = NO synergy.

**Why are echinocandins (e.g., caspofungin) so safe?** Their mechanism, inhibiting 1,3 glucan linkages in fungi, does not exist in human cells.

**What is the mechanism of daptomycin failure in pneumonia?** Inactivation by surfactant

## Follow-up Management and Prevention

- Stabilize the CNS bleed with platelet transfusions
- Treatment with cytosine arabinoside (ARA-C) and daunorubicin or idarubicin
- All-trans-retinoic acid (ATRA) is added just for M3 promyelocytic leukemia
- Add voriconazole or caspofungin if still febrile 2–3 days after addition of vancomycin
- Allogenic bone-marrow transplantation in those with high-risk disease or those who relapse after induction chemotherapy

## Final Diagnosis

Acute myeloblastic leukemia/acute promyelocytic leukemia/disseminated intravascular coagulation

# CASE 2

## Chief Complaint

Fatigue

## History and Physical Examination

A 75-year-old man comes to the office because of progressive fatigue over the last 3 months, as well as several episodes of upper respiratory infection over the last year. He also feels "fullness" in his abdomen and states that his appetite has deteriorated, although he has not lost any weight. He denies chronic fevers, chills, cough, and a history of abnormal bleeding.

Physical examination shows bilateral adenopathy in the cervical and supraclavicular chain. The lymph nodes are hard and nontender; the largest is approximately 3 cm. The chest is clear and the heart has a RRR with normal S1 and S2. The abdomen is soft and nontender; a splenic edge is palpated 5 cm below left costal margin, and bilateral inguinal adenopathy is present. Rectal examination is negative for fecal occult blood.

## Differential Diagnosis

1. Chronic lymphocytic leukemia
2. Chronic myeloid leukemia
3. Hodgkin's or non-Hodgkin's lymphoma
4. Infectious mononucleosis
5. Cytomegalovirus infection

## Initial Management

**Setting:** outpatient

## Diagnostic/Therapeutic Plan

- CBC
- Differential
- Chest x-ray
- BUN/creatinine
- Heterophile antibodies (monospot test)

## Test Results

- WBCs 75,000/$mm^3$ (normal 4,000–11,000/$mm^3$), hemoglobin 10 mg/dL (normal: 13–17 mg/dL), platelets 70,000/$mm^3$ (normal 150,000–400,000/$mm^3$)
- 80% mature lymphocytes, 15% granulocytes, 5% monocytes
- Chest x-ray: normal
- BUN/creatinine: 20 mg/dL, 1.0 mg/dL
- Monospot and CMV antibodies: negative

### Assessment

The patient presents with diffuse lymphadenopathy, splenomegaly, and a history of fatigue and frequent infections. A primary malignancy of the lymphocytes needs to be excluded.

The subacute presentation here is more consistent with a lymphoma or chronic leukemia rather than acute leukemia. Infectious etiologies causing generalized adenopathy and splenomegaly include cytomegalovirus and Epstein-Barr virus-related illness. The thrombocytopenia and hemolytic anemia are likely autoimmune in nature and related to the primary disease.

**CCS NOTE**

Normal lab values are routinely provided with test results on CCS.

### Further Management Plan/Results

| | |
|---|---|
| 1. Bone marrow biopsy | Diffuse infiltration with mature-appearing lymphocytes (10% of total); myeloid and erythroid maturation appear normal; increased numbers of megakaryocytes are seen |
| 2. Direct Coombs test | Positive |
| 3. Lymph node biopsy | No lymphoma |
| 4. Flow cytometry of peripheral blood | Positive for CD5 and CD20 |
| 5. Cytogenetics | Normal |

### Discussion

Chronic lymphocytic leukemia (CLL) is the most common (30%) adult leukemia.

- Primarily affects people age >50
- Characterized by prominent peripheral lymphocytosis of mature-appearing lymphocytes of B-cell lineage; the cells typically infiltrate the lymph nodes diffusely, the spleen, and the bone marrow
- Not associated with prior exposure to radiation or chemicals
- In some the disease is indolent and detected coincidentally on routine blood work, while in others it can progress more rapidly

Presentation may include:

- History of recurrent infections
- Decrease in cell-mediated immunity
- Hypogammaglobulinemia (common)
- Autoimmune antibodies to hematopoietic cells
- Autoimmune hemolytic anemia (15% of cases)
- Immune-based thrombocytopenia and granulocytopenia

Several staging systems exist, most notably the Rai and Binet systems. In Rai system:

- **Low risk**: patients with lymphocytosis alone (stage 0)
- **Intermediate risk**: patients with lymphadenopathy (stage 1) or splenomegaly (stage 2)
- **High risk**: patients with anemia and thrombocytopenia (stage 3 or 4)

Low-risk disease is associated with survival >10 yrs, whereas high-risk disease is associated with survival <5 yrs. Like most chronic hematologic malignancies, patients can go into remission for long periods of time with treatment, but curing the disease is difficult.

Treatment initially involves observation over time, unless patient is symptomatic with extensive fever/chills/sweats, recurrent infections, or profound anemia/neutropenia/thrombocytopenia. Indications for treatment include:

- Systemic symptoms
- Bone marrow failure
- Autoimmune manifestations
- Massive splenomegaly
- Bulky lymph node disease
- Recurrent infections

There is no clear evidence that a specific treatment for CLL is more effective than another. Treatment may look like the treatment for non-Hodgkin's lymphoma, as CLL is really a form of lymphoma that is circulating in the blood.

- Fludarabine/cyclophosphamide/rituximab (FCR) is given to younger, fit patients. (Fludarabine can be used as a single agent or combined with an anti-CD20 agent such as rituximab. Cyclophosphamide is often used.)
- Bendamustine/rituximab (B/R) is given to less fit or older patients.
- Prednisone is sometimes added in the presence of autoimmune manifestations, e.g., anemia or thrombocytopenia.

### Follow-up Management and Prevention

- Fludarabine or bendamustine
- Add rituximab for those CD20-positive (most)
- Cyclophosphamide (often used with fludarabine and rituximab)
- Chlorambucil in older, more fragile persons

### Final Diagnosis

Chronic lymphocytic leukemia

### CLINICAL PEARL

CLL patients are usually asymptomatic, with increased infections. WBCs are increased with a predominance of mature lymphocytes. Hemolytic anemia is common.

- **Asymptomatic patients; stage 0-1**: observe without chemotherapy
- **Symptomatic patients or those with bone marrow failure; stage 2-4**: treat with FCR (fludarabine, rituximab, and cyclophosphamide) or bendamustine/rituximab (B/R)

# CASE 3

## Chief Complaint

"My shoulder hurts."

## History and Physical Examination

A 75-year-old woman comes to the emergency department with severe pain in her left shoulder. She states that she was leaning against a wall with her left arm when suddenly she felt "something snap" in that arm. She states that over the last several months, she has experienced intermittent back and rib pain but didn't seek medical attention. She denies fever and chills. There is no history of weight loss.

Her T is 37.0 C (98.6 F), BP 110/68 mm Hg, and pulse 76/min. She is unable to lift her left arm. Physical examination is otherwise unremarkable.

## Differential Diagnosis

1. Traumatic fracture
2. Pathologic fracture (e.g., multiple myeloma, osteoporosis)
3. Metastatic cancer (breast, lung, ovary)

**CCS NOTE**

In the ICU, examine only the areas surrounding the chief complaint in acutely ill patients. You can always do a complete physical examination later.

## Initial Management

**Setting:** emergency department

## Diagnostic/Therapeutic Plan

- Plain film of the left shoulder
- BUN, creatinine
- Total protein/albumin
- LFTs
- CBC
- Serum calcium

## Test Results

- Fracture of proximal humerus with multiple lytic lesions
- BUN, creatinine: 28, 2.0 mg/dL
- Total protein/albumin: 9.0 g/dL (elevated), albumin 3.5 g/dL (normal)
- LFTs normal
- WBC 5,000/mm$^3$ (normal: 4,000–11,000/mm$^3$), Hgb 11 mg/dL (normal 12–16 mg/dL), platelets 120,000/mm$^3$
- Serum calcium 11.5 mg/dL (normal 8.5–10.2 mg/dL)

## Assessment

The presence of elevated serum protein/albumin ratio in the setting of pathologic fracture raises concern for multiple myeloma. In addition, the patient has symptoms in other bony areas and evidence of renal failure. The most common presentation of myeloma is bone pain.

### Basic Science Correlate

**Mechanism of renal failure in myeloma:**

- IgG clogs up glomeruli
- Uric acid damages tubules
- Hypercalcemia toxic to tubules
- Amyloid
- Bence-Jones protein toxic to tubules

**Mechanism of hyperuricemia:**

- Purines and pyrimidines from plasma cell nuclei transform into uric acid

Why don't myeloma bone lesions light up on a nuclear bone scan?

- Technetium nuclear isotope is deposited by osteoblast. Myeloma lesions are purely lytic

## Further Management Plan/Results

| | |
|---|---|
| 1. Normal saline bolus | |
| 2. Pamidronate | |
| 3. SPEP | Presence of monoclonal spike immunoglobulin G: 6 g/dL |
| 4. Urine protein electrophoresis | Positive for Bence-Jones protein |
| 5. Skeletal survey | Multiple lytic lesions in the ribs and vertebrae |
| 6. Bone marrow | 35% plasma cells |
| 7. Beta 2 micro globulin | Elevated |

## Discussion

The patient requires an orthopedic procedure to correct the fracture. Radiation therapy to the arm may be required for pain control. Ideally, radiation therapy should be limited initially so that chemotherapy is not compromised by the depletion of bone marrow reserves.

There are numerous treatment options for chemotherapy and there is no one clear "best choice." Options are a combination of 2 or 3 of the following, such as bortezomib, prednisone, or melphalan when age >70. Combination regimens, including other alkylating agents, vincristine, doxorubicin, and prednisone, may yield a more rapid response with greater adverse effects. Hypercalcemia should be initially managed with hydration and bisphosphonates.

Multiple myeloma is primarily a disease of older patients. An elevated monoclonal immunoglobulin spike characterizes it. It is differentiated from the more common monoclonal gammopathy of unknown significance by the height of the M spike (>3 g protein), the presence of bony lesions, or marrow infiltration with >10% plasma cells.

Multiple myeloma most commonly presents as bone pain involving the ribs and back. Bony lesions are caused by infiltration of plasma cells and activation of osteoclasts that are responding to a hormonal factor made by the myeloma cells. Bony lesions are almost exclusively lytic, so bone scans are usually negative. Plain films diagnose bony lesions. Hypercalcemia is often a problem because of mobilization of calcium from bone. Patients may also suffer from cord compression because of involvement of vertebrae.

Patients with multiple myeloma are at increased risk for bacterial infections because of associated diffuse hypogammaglobulinemia. This is caused by suppression of antibody production aside from the monoclonal spike.

Staging relates to the presence of anemia, the height of the M spike, the presence of hypercalcemia, and the degree of skeletal involvement. These, and beta-2 microglobulin, act as prognostic indicators.

Multiple myeloma is usually responsive to but not curable with standard chemotherapy. A variety of regimens involving steroids, alkylating agents, and thalidomide-derivatives have been developed. Combination regimens usually lead to a more rapid response without improving survival. Bortezomib is a proteasome inhibitor that is commonly used.

Once a patient is moved to a minimal disease state without symptoms, observation is sufficient until problems later arise. Bony lesions can be treated with radiation therapy for pain control. Autologous stem-cell transplantation is used in those age <70 in an attempt to drive the disease into deeper remission.

## Follow-up Management and Prevention

- Surgical repair of humerus
- Chemotherapy for myeloma with prednisone, melphalan, and possibly bortezomib initially (in older patients for palliation)
- Thalidomide or lenalidomide
- Autologous bone-marrow transplantation in those age <70
- Pamidronate (bisphosphonates)

### Basic Science Correlate

What is the mechanism of massive volume depletion in hypercalcemia?

- High calcium inhibits ADH effect on V2 receptors in collecting duct, causing nephrogenic diabetes insipidus
- Osmotic diuresis

How come hemolysis does not cause hyperuricemia?

- Mature red cells have no nuclei and therefore no nucleic acids

How come autologous stem cell transplantation can be done at a much older age (up to age 70) than allogeneic transplantation?

- No rejection with autologous transplantation
- No graft versus host disease
- Stem cells grow to mature cells faster
- Much shorter duration of neutropenia

### CLINICAL PEARL

Multiple myeloma

- Clinically: bone pain and fractures, infections, anemia
- Protein electrophoresis: monoclonal spike (M protein)
- M protein >3 g
- Renal insufficiency
- Urine: Bence-Jones protein
- Plasma cells >10% in the marrow (usually >30%)

## Final Diagnosis

Multiple myeloma

# CASE 4

## Chief Complaint

Enlarged lymph node in the neck

## History and Physical Examination

A 25-year-old woman comes to the office with a history of enlarged lymph nodes in her neck. The nodes are in the cervical area and have been enlarged over the last several weeks. She denies fever or weight loss. She is not on any medication.

Physical examination of the eyes, ears, nose, and throat is normal. There are several 2- to 3-cm firm, freely mobile lymph nodes in the right anterior cervical chain. The nodes are not warm, red, or tender. The chest is clear and heart is normal without murmurs. The abdomen is soft and non-tender with no hepatosplenomegaly. There is no peripheral edema noted.

## Differential Diagnosis

1. Hodgkin's lymphoma
2. Non-Hodgkin's lymphoma
3. Tuberculosis
4. Epstein-Barr virus infection
5. HIV
6. Acute lymphocytic leukemia
7. Sarcoidosis

## Initial Management

**Setting:** outpatient

## Diagnostic/Therapeutic Plan

- CBC
- LFTs
- Chest x-ray
- Cervical lymph node biopsy (excisional biopsy)

## Test Results

- CBC normal
- LFTs normal
- Chest x-ray normal
- Cervical lymph node biopsy: nodular sclerosis Hodgkin's lymphoma

### CCS NOTE

Each part of the physical exam takes 1 minute when ordered individually, except for the HEENT and pelvic and rectal exams. For each of those, give 2 minutes.

### Assessment

Rapidly enlarging, firm, nontender, cervical lymph nodes suggest lymphoma. Adenopathy, fevers, night sweats, and cough are also suggestive of lymphoproliferative disease. Tuberculosis and Epstein-Barr virus should also be considered when these occur.

Although a history of sweating may be suggestive of lymphoma, there is no definitive way to distinguish tuberculosis from lymphoma or to differentiate the types of lymphoma without a biopsy. No further testing is required to confirm diagnosis after this. The remainder of the tests is to determine the stage.

The main point of staging is to determine who needs extensive combination chemotherapy and who can be safely treated with localized radiation and a lower dose of radiation. Any patient with "B" symptoms, such as fever, weight loss, or night sweats, should receive predominantly chemotherapy. This patient seems, so far, to have lymphoma limited to a single lymph node group. If further testing confirms that the disease is localized, she can be treated primarily with radiation.

Although most Hodgkin's lymphoma is localized to 1 or 2 lymph node groups in 80–90% of patients, and non-Hodgkin's lymphoma disease is more widespread, the only way to be truly certain which one the patient has is with an excisional lymph node biopsy.

### Further Diagnostic Plan/Results

| | |
|---|---|
| 1. CT scan of abdomen and pelvis | No adenopathy; liver and spleen WNL |
| 2. PET scan (occasionally) | No abnormalities |
| 3. Bone marrow biopsy | Negative |

### Discussion

Hodgkin's disease is a common form of lymphoma whose peak occurrence is in a bimodal pattern. It occurs at age 15–35 and age >50. Diagnosis rests on identification of Reed-Sternberg cells in the pathologic specimen.

**Four histologic patterns exist:**

- Lymphocyte predominant
- Nodular sclerosing
- Mixed cellularity
- Lymphocyte depleted

When staged accurately, histologic pattern is not an independent predictor of response to treatment or prognosis.

Patients have documented defects in cell-mediated immunity. They are often anergic and are more susceptible to herpes zoster. Hodgkin's disease spreads in a stepwise fashion to contiguous lymph node chains. Prognosis is related to the number of involved sites. In some cases, lymph node sites are "skipped." Patients often present with constitutional symptoms. These include fever, night sweats, and weight loss of >10% of body weight. Pruritus is not considered a B symptom, although it commonly occurs.

**Staging is as follows:**

| | |
|---|---|
| **Stage I** | 1 lymph node chain |
| **Stage II** | ≥2 chains on one side of diaphragm |
| **Stage III** | Involvement of both sides of diaphragm; may include spleen |
| **Stage IV** | Liver, bone marrow, or extranodal involvement |

Staging evaluation should be directed at determining different treatment plans.

- Stages I/II: treat with chemotherapy combined with involved field radiation therapy
- Stages III/IV: treat with higher-intensity chemotherapy
- The presence of bulky disease (i.e., >1/3 mediastinal diameter) requires both chemotherapy and radiation to shrink the lesion so as to make it more likely for response.
- CT of the abdomen is used to exclude stage III disease; if it is normal, PET scan is used to rule out lymph nodes of normal size, which may have distorted architecture from involvement.
- Staging laparotomy is no longer the standard of care.
- Stages III/IV and those with B symptoms: treat with high-dose chemotherapy with ABVD alone (doxorubicin, bleomycin, vinblastine, dexamethasone)
  - MOPP combination chemotherapy is no longer used due to association with leukemia later in life.
  - Prognosis ranges from >90% disease-free survival for early disease to 50–60% with more advanced stage disease.
  - The presence of systemic symptoms is a negative prognostic indicator.
  - Patients who relapse after radiation therapy alone can often be cured with chemotherapy. Those who relapse >1 yr after chemotherapy are often still sensitive and can be retreated. Those who relapse <1 yr after chemotherapy or are not achieving remission have an extremely poor prognosis.

One late concern is the development of secondary malignancies that appear to be treatment-related. Secondary acute myelocytic leukemia is seen in patients treated with chemotherapy and particularly with chemotherapy/radiation therapy. These are seen predominantly in the first 10 yrs. Solid tumors are seen with increased frequency in the radiation field at >10 yrs after treatment. Coronary artery disease and valvular abnormalities are often seen 20–30 yrs after radiation therapy for Hodgkin's disease.

**CLINICAL PEARL**

Hodgkin's lymphoma

- Clinically: night sweats, weight loss, fatigue
- Lymphadenopathy
- Chest x-ray shows mediastinal lymphadenopathy (unilateral or bilateral).
- Lymph node biopsy shows Reed-Sternberg cells

### Follow-up Management and Prevention

Follow up with combined modality therapy: specifically, 3 to 4 cycles of chemotherapy (ABVD) and radiation to the cervical nodes. Know the long-term adverse effects:

- Radiation: thyroid disease, lung and breast cancer
- Radiation markedly accelerates coronary artery disease
- Vincristine: peripheral neuropathy
- Bleomycin: pulmonary fibrosis
- Adriamycin (doxorubicin): cardiomyopathy

Chemotherapy frequently causes infertility.

### Final Diagnosis

Hodgkin's disease, stage IA

# CASE 5

## Chief Complaint

"I have a cough, fever, and headache."

## History and Physical Examination

A 55-year-old man comes to the office with a recurrent cough productive of yellow sputum and fever. He was recently treated with 2 weeks of antibiotics for pneumonia. He had bloody sputum 3 days ago. He has a decrease in appetite and weight loss of 12 lb over the past month. He smoked 2 packs of cigarettes a day for the past 30 years.

He is ill-appearing. BP 150/90 mm Hg, pulse 100/min, T 37.8 C (100.0 F). He has facial edema and plethora. His neck is supple without adenopathy, with prominent jugular venous distention. There is marked dilatation of peripheral veins across the anterior chest. Chest is clear. Abdomen soft and nontender, with no hepatosplenomegaly. There is mild edema of upper extremities. Neuro exam nonfocal.

## Differential Diagnosis

1. Lung cancer/superior vena cava syndrome
2. Lymphoma/superior vena cava syndrome
3. Tuberculosis
4. Infectious pneumonia

## Initial Management

**Setting:** emergency department

## Diagnostic/Therapeutic Plan

- Chest x-ray
- CBC
- Calcium level
- LFT
- Normal saline
- Oximeter
- Oxygen

## Test Results

- Chest x-ray: large perihilar mass extending into mediastinum; normal cardiac silhouette; right-sided infiltrate distal to the mass
- CBC normal
- Calcium level: 13 mg/dL (normal 8.5–11.5 mg/dL)
- LFT normal

### Further Management

- CT scan of chest
- Pamidronate
- Continue normal saline
- Bronchoscopy with biopsy

### Test Results

- CT scan of chest: large hilar mass extending into mediastinum with compression of superior vena cava
- Bronchoscopy: squamous cell cancer

### Assessment

This patient has a pulmonary mass extending into the mediastinum with superior vena cava syndrome and hypercalcemia. The evidence for the superior vena cava syndrome on examination is the facial fullness (or plethora), dilation of chest veins, and upper extremity edema. Diuretics are not needed for hypercalcemia management unless there is no urine output with fluid administration. Patients with hypercalcemia have a massive volume depletion.

#### CCS NOTE

Significant procedures that take time, such as a bronchoscopy, will require you to advance the clock. A note will pop up, asking if you are sure that you want to advance the time. This does not mean you have made a mistake!

### Discussion

Lung cancer is the leading cause of cancer death in the United States for both men and women. Asbestos exposure is associated with a tenfold increase in risk that is further amplified by concurrent smoking. Roofers and workers with tar, nickel, hydrocarbons, and uranium are at increased risk.

The main histologic subtypes include adenocarcinoma, squamous cell, small cell, and large cell. Bronchoalveolar carcinoma is seen in <5%. Patients may present with hemoptysis from an ulcerating lesion or recurrent pneumonia caused by an obstructing lesion and the development of postobstructive pneumonia. Dyspnea may develop from lymphangitic spread or from the development of a malignant pleural or pericardial effusion. Hoarseness may result from injury to the recurrent laryngeal nerve. Tumor involving the upper lobes can produce Pancoast syndrome, which is associated with infiltration of the brachial plexus and sensory and/or motor findings in the upper extremity. Squamous and large-cell carcinomas tend to present with central lesions, with the latter more likely to metastasize to distant sites.

Adenocarcinoma more commonly presents with peripheral lesions, making sputum cytology less reliable. It can arise in areas of former scars and tends to cause symptoms by metastasizing. Bronchoalveolar carcinoma is often multifocal, due to transbronchial spread, and is associated with significant bronchorrhea.

This patient shows signs of superior vena cava syndrome. This is the result of a tumor invading the mediastinum and compression on the superior vena cava with resultant increased venous pressure transmitted to the neck, head, and upper extremities. Physical findings include facial and upper extremity edema, distended neck veins, and engorged collaterals on the chest wall. Neurologic symptoms include mood disturbance and irritability. When this condition is severe, cardiac output is compromised because of poor venous return, and this constitutes an oncologic emergency that requires emergency radiation therapy.

A variety of paraneoplastic syndromes are associated with lung cancer. These include syndrome of inappropriate antidiuretic hormone secretion (SIADH: associated with small-cell carcinoma), Cushing syndrome (associated with production of adrenocorticotropic hormone; ACTH), and hypercalcemia caused by parathyroid-like hormone production seen in conjunction with squamous cell carcinoma.

Staging relates to tumor size, lymph node involvement, and evidence of metastatic disease.

Stage I and II are generally treated with surgical resection with or without post surgical (adjuvant) chemotherapy. Surgery for stage IIIA is controversial, and studies are ongoing regarding the efficacy of presurgical (neoadjuvant) chemotherapy in this setting. Stage IIIB is treated with radiation therapy. The role of chemotherapy for stages IIIB or IV is for palliation and can increase the quality and quantity of a patient's life.

### NOTE

The staging system often changes and so is not often tested on the USMLE. In general, though, as the size of the tumor and the number of involved lymph nodes increase, the stage becomes higher and the overall prognosis worsens.

### Follow-up Management

- Radiation of tumor mass
- Repeat calcium level
- Continue normal saline and bisphosphonates (e.g., pamidronate)

### Final Diagnosis

Squamous cell lung cancer/superior vena cava syndrome

## CASE 6

### Chief Complaint

"I feel a lump in my left breast."

### History and Physical Examination

A 52-year-old nulliparous woman finds a lump in the left breast while doing a self-exam. The mass is hard but not tender. She had her first menstrual period at age 12 and has been postmenopausal for 3 years. Her last mammogram was 1 year ago. Her mother had a history of breast cancer diagnosed at age 70. She has 3 sisters, all of whom are in good health.

Physical examination shows a 3-cm movable mass in the retroareolar region of the left breast. The mass is nontender. There is no nipple discharge, retraction, or dimpling. The skin above the lesion appears normal. Axillary examination on the left reveals a few small lymph nodes that are freely movable. The right breast is free of masses. Her lungs are clear, and her abdomen is soft without hepatosplenomegaly. Neurologic examination is nonfocal.

### Differential Diagnosis

1. Benign cystic disease
2. Breast carcinoma
3. Metastatic disease to the breast
4. Fibroadenoma of the breast
5. Intraductal papilloma

### Initial Management

**Setting:** outpatient

### Diagnostic/Therapeutic Plan

- Mammography
- Needle biopsy

**CCS NOTE**

Always ask for an oncology consult when you have an oncology patient needing chemotherapy.

### Test Results

- 3.5-cm mass with irregular borders in retroareolar region of left breast; no other lesions seen in either breast
- Needle biopsy: invasive ductile carcinoma; estrogen receptor; progesterone receptor-positive

### Assessment

The routine detection of breast mass on examination is the most common presentation of breast cancer. Differentiation between malignant and benign disease is crucial. Malignant disease is characterized on examination by irregular borders, being fixed to fascia, skin dimpling, and nipple discharge. Bloody cysts should always be investigated. Mammograms are used to rule out other lesions that are not palpable. A normal mammogram does not obviate the need for biopsy of a suspicious solid mass.

Mammography should be done even though you need a breast biopsy for 2 reasons. The first is to see if there is bilateral disease. The second is to see if there is more than 1 location of breast cancer in the same breast. Multifocal breast cancer means you cannot do a lumpectomy with radiation. Mammography should be done before the breast biopsy because the biopsy damages the architecture of the breast.

### Further Management

- Sentinel lymph node biopsy
- HER2/Neu antigen

**CLINICAL PEARL**

Do mammogram first, then biopsy next. The mammogram comes before the biopsy because biopsy would alter the mammogram.

### Test Results

- Sentinel lymph node biopsy: positive
- HER2/Neu antigen: positive

### Discussion

Breast cancer will affect approximately 12% of women in the United States, and 3.5% will die of the disease. It is the leading cause of death among American women age 40–55.

Family history is an important risk factor. Its significance increases with the number of immediate relatives involved, bilateral disease, and their age at onset. The risk may approach 50% if both mother and sister had disease age <50. However, 75% of breast cancer patients do not have a relative with a history of breast cancer.

Another major risk factor is number of ovulatory cycles a woman undergoes. Early menarche and late menopause are associated with increased risk due to increased lifetime exposure to estrogen. High-dose oral contraceptives and estrogen replacement may be associated with increased risk because of estrogen exposure, but lower-dose estrogen preparations are not clearly shown to increase risk. Nulliparity also carries increased risk.

A history of fibrocystic disease is not considered a risk factor.

Screening has shown to be of greatest benefit in women age >50, but whether to start screening at age 40 or 50 is still considered controversial and many physicians recommend this to their patients.

| | |
|---|---|
| **Stage I** | Tumors <2 cm without lymph node disease |
| **Stage II** | Lesions >2 and/or lymph node involvement |
| **Stage III** | Locally advanced disease including inflammatory breast cancer |
| **Stage IV** | Metastatic disease; primary sites of metastases include bone, lung, pleura, liver, and the CNS |

Sentinel lymph node biopsy is performed to see if an axillary dissection is necessary. A dye is injected into the operative site. The first node to pick up the dye is the "sentinel" node. If there is no cancer in it, then a further lymph node dissection is not needed.

Treatment for local disease is modified radical mastectomy and axillary dissection or lumpectomy and axillary dissection followed by radiation therapy to the involved field. These 2 options are associated with the same overall survival. For tumors >1 cm, adjuvant chemotherapy is given to reduce the risk of recurrence by approximately 30%. The most common regimen is doxorubicin, cyclophosphamide, docetaxel. Stage II disease is more difficult to manage and usually requires preoperative (neoadjuvant) chemotherapy/radiation therapy to create a resectable disease. Stage IV disease is incurable with standard chemotherapy. Research has shown that high-dose chemotherapy with autologous bone marrow rescue actually worsens survival. Chemotherapy and radiation therapy are used in this setting for palliative purposes.

**Therapies which lower mortality in breast cancer:**

- Surgical removal: either mastectomy or lumpectomy with breast radiation
- Tamoxifen or raloxifene (selective estrogen receptor modifiers) for premenopausal women
- Aromatase inhibitors (anastrazole, letrozole) for postmenopausal women
- Anti-HER2/Neu (trastuzumab +/– pertuzumab)
- Chemotherapy

### CLINICAL PEARL

- Screening with mammography has been shown to be most effective age >50; however, this is a controversial topic among various groups. Many physicians still initiate screening at age 40. You will not be tested on controversial topics because there is no one right answer.
- Lumpectomy with radiation is equally as effective as modified radical mastectomy.
- There is a higher rate of focal recurrence when lumpectomy is used, but overall outcomes are unchanged.
- Adjuvant therapy:
  - Breast cancer in premenopausal women is aggressive; therefore, treatment is usually chemotherapy after removal of the tumor
  - Breast cancer in post-menopausal women should be treated with aromatase inhibitors if estrogen-receptors are positive; if receptors are negative, chemotherapy is used as adjuvant treatment

## Follow-up Management

- Lumpectomy with lymph node dissection with radiation (breast and axillary area)
- Adjuvant chemotherapy
- Trastuzumab with HER2/Neu positive persons
- Tamoxifen or aromatase inhibitors for either ER or PR positive persons for 5–10 yrs

## Final Diagnosis

Breast cancer, stage II

# CASE 7

## Chief Complaint

"I want to be checked out for cancer."

## History and Physical Examination

A 52-year-old woman comes to the office stating that her sister was recently diagnosed with breast cancer and so she wants to be tested for cancer. She reached menarche at age 10 and is now premenopausal. She has had no pregnancies. In addition to her younger sister, an aunt was diagnosed with breast cancer. Her mother died secondary to ovarian cancer, and a grandfather had a history of colon cancer.

Upon examination her BP is 110/70 mm Hg and pulse 80/min. She is anxious. Rectal exam shows guaiac-negative stool. Breast exam shows no palpable masses and no axillary adenopathy.

## Initial Management

**Setting:** outpatient

### CCS NOTE

The case simulations will likely focus more on the prevention of cancer than on the specific treatment of individual cancers.

## Diagnostic/Therapeutic Plan

- Screening mammography
- Colonoscopy
- Pap smear

## Test Results

- No abnormalities
- Colonoscopy: single polyp removed, 1 cm, benign pathology
- Pap: low-grade squamous intraepithelial lesion (SIL)

## Assessment

In patients who have several family members with breast or ovarian cancer, the possibility of a familial cancer syndrome is raised. **BRCA-1** refers to a genetic mutation in a DNA repair gene that is associated with increased risk for both breast and ovarian cancer; it is transmitted in an autosomal dominant fashion. It is associated with early-onset disease with a penetrance of 85% by age 70.

The management of what to do when the BRCA gene is positive is not clear. Prophylactic tamoxifen reduces the risk of cancer by 50% and should be considered where there are 2 first-degree relatives with breast cancer. An overall survival advantage for prophylactic bilateral mastectomy over rigorous screening in BRCA-1 mutated patients has yet to be shown.

**CCS NOTE**

The exam will likely expect you to follow the U.S. Preventive Health Services Task Force (USPSTF) recommendations for standard of care, but these sometimes differ from individual specialty guidelines. The exam does not follow individual recommendations from private or for-profit organizations.

Lynch syndrome is associated with hereditary non-polyposis colorectal cancer (HNPCC), endometrial cancer, and ovarian cancer. Li-Fraumeni syndrome is related to inherited abnormalities in the p53 tumor-suppressor gene and is associated with early breast cancer, soft-tissue sarcoma, brain tumors, adrenal cortical cancer, and leukemia. There are guidelines in place for how to screen patients with a strong family history of HNPCC (Amsterdam criteria), but these are beyond the scope of USMLE testing.

The patient described here has several risk factors for breast cancer. In addition to her family history, she has a history of early menarche, late menopause, and nulliparity. Her examination and mammogram do not suggest the presence of a malignancy. A Pap smear of low-grade SIL usually requires immediate colposcopy to evaluate a possible lesion. However, because many of these lesions spontaneously regress, some physicians favor a repeat Pap smear in 6 mos. If several repeat tests are normal, then the Pap is done every 2–3 yrs.

### Further Management Plan/Results

- Colposcopy: normal

### Discussion

There is general agreement that women age >50 should undergo mammography yearly, but many physicians will still initiate screening at age 40.

Cervical cancer is associated with multiple sexual partners and early promiscuity. The etiologic agent is HPV virus. Pap smear screenings and vaccination strategies have shown a major impact on incidence and mortality. Screening should start at age 21 and be performed yearly. Following 3 normal examinations, in some settings, Pap can be performed every 3 yrs and can generally be discontinued age >65.

The interval between screenings can be increased to every 5 yrs at age 30–65 if HPV testing is also done. The age of onset of sexual activity no longer matters.

Prostate-specific antigen (PSA) testing is no longer recommended routinely. PSA screening in the average-risk patient does not improve mortality and may even worsen it because of the morbidity derived from biopsy and surgical management.

| | Starting Age | Frequency | Ending Age |
|---|---|---|---|
| **Mammography** | 50 | Yearly | 70 |
| **Pap Smear** | 21 | Every 3 yrs or every 5 yrs with HPV testing | 65 |
| **Colonoscopy** | 50 | Every 10 yrs | None |

### Follow-up Management

- Repeat Pap smear in 6 mos
- Follow up colonoscopy in 3 to 5 yrs
- Repeat mammogram in 1 year

### Final Diagnosis

Cancer screening in average risk patients

# CASE 8

## Chief Complaint

"I have blood in my stool."

## History and Physical Examination

A 76-year-old man comes to the office for pre-operative evaluation of a mass found on the left side of his colon. The patient came to attention several weeks ago because of fever. His blood cultures grew *Clostridium septicum*, which elicited referral for colonoscopy, the results of which showed the left-sided mass. Biopsy of the mass showed adenocarcinoma of the colon.

Physical examination reveals an alert older man in no distress. T is 98° F, pulse 86/min, BP 112/72 mm Hg. Chest is clear and abdomen is soft and non-tender. Cardiovascular exam is normal.

## Differential Diagnosis

1. Colon cancer: local
2. Colon cancer: metastatic
3. Hereditary non-polyposis colorectal cancer (HNPCC)

## Initial Management

**Setting:** outpatient

## Diagnostic/Therapeutic Plan

- Abdominal CT
- Carcinoembryonic antigen (CEA)
- Surgical consultation
- Oncology consultation
- CBC
- PT and aPTT

## Test Results

- Abdominal CT: lesion limited to colon, no invasion of surrounding tissue; no liver or lung metastases; surrounding nodes are normal in size
- CEA: elevated
- CBC: hematocrit 32%, MCV 76 fl (low)
- PT and aPTT: normal

### Assessment

When you find colon cancer that is local to the colon without metastases, you have a definite chance of a real cure. Colonoscopy is meant to find cancers before they either spread locally into the surrounding lymph nodes or more distantly into the liver, lungs, brain or bone. When cancer is found early without spread to the nodes, cure by primary resection is possible without the need for diverting colostomy.

*Clostridium septicum* and *Streptococcus bovis* are 2 organisms frequently associated with colonic pathology, and when they are found, should always lead to an automatic colonoscopy. The CEA in this case is not to diagnose colon cancer, but to be used to follow the response to treatment. Resection of the cancer and adjuvant chemotherapy should result in a decrease in the CEA level.

It is understandable that the person has microcytic anemia when presenting with blood in the stool. Although you should order surgical and oncologic consultation on CCS, do not expect any consultant to make a specific recommendation.

### Further Management

- Colectomy (partial or complete)
- Screening of family members

### Discussion

With a family history of colon cancer, perform colonoscopy in the children by age 40 or 10 yrs earlier than the age at which the cancer occurred in the source patient. The interval should be every 10 yrs when the family member was age ≥60 when they developed the cancer. If the source patient had the cancer age <60, the family members should be screened every 5 yrs.

HNPCC is when there are 3 family members with colon cancer in at least 2 generations and one person had it prematurely (which is age <50). In HNPCC, screening colonoscopy should start at age 25 and be done every 1 to 2 yrs.

Risks for colon cancer also include the presence of a family history or a familial syndrome, such as familial adenomatous polyposis (FAP) where the incidence for malignancy approaches 100% by age 50. In FAP screening, sigmoidoscopy should begin at age 12, and when malignancy is seen a total colectomy is recommended. Current recommendations for normal risk patients include yearly testing for fecal occult blood, which reduces mortality by 30 to 40%, and flexible sigmoidoscopy every 3–5 yrs. Sigmoidoscopy can miss up to 50% of cancers that are more proximal. Colonoscopy can be used instead of the sigmoidoscopy every 10 yrs. Patients with a polyp identified should undergo a colonoscopy with a repeat 3 to 5 yrs later. Stool heme testing should start at age 50 and be performed every year.

With IBD, screening colonoscopy should be done after 8 yrs of involvement of the colon. This is with either Crohn's disease or ulcerative colitis.

**CCS NOTE**

On CCS, you cannot physically move the patient to the operating room, but you can order the procedure you feel is needed. USMLE Step 3 is a test of general medicine. It will consider that you know to screen the family members as a more important action step than a specific operative technique. The patient's children should all be screened by age 40.

### Follow-up Management and Prevention

**Summary of colon cancer screening:**

- **General population:** begin age 50, every 10 yrs colonoscopy
- **One family member:** begin age 40, every 10 yrs colonoscopy
- **Three family members:** (HNPCC) begin age 25, yearly
- **FAP:** begin age 12, yearly

Adjuvant chemotherapy after colectomy to remove micrometastases

Repeat CEA

### Final Diagnosis

Colon cancer

# CASE 9

## Chief Complaint

"I'm tired and my belly hurts."

## History and Physical Examination

A 55-year-old, generally healthy man comes to the office for a follow-up visit of fatigue and left upper quadrant abdominal pain. The fatigue has been slowly progressive over several weeks. On his last visit, CBC showed WBC 157,000 $mm^3$, hematocrit 31%, and slightly elevated platelet count.

His BP is 110/70 mm Hg and pulse 75/min. He is afebrile. The chest is clear to auscultation. Cardiovascular examination is normal. The abdomen shows fullness in the left upper quadrant.

## Differential Diagnosis

1. Chronic lymphocytic leukemia (CLL)
2. Chronic myelogenous leukemia (CML)
3. Acute leukemia

## Initial Management

**Setting:** outpatient

## Diagnostic/Therapeutic Plan

- Differential of WBC
- Peripheral smear
- Abdominal U/S
- PCR for BCR/ABL (Philadelphia chromosome translocation of 9:22)

## Test Results

- 95% neutrophils
- Peripheral smear normal, no blasts
- Enlarged spleen
- PCR for BCR/ABL present

## Assessment

Chronic fatigue is a nonspecific finding, and a CBC to exclude anemia is always a good place to start. Elevated WBC in an afebrile, generally healthy person can be CML, CLL, or on occasion a reactive elevation to another infectious/inflammatory condition.

Acute leukemia can cause a high, low, or normal WBC. It would be highly unlikely for acute leukemia to be the cause of an isolated elevation in WBC without abnormalities of the other cell lines. CLL is usually seen in patients age >60, and it is easy to diagnose with the differential on the CBC. The smear is great to exclude acute leukemia when there are no blasts seen. The smear CML often shows a left-shifted pattern, with myelocytes at various stages of maturation (myelocytes, metamyelocytes, etc.).

Sonography of the abdomen is important with the abdominal pain. CML often causes LUQ abdominal pain from spleen enlargement (splenomegaly). Oftentimes, the patient 'feels full' even though a small meal has been eaten. This is caused by the spleen pressing on the stomach.

The leukocyte alkaline phosphatase (LAP) score is not typically needed to tell the difference between leukemia and a reactive high WBC. LAP is elevated in a high WBC count that is caused by infection. LAP score is low in leukemia because the cells are abnormal. Instead of LAP score, we can do the PCR for the BCR/ABL mutation.

### Further Management Plan/Results

| | |
|---|---|
| Bone marrow biopsy | Infiltration with large numbers of normal-appearing neutrophils (<20% of total) |

### Discussion

CML is treated with imatinib, a highly effective tyrosine-kinase inhibitor. Imatinib has largely eliminated the need for bone marrow transplantation. It is one of the great miracles of medicine for those with CML. It takes death and transforms it to life.

CML had formerly been a disease with near 100% need for transplantation by 5 yrs after diagnosis. CML has the highest rate of transformation to acute leukemia of any form of leukemia.

Imatinib is a pill with minimal adverse effects. It has the ability to eliminate the Philadelphia chromosome entirely in 60% of patients. Some 98% of patients achieve hematologic control with imatinib, so bone marrow transplant is seldom used. (Thus, bone marrow transplant is never the best initial therapy.)

The fundamental defect in CML is the Philadelphia chromosome, which is a translocation in genetic material between chromosomes 9 and 22. When they fuse into a new chromosome, the junction point is known as the BCR/ABL region. These are the most specific tests for CML. The BCR/ABL produces tyrosine kinase, which drives the proliferation of the malignant cells. Imatinib inhibits the tyrosine kinase produced by the Philadelphia chromosome or BCR/ABL and usually puts the patient into remission. Other, newer agents such as dasatinib, nilotinib, and ponatinib exist, but the first-line treatment is currently imatinib.

### Follow-up Management

- Imatinib (Gleevec)
- Bone marrow transplantation (curative but generally done only for the few patients not controlled by imatinib or another tyrosine kinase inhibitor)
- If acute leukostasis reaction develops, e.g., shortness of breath, blurry vision, or confusion, then leukapheresis can be used.

### Final Diagnosis

Chronic myelogenous leukemia

#### CLINICAL PEARL

**CML**

- High WBC with normal-appearing neutrophils and maturing neutrophils in peripheral blood
- Philadelphia chromosome and BCR/ABL are present
- Treat with the tyrosine kinase inhibitor, imatinib
- Bone marrow transplantation is curative if non-responsive to tyrosine-kinase inhibitors

#### CLINICAL PEARL

**CLL**

- Exclusively in older patients
- High WBC count that is all lymphocytes
- Smear is generally normal, except for "smudge" cells, which are essentially an artifact
- Treat with fludarabine, rituximab, cyclophosphamide, bendamustine, or chlorambucil

# Endocrinology 8

## CASE 1

### Chief Complaint

Lower abdominal pain, dysuria, weakness, and lethargy for 2 days

### History and Physical Examination

A 17-year-old girl comes to the emergency department with lower abdominal pain, increasing weakness, and lethargy for 2 days. Her family has noticed a decreased appetite, nausea, and vomiting. For the last month they have also noticed that the patient has been complaining of being thirsty, going to the bathroom to urinate constantly, and losing weight.

Her T is 37.8 C (100.0 F), BP 100/70 mm Hg, pulse 130/min, and respirations 32/min. She is ill appearing and lethargic. She answers questions with difficulty but appropriately. Physical examination shows a fruity odor on her breath, dry oral mucosa, a supple neck, no jugular venous distension, equally round and reactive pupils, and clear lungs. The heart has a regular rhythm and is tachycardic. The suprapubic abdomen is tender to deep palpation. Neurologic examination shows no obvious focal deficits.

### Differential Diagnosis

1. Diabetic ketoacidosis (DKA): patient has signs and symptoms of diabetes mellitus (DM), including polydipsia, polyuria, and weight loss; DKA is often the initial presentation of type 1 DM in young adults; it can present with intravascular volume depletion and altered mental status
2. Meningoencephalitis: presents with altered mental status and fever; most common causes in United States are herpes simplex virus and West Nile virus; the presence of polyuria, polydipsia and weight loss in preceding month argue against this diagnosis
3. Sepsis secondary to UTI: can present with fever and altered mental status, but seen almost exclusively in older adult patients
4. Abdominal infection: appendicitis can present with fever, nausea/vomiting, and abdominal pain; the presence of other symptoms for the past 1 month makes this acute diagnosis less likely
5. Drug overdose: usually does not present with fever, however should always be ruled out in young adults presenting with altered mental status

**CLINICAL PEARL**

Breath that has a fruity odor is caused by acetone and suggests ketoacidosis.

### Initial Management

**Setting:** emergency department

### CCS NOTE

The Step 3 exam requires you to learn diagnostic tests **and** treatment plans, as well as the order in which they are performed. In a tachycardic patient with nausea and vomiting, IV fluids should always be included in the initial set of orders.

### Diagnostic/Therapeutic Plan

- Plasma glucose, serum electrolytes, serum creatinine and BUN; CBC with differential
- Urine studies: urinalysis, urine culture, urine ketones, beta hCG
- Arterial blood gas
- EKG
- Toxicology screen
- Monitor vital signs; start $O_2$ via nasal cannula; start IV hydration with normal saline +/− IV antibiotics
- CT abdomen/pelvis (but not needed in this case)
- Lumbar puncture no longer needed

### Test Results

- Biochemical profile: sodium 130 mEq/L (normal: 135–145 mEq/L), potassium 5.5 mEq/L (normal: 3.5–5.2 mEq/L), chloride 100 mEq/L (normal: 96–108 mEq/L), bicarbonate 7.5 mEq/L (normal: 20–24 mEq/L), BUN/creatinine 65 mg/dL / 2.5 mg/dL (normal: 10–20 mg/dL / 0.6–1.2 mg/dL), glucose 490 mg/dL (normal: 80–120 mg/dL)
- CBC: WBC 15.9 with 90% neutrophils on differential
- Urinalysis: WBCs 60, +leukocyte esterase, +glucose, +ketones; beta hCG negative; urine culture pending
- Arterial blood gas: pH 7.26, $pCO_2$ 16 mm Hg, $pO_2$ 128 mm Hg, $HCO_{3-}$ 7.5 mm Hg
- EKG: sinus tachycardia
- Toxicology screen: negative

### Assessment

### CCS NOTE

Severe metabolic acidosis with a very low serum bicarbonate is an indication for placing the patient into the ICU.

The history suggests that the patient has new onset diabetes. She has polyuria, polydipsia, and weight loss for 1 month. The patient now presents to the ED because the disease has suddenly progressed to acute illness with abdominal pain and altered mental status. Labs show a severe anion gap metabolic acidosis with urinary ketones, supporting a diagnosis of ketoacidosis. The patient also has hyperglycemia and glucosuria, supporting a diagnosis of diabetes, likely type 1. As a result of the hyperosmolar diuresis and nausea/vomiting, the patient also has intravascular volume depletion, which induced acute kidney injury.

The patient is in DKA, life-threatening condition.

A common precipitant of DKA is an infection, which increases the body's insulin requirement. In this case, the patient's UTI was likely the cause. Symptoms of severe diabetic ketoacidosis include altered mental status which can progress to coma, as well as nausea, vomiting, abdominal pain, and hyperventilation.

The differential diagnosis for altered mental status is broad and includes metabolic, infectious, toxic, endocrine, and neurologic causes. A careful history and physical exam can aid in narrowing down which tests are initially ordered in the workup.

### Basic Science Correlate

DKA is primarily a complication of type 1 DM. It can result from omission of insulin or medical illness. The condition can develop in a matter of hours if a patient has complete insulin deficiency. Because it occurs rapidly, glucose levels are typically lower than those seen in hyperosmolar nonketotic coma, which occurs in uncontrolled type 2 DM and may be subacute in presentation. Insulin normally inhibits hormone-sensitive lipase. Uninhibited, hormone-sensitive lipase releases fatty acids, which are then converted to acetyl CoA, which is converted to ketone bodies in the liver. Even a small amount of endogenous insulin can prevent this process. (Since type 2 DM patients usually have some degree of endogenous insulin production, DKA is rarely a complication for them.)

However, ketosis-prone type 2 diabetes ("Flatbush diabetes") is increasingly recognized. Patients are type 2 diabetics who present with DKA due to glucose toxicity of the beta-cells from severe hyperglycemia. They have variable periods of insulin-dependence and independence, and can go into DKA when they have severe insulin deficiency. Insulin therapy is required until the DKA is resolved to suppress lipolysis and ketogenesis and the beta cells are no longer toxic. Antibodies for type 1 diabetes should be sent for assessment, as should beta cell reserve with c-peptide weeks to months after the DKA. If the c-peptide is more than 1 ng/mL, beta-cell function is preserved; insulin should be stopped and metformin and lifestyle modification started.

Late autoimmune diabetes in adults can be seen. Think of this in lean patients age 35-50 with a personal or family history of autoimmune disease. Glutamic acid decarboxylase (GAD65), tyrosine phosphatases IA-2, islet cell, insulin, and zinc transporter antibodies should be checked to confirm the diagnosis. Many patients with type 1 DM have celiac sprue, vitiligo, primary adrenal failure, or thyroid disease.

- The primary mechanism for hyperglycemia is increased hepatic gluconeogenesis. Glucagon and epinephrine are the hormonal signals that increase gluconeogenesis. In an insulin-deficient state, glucagon and epinephrine are increased. There is also some degree of glycogenolysis from the liver, but this is short lived.
- Acidosis and electrolyte abnormalities can be life-threatening by inducing cardiac arrhythmias. Total body potassium is usually low, though initially the serum potassium may appear normal to high because of the metabolic acidosis (transcellular shift of K+ out of cell for H+ into cell). Phosphorus and magnesium may also be depleted.

### CLINICAL PEARL

A mnemonic to recall the differential diagnosis of altered mental status without focal neurological deficits in decreasing order of frequency is **DIM**:

- **D**rugs (adverse effects or overdose)
- **I**nfections
- **M**etabolic (sodium, glucose, calcium, renal)

## Further Management

- Admit patient to ICU
- Use aggressive fluid resuscitation with crystalloids (0.9% normal saline); change fluids to D5 1/2NS once glucose level falls to <250 mg/dL
- Give bolus of regular insulin, then start insulin drip and continue until anion gap is closed; then give dose of subcutaneous insulin before stopping drip and continue with subcutaneous insulin
- Monitor glucose and electrolytes ($K^+$, $Mg^{2+}$, $PO^{4-}$) every 2–4 hours and replete as needed; add $K^+$ to fluids to keep up with replacement; if serum K <3.3 mEq/L, do not start insulin but rather give IV potassium chloride 20-30 mEq/L until ≥3.3 mEq/L; if K normal (3.3-5.2 mEq/L), add K to the IVFs to prevent hypokalemia

### CCS NOTE

With severe hyperglycemia, the osmolality of the extracellular fluid rises and water shifts to the extracellular space, causing a decrease in the sodium concentration. Serum sodium decreases by 1.6 mEq/L for every 100 mg/dL of glucose **above normal**. There is no net change in total body water, and when the glucose is corrected, the sodium concentration will return to normal.

- Check blood cultures
- Check blood for ketones
- Check hemoglobin A1c (so there is a baseline)
- Start antibiotics for UTI

**CLINICAL PEARL**

Insulin will move glucose and phosphate into the cell simultaneously. Additionally, as the acidosis improves, serum $K^+$ will decrease. Severe hypokalemia or hypophosphatemia can cause respiratory paralysis. Monitor and replace these electrolytes aggressively.

### Discussion

Type 1 DM compromises 5% of all diabetes. It is caused by autoimmune destruction of the insulin secreting pancreatic beta cells, possibly triggered by a viral infection. Additionally, HLA susceptibility genes found in regions on chromosome 6 may play a role. It usually presents with DKA.

Type 1 DM usually presents with DKA. The patient may have an antecedent history of fatigue, polyuria, polydipsia, polyphagia, dehydration, and blurry vision. DKA can be precipitated by an acute infection or severe stress. Symptoms include nausea/vomiting, altered mental status, and abdominal pain (but do serial abdominal exams first, and a CT only if tenderness and pain persist after the DKA has resolved).

DKA is a life-threatening complication of type 1 DM and it is usually managed in an ICU setting. Management involves aggressive fluid resuscitation, replacement of insulin and electrolytes, and treatment of any underlying infection.

**CCS NOTE**

When there is evidence of infection (e.g., fever) and WBC in the urine, always begin antibiotics before obtaining the results of the urine culture.

### Follow-up Management and Prevention

Long-term treatment for type 1 DM is insulin. This usually consists of long-acting basal insulin administered 1× a day and ultra-short-acting insulin given prior to meals. Alternatively, a subcutaneous insulin pump may be used for continuous infusion, with the ability to bolus for meals or during increased periods of stress.

These regimens allow for more precise control of blood glucose and avoidance of hypoglycemia. Fasting and pre-meal target glucose is 80–130 mg/dL. Postprandial levels should not exceed 180 mg/dL. Goal $HgA_1C$ is <7% in nonpregnant adults with a long-life expectancy, and should be monitored at 3–6 month intervals.

Of note, the "honeymoon" period (in insulin-dependent DM patients) is an initial episode of ketoacidosis followed by a symptom-free interval. Although the patient's insulin requirement during this phase may be minimal, a small amount of insulin should be continued as the disease will progress.

Euglycemic DKA has been seen in patients taking SGLT2 inhibitors. There will be an anion gap metabolic acidosis and ketosis with glucose <250 mg/dL. If ketones are negative, check beta-hydroxybutyrate (BHB) (a common ketone but is not tested in serum or urine ketones). In high stress states, catecholamines can convert ketones to BHB.

### Final Diagnosis

Diabetic ketoacidosis

# CASE 2

## Chief Complaint

Confusion

## History and Physical Examination

A 49-year-old obese man is brought to the emergency department by his wife because he is "not himself." He was very drowsy and not eating much for the last 4 days. He was making urine every hour and was drinking water because he felt thirsty. His wife had not noticed any fever, chills, nausea, or vomiting. He was known to be hypertensive for 10 years and takes hydrochlorothiazide. About 2 years ago he was told by his doctor that he had borderline diabetes mellitus and was started on a diet. No medications were prescribed at that time.

On examination today his T is 37.7 C (99.9 F), BP 100/60 mm Hg, pulse 110/min with orthostasis, and respirations 20/min. $SpO_2$ is 98% on room air. He appears very lethargic. He is arousable but responds incoherently to questions. He orients only to his name, and has no idea where he is or who his wife is. Lung examination is normal with good air entry. Heart exam shows tachycardia, but a normal rhythm without a murmur. There are no focal neurologic signs, and the rest of the physical examination is unremarkable.

## Differential Diagnosis

1. Hyperosmolar hyperglycemic nonketotic syndrome (HHNS)
   - A complication of type 2 DM; presents with altered mental status and intravascular volume depletion; plasma osmolality is typically >320 mosm/kg and plasma glucose >600 mg/dL in the absence of serum ketones and metabolic acidosis
2. Other metabolic etiologies: electrolyte disorders: hypercalcemia and hyper/hyponatremia
   - In particular, severe hypercalcemia also presents with altered mental status and profound volume depletion; other diagnoses include hypoxia/hypercapnia, hyper/hypothyroidism, hepatic encephalopathy, uremic encephalopathy, and drug intoxication or withdrawal.
3. Infections: sepsis secondary to a UTI, pneumonia and encephalitis/meningitis
   - Oftentimes, an infection alone can present with altered mental status but infection can also precipitate HHNS; an infectious workup should always be pursued
4. Stroke
   - Less likely given altered mental status without other focal abnormalities
5. Structural lesion: brain tumor or abscess

### CCS NOTE

The **least crucial part** of the CCS is the Final Diagnosis. A correct clinical process is preferred over a correct but rushed diagnosis. You will never lose points for getting a sodium, glucose, or calcium level in a delirious patient.

### Initial Management Plan

**Setting:** emergency department

### Diagnostic/Therapeutic Plan

- Electrolytes, glucose, BUN, creatinine, serum osmolality, LFTs, thyroid function tests, ammonia level
- CBC with differential
- Urinalysis
- Lumbar puncture
- Chest x-ray
- CT head without contrast
- Urine drug screen

### Test Results

- Sodium 130 mEq/L, potassium 5.2 mEq/L, chloride 95 mEq/L, bicarbonate 24 mEq/L, BUN/creatinine 58 mg/dL/2.2 mg/dL, glucose 998 mg/dL, serum osmolality 336 mOsm/kg, calcium 9.8 mg/dL, total protein 7.3 g/dL, albumin 4.2 g/dL, AST 13 u/mL, ALT 20 u/mL, total bilirubin 0.3 mg/dL, alkaline phosphatase 71 u/mL, TSH 0.86 mIU/L, ammonia 30 mcg/dL
- WBC 15,000/mm$^3$, hemoglobin 15.5 gm/dL, platelets 354 k/uL; unremarkable differential
- Urinalysis: specific gravity 1.029, 4$^+$ glucose, 2$^+$ protein, no WBCs
- Lumbar puncture normal
- Chest x-ray normal
- CT head non-contrast normal
- Urine drug screen negative

### Assessment

Both diabetic ketoacidosis (DKA) and HHNS are complications of DM, typically type 1 DM and type 2 DM, respectively. Both DKA and HHNS may be associated with altered mental status and dehydration. Patients with DKA have ketones in the serum and urine, an anion gap metabolic acidosis, and a blood pH <7.3. In HHNS, serum and urine ketones are absent, there may be a mild metabolic acidosis (usually none at all), and blood pH is >7.3. Additionally, patients with HHNS have very high blood sugars, often above 600 mg/dL, which cause an osmotic diuresis inducing severe intravascular volume depletion.

The patient's lab results support the diagnosis of HHNS. His antecedent history of borderline DM is the key historical clue. He has acute kidney injury, likely pre-renal in origin from extremely high glucose levels. In turn, the high serum glucose has elevated his serum osmolality and is the driver of both the intravascular volume depletion and altered mental status.

The other diagnoses on the differential are effectively ruled out given normal LFTs, calcium, TSH, ammonia, lumbar puncture, CXR, and CT head. Patient does have low serum sodium, but this is falsely low because of hyperglycemia.

#### CCS NOTE

With severe hyperglycemia, the osmolality of the extracellular fluid rises and water shifts to the extracellular space causing a decrease in the sodium concentration. The serum sodium level decreases by 1.6 mEq/L for every 100 mg/dL of glucose above normal.

### Basic Science Correlate

Pre-renal azotemia is characterized by an increase in BUN and plasma creatinine due to decreased blood flow to the kidneys. The decreased blood flow to the kidneys causes increased renin secretion via RAS axis, which in turn increases aldosterone secretion. Aldosterone causes reabsorption of sodium and wasting of potassium and hydrogen ions. This mechanism aims to preserve sodium in order to stabilize the loss of intravascular volume.

## Further Management Plan/Results

1. Initial fluid resuscitation in the ED with large volumes of normal saline intravenously. Admission to general medical ward or ICU depending on patient's status after initial volume resuscitation. Fluid replacement is the cornerstone of HHNS management.
2. Insulin
3. Monitor vital signs and labs closely, especially fingerstick, serum electrolytes, and renal function. Replete electrolytes as needed. Often, potassium can be added to fluids as total body potassium is low from the osmotic diuresis.
4. Search for and treat the underlying cause of the HHNS. As is often the case with DKA, HHNS usually has a precipitating factor (infection, infarction, intoxication, medical noncompliance).
5. Collect blood and urine cultures
6. Check EKG

## Discussion

Type 2 DM is associated with obesity and insulin resistance. It has a strong genetic predisposition. It accounts for approximately 90% of DM cases in the United States. Secondary causes of type 2 DM include Cushing's syndrome, exogenous steroid administration, other medications (thiazides, phenytoin, pentamidine), cystic fibrosis, and chronic pancreatitis.

HHNS is an acute complication of DM that occurs predominantly in patients with type 2 DM. It is characterized by severe hyperglycemia in the absence of significant ketosis. Precipitating factors include noncompliance with treatment, infection, infarction, and other stressors. The pathogenesis is hyperglycemia causing an osmotic diuresis followed by the inability to drink sufficient water to keep up with urinary losses. It is clinically manifested by weakness, polyuria, polydipsia, lethargy, confusion, and coma. From an epidemiological standpoint, the patient is usually an older adult type 2 diabetic.

The diagnosis of HHNS is suggested by profoundly elevated blood glucose (1,000 mg/dL) and serum osmolality (serum osmolality in mOsmol/kg $H_2O$ = 2 [sodium] + BUN/2.8 + serum glucose/18). Acute kidney injury may also be present if the patient is extremely volume-depleted. Serum bicarbonate levels are usually normal (or a mild metabolic acidosis in some cases) and blood pH is >7.3. Serum and urine ketones will be absent.

### CLINICAL PEARL

Coronary artery disease may present in a typical fashion or may be silent in patient with diabetes. 'Silent ischemia' has been associated to cardiac autonomic neuropathy. New-onset uncontrolled hyperglycemia and hyperosmolar hyperglycemic state (with or without the presence of dyspnea) may be a presentation of an acute coronary syndrome in patients with diabetes.

### CCS NOTE

The case simulations do not ask for specific levels of fluids. You can specify either bolus or continuous only. You can repeat the bolus and recheck vital signs.

Chronic complications of DM involve both the micro- and macrovasculature.

- Microvascular complications: retinopathy, nephropathy, neuropathy
- Macrovascular complications: increased risk of MI, stroke, and peripheral vascular disease (treatment is risk-factor control with BP and cholesterol-lowering medications, plus prophylaxis with anti-platelet agents)

Evidence shows that lowering the hemoglobin A1c prevents microvascular complications, but may not prevent macrovascular complications.

Treatment for type 2 DM primarily involves oral hypoglycemic agents. Metformin is considered first-line therapy in all type 2 diabetics. Insulin is usually reserved for patients that remain uncontrolled on multiple oral hypoglycemic agents.

### Follow-up Management and Prevention

Diabetes is a chronic disease. It requires regular monitoring to prevent acute complications (as in this case) as well as micro- and macrovascular complications.

- Monitor hemoglobin every 3–6 mos (goal A1c <7%)
- Monitor BP at every office visit (JNC 8 guidelines suggest goal BP <140/90 mm Hg)
- Statin for all diabetic patients, plus annual lipid monitoring (as per newer cholesterol guidelines)
- Annual dilated eye exam and foot exam
- Annual urine check for the presence of microalbumin (if detected, start an ACEI or ARB should be initiated
- Annual influenza vaccine
- One-time pneumococcal vaccine (repeat 1× if first dose given age <65 and >5 yrs ago)

### Final Diagnosis

Hyperosmolar hyperglycemic nonketotic syndrome

# CASE 3

## Chief Complaint

Increased serum calcium on routine medical evaluation

## History and Physical Examination

A 30-year-old man comes to your office for the evaluation of hypercalcemia, noted on routine tests performed at his workplace. He denies any specific complaints and is not taking any medications. His past medical history is significant for several episodes of renal stones 2 to 3 years ago. Physical examination is unremarkable.

## Differential Diagnosis

1. Primary hyperparathyroidism
2. Malignancy
3. Sarcoidosis
4. Familial hypocalciuric hypercalcemia

## Initial Management

**Setting**: outpatient

## Diagnostic/Therapeutic Plan

- Basic metabolic panel (sodium, potassium chloride, bicarbonate)
- Serum calcium
- Chest x-ray
- Urine calcium

## Test Results

- Basic metabolic panel WNL
- Serum calcium 11.3 mg/dL (normal: 8.5–10.3 mg/dL)
- Chest x-ray normal
- Urine calcium elevated

## Assessment

Most cases of asymptomatic hypercalcemia in young ambulatory patients are caused by primary hyperparathyroidism. Given the history of renal stones 2 years ago, the patient probably has had increased serum calcium for a long time without any other problems. The age of the patient and the benign course of his hypercalcemia make a diagnosis of malignancy less likely, but malignancy should always be ruled out in cases where History and Physical Examination suggest it.

**CCS NOTE**

Asymptomatic patients should always remain out of the hospital. Such patients should be sent home between office visits.

Malignant diseases can lead to hypercalcemia via parathyroid hormone-related proteins or by bone metastases. Other causes of hypercalcemia include drugs (thiazides, lithium), granulomatous diseases (sarcoidosis), thyrotoxicosis, and immobilization.

Familial hypocalciuric hypercalcemia is a benign condition that can be diagnosed by checking urinary calcium levels (<200 mg/24 h) combined with a family history of similar conditions and normal parathyroid hormone levels.

### Further Diagnostic Plan/Results

| | |
|---|---|
| Immunoassay for serum parathyroid hormone | 22 mEq/mL (normal: 4–9 mEq/mL) |

### Treatment Plan

- Parathyroidectomy (because of young age and history of kidney stones)

### Discussion

The higher level of parathyroid hormone is in favor of primary hyperparathyroidism. About 85% of cases are caused by adenoma of a single gland, 15% are caused by hyperplasia of all 4 glands, and <1% are caused by parathyroid carcinoma.

In an older asymptomatic patient with serum calcium <12 mg/dL, conservative management is an option. The only effective treatment for primary hyperparathyroidism is parathyroidectomy. Many patients have a benign course over the years, but a major concern is the possibility of progressive bone loss, increased risk of fractures, and recurrent nephrolithiasis.

Because this patient has a history of nephrolithiasis and persistently high calcium, surgery is indicated. Surgery has high success rate with low morbidity and mortality. Other indications are age <50, GFR <60 mL/min, urine calcium >400, osteoporosis, and calcium >11.5 mg/dL.

Patients with primary hyperparathyroidism are at high risk for pseudogout. On the exam, if you are asked about a knee effusion, the cause is likely pseudogout.

Acute management of hypercalcemia is warranted when serum calcium >12 mg/dL or when severe symptoms are present. The goal is to alleviate symptoms; it is not necessary to achieve normal serum calcium levels. These measures allow time to complete diagnostic studies and begin treatment of underlying conditions.

Initial management of a patient with very high serum calcium is as follows:

- Replace extracellular fluid volume with 0.9% saline (3–6 L/d in first 24 hrs) to restore glomerular filtration rate and promote calcium excretion
- Once extracellular fluid volume is restored, give IV furosemide 2–4x per day if and only if there is evidence of fluid overload or heart failure
- Closely monitor fluid balance and electrolytes. (Avoid thiazides because they impair calcium excretion and increase serum calcium.).

If hypercalcemia does not improve with fluids, alternative therapies:

- Calcitonin (immediate-acting) if there is decreased CNS function
- Bisphosphonates (longer-acting but long-lasting): zoledronic acid (most potent) and pamidronate
- Dialysis if the hypercalcemia with acute kidney injury

### Further Follow-up

One week later the patient is admitted to the hospital and has successful removal of a single parathyroid adenoma. He is doing well after the surgery and is transferred to the surgical wards. The nurse contacts you 12 hours after the surgery and tells you that the patient has developed facial spasm. You immediately order a calcium level and find it to be 6.4 mg/dL.

**What is the likely diagnosis of the hypocalcemia and what would you do next?** Likely diagnosis is hungry bone syndrome; treatment of hypocalcemia is IV calcium. It is important to check 25-hydroxyvitamin D levels to look for and correct vitamin D deficiency before surgery (to minimize hypocalcemia). Vitamin D deficiency is common. Also, pseudogout is seen after a parathyroidectomy.

### Final Diagnosis

Hypercalcemia secondary to parathyroid adenoma

# CASE 4

## Chief Complaint

"I feel tired all the time."

## History and Physical Examination

A 64-year-old woman comes to your office with complaints of feeling tired all the time for the past 6 months. She was planning to visit you for a while, but has put it off until now. She has gained about 8 pounds over the last 6 months. She does not feel like doing much of anything. She complains of feeling cold and has been using heavy blankets even in the summer. She is constipated, gets frequent headaches, and is experiencing severe muscle cramps. The only good thing she has to report is that her anginal chest pains are less frequent than they used to be. She had only 2 episodes of chest pain in the last 6 months and none in the last 4 months. For her angina she was taking isosorbide dinitrate and a beta-blocker. Her cardiologist had recommended coronary artery bypass graft after cardiac catheterization showed more than 70% obstruction of the left main artery.

Today her BP is 150/100 mm Hg and pulse 50/min. Her skin is dry. There is no thyromegaly. The deep tendon reflexes have a delayed relaxation phase. The rest of the physical examination is unremarkable.

### CCS NOTE

The amount of physical examination performed is initially determined by the history. Examine any area that the patient describes as symptomatic. You can always go back and examine the patient further, such as looking at other organ systems.

## Differential Diagnosis

1. Hypothyroidism

## Initial Management

**Setting:** outpatient work up and treatment

## Diagnostic/Therapeutic Plan

- TSH
- Free T4

## Test Results

- TSH: 49 mU/mL (normal 0.1–5 mU/mL)
- Free T4: 1.5 mg/mL (normal 5–12 mg/mL)

## Assessment

This older adult patient has typical symptoms of hypothyroidism. The weight gain, cold intolerance, and complaint of feeling tired all the time are highly suggestive of hypothyroidism. Cognitive deficits may be seen in the older adult.

The seemingly improving anginal history is not uncommon in hypothyroidism. As the demand for oxygen by the myocardium is diminished, the angina "improves." Dry skin and a puffy face are signs of long-standing hypothyroidism. The diastolic hypertension and the delayed relaxation phase are classical signs of hypothyroidism. The lab tests are diagnostic of primary hypothyroidism.

**Primary hypothyroidism** (cause of hypothyroidism in >95% of cases) is caused by:

- Chronic thyroiditis (Hashimoto's disease), associated with antimicrosomal antibodies (**most common**)
- Post-ablative surgery or radioactive iodine, heritable biosynthetic defects, and iodine deficiency
- Drugs such as lithium and acetylsalicylic acid

Suprathyroid causes of hypothyroidism include pituitary-induced hypothyroidism (**secondary hypothyroidism**) or hypothalamic-induced hypothyroidism (**tertiary hypothyroidism**).

## Further Management Plan

1. Consider bypass surgery **before** correcting thyroid dysfunction
2. Thyroxine replacement

### CCS NOTE

Consultations can be requested at any point in the case simulation, but you will need to provide a reason for the consultation in ≤10 words. The consultants do not tell you how to manage the case; they arrive promptly but say almost nothing.

## Discussion

The presence of CAD here makes this situation more complex. In patients with hypothyroidism, it is preferable to get coronary artery bypass graft done before correcting the thyroid dysfunction with levothyroxine. (Studies have shown that correction with levothyroxine before a graft is not only unnecessary, it is also potentially dangerous. Levothyroxine will increase the heart rate and can potentially aggravate angina/precipitate myocardial infarction.) T3 should never be used. Theoretically, it is more dangerous than levothyroxine. If the patient had no history of angina, she would have been started on 25 mcg of levothyroxine and gradually increased over weeks until she became clinically and biochemically euthyroid.

The normal function of the thyroid gland is directed toward the secretion of L-thyroxine (T4) and triode-L-thyroxine (T3), which regulate metabolic processes. The main secretory hormone of the thyroid is T4, and it is only the free, nonbound-to-protein fraction of T4 and T3 that affects metabolism. This free hormone is <0.01% of the total. Over 99% of the total hormones are bound to thyroid-binding globulin.

Lab tests to measure free T4 and free T3 are now more accessible and give a direct measurement of the metabolic active percentage of the hormone. These are the measurements to look for when assessing thyroid function.

Total T4 or T3 is not always accurate because it measures protein-bound and unbound thyroid hormones. Increased thyroid-binding globulin levels, and thus total T4 levels, are seen in pregnancy and with the use of oral contraceptives (but free or active T4 level is normal). In pregnancy with hypothyroidism, increase levothyroxine by 30% and check TSH every 2 weeks.

Start levothyroxine 25 mcg in patients age >60 and 12.5 mcg in patients with ischemic heart disease.

Decreased thyroid-binding globulin levels, and thus total T4 levels, are also seen in nephrotic syndrome and cirrhosis (but free or active T4 level is normal with the patient being euthyroid).

TSH is probably the most useful test in the diagnosis of hypothyroidism, and should be the first test first when assessing thyroid hormone function, i.e., it is the best screening test for both hyper- and hypothyroidism. Overall, if TSH is normal, then likely the patient is euthyroid. It is also the best test to do when following treatment of thyroid diseases.

In patients with suspected secondary hypothyroidism (e.g., radiation to the head, Sheehan syndrome or hemochromatosis), TSH alone is not enough because they can have a normal TSH, so T4 must also be checked. (On the exam, look for these hints in the question.)

## Final Diagnosis

Hypothyroidism

# CASE 5

## Chief Complaint

Weight loss

## History and Physical Examination

A 44-year-old woman comes to the office complaining of 15-lb weight loss over 3 months. She gives a history of feeling hot and sweaty, and of difficulty sleeping and easy arousability. She also complains of muscle weakness, especially when she tries to climb stairs. She admits to moving her bowels 2–3 times per day for the last 4 months. She has also noticed that her hands tremble all the time and her heart is racing. She is afebrile, blood pressure is 150/90 mm Hg, pulse 112/min, and respirations 16/min.

Upon physical examination she is thin and is very restless. She has a pronounced stare. There is a diffusely enlarged thyroid without any bruit. A very fine tremor of both hands is noted. She is unable to get up from a squatting position without assistance.

### CCS NOTE

The amount of physical examination you choose to perform is based on what you might consider as abnormal. You do not lose points if a test result is normal.

## Differential Diagnosis

1. Grave's disease
2. Toxic multinodular or nodular goiter
3. Subacute thyroiditis

## Initial Management

**Setting:** outpatient work up and treatment

## Diagnostic/Therapeutic Plan

- Serum TSH
- Serum free T4

## Test Results

- TSH <0.1 mU/mL (normal 0.5–5 mU/mL)
- Free T4 6 ng/dL (normal 0.8–2 ng/dL)

## Assessment

This patient has all the symptoms and signs of primary hyperthyroidism due to Grave's disease.

## Further Management Plan/Results

| | |
|---|---|
| 24-hour radioactive iodine uptake scan | 68% (normal: 25–35%) diffuse uptake |

## Treatment Plan

- Beta-blocker and antithyroid drugs (propylthiouracil or methimazole) initially, to suppress the hyperactive thyroid
- After the patient is euthyroid, radioactive iodine ablation for permanent treatment

## Discussion

Treatment for acute thyrotoxicosis is antithyroid medication plus a beta-blocker, to make the patient clinically euthyroid. Once the patient is less toxic, radioactive iodine can be used for permanent resolution of hyperthyroidism.

If radioactive iodine is given during severe hyperthyroidism, that could induce radiation thyroiditis and thus release more thyroxine into the circulation (and here, worsen her condition). Surgery is not an option in the initial treatment of Grave's disease; it is useful only for patients who have a large goiter (causing tracheal compression), who refuse to take radioactive iodine; and who are pregnant.

Radioactive iodine is the main therapeutic option for Grave's disease.

In the United States, the most common cause of hyperthyroidism in young people is Grave's disease. Those with Grave's disease have diffuse thyromegaly and may also have vascular bruit on auscultation because of increased blood supply to the gland. Up to 70% of patients with Grave's have exophthalmos, which is not a feature of any other thyroid disease. The presence of exophthalmos makes the diagnosis certain.

The myopathy described in the patient here is proximal myopathy, which is the most common myopathy in Grave's and in all thyroid disease.

- Plummer's disease patients have long-standing multinodular goiters, which become thyrotoxic later.
- Toxic multinodular goiter patients have a hyperfunctioning solitary nodule, which is not present in this patient.
- Subacute thyroiditis patients have diffuse thyromegaly like our patient, but the thyroid is tender. Subacute thyroiditis patients are differentiated by their short duration of symptoms and low 24-hour radioactive iodine uptake (usually <5%).

## Final Diagnosis

Grave's disease

### CCS NOTE

Organ system-specific consultations should be requested for complex cases. Do not worry if the consultant doesn't offer advice; it still shows that you know when to ask for assistance.

# CASE 6

## Chief Complaint

"I feel thirsty, and I'm urinating a lot."

## History and Physical Examination

A 56-year-old woman with no past medical history comes to your office complaining of polyuria and polydipsia of 4 days duration. She denies dysuria and has no fever or chills. She also admits to a 13-lb weight gain, severe fatigue and depression for the past 4 months. Her skin has also been bruising easily. She denies shortness of breath or chest pain. She takes no medications.

On exam she is afebrile. Her blood pressure is 160/98 mm Hg, pulse 78/min, and respirations 14/min. She is obese and her face is remarkably round and ruddy. There are several purple striae over the abdomen and the thighs. Heart and lung examinations are WNL. Neurologic examination reveals mild bilateral upper extremity weakness. There is mild edema of the lower extremities.

### CCS NOTE

Do not administer emergency therapy to lower BP unless there are symptoms such as shortness of breath, blurred vision, chest pain, or confusion. This patient's BP does not need urgent therapy because the symptoms are unrelated to it.

## Differential Diagnosis

1. Cushing's syndrome: due to prolonged exposure to supraphysiologic levels of cortisol; patients typically have truncal obesity, moon facies, violaceous striae, new onset DM, and hypertension; this patient's presentation strongly suggests hypercortisolism
2. Hypothyroidism: characterized by many of the symptoms this patient displays, including weight gain, fatigue and depression
3. New onset DM: obesity, polyuria and polydipsia suggest diabetes; however, DM does not present with skin bruising

## Initial Management

**Setting**: outpatient work up and treatment

## Diagnostic/Therapeutic Plan

- Glucose level, electrolytes, kidney function, calcium
- CBC
- TSH
- Hemoglobin A1c
- 24-h urine free cortisol excretion
- Overnight 1-mg dexamethasone suppression test (has a lot of false-positives, e.g., with patients who have depression or alcoholism, who are on OCPs, and who are taking carbamazepine)
- Midnight salivary cortisol measurement
- Plasma ACTH
- MRI pituitary gland

### Test Results

- Glucose: 356 mg/dL, sodium: 138 mEq/L, potassium: 3.1 mEq/L, chloride: 95 mEq/L, bicarbonate: 34 mEq/L, BUN: 13 mg/dL, creatinine: 0.7 mg/dL, calcium: 9.8 mg/dL
- CBC: normal
- TSH: normal
- Hemoglobin A1c 8.1%
- 24-h free cortisol secretion: 650 ug/24 hr (normal: <200 ug/24 hr) elevated
- Overnight dexamethasone suppression test: 28 μg/dL (normal: <5 μg/dL) non-supressable
- Midnight salivary cortisol measurement: 24 nmol/mL (normal <4 nmol/L) elevated
- Plasma ACTH: 18 mg/L (normal <5 ng/L)

### Assessment

The patient presents with symptoms suggestive of hypercortisolism. Clinical features include:

- Truncal obesity
- Moon facies (round-shaped face)
- Dorsocervical fat pad (buffalo hump)
- Skin changes such as striae, acne, and bruising
- Osteopenia
- Neuropsychiatric symptoms (emotional lability, depression, psychosis)
- Menstrual irregularities
- Impotence
- Possible new onset DM and hypertension as well

These symptoms and signs are all suggestive of Cushing's syndrome. The diagnostic workup aims to confirm excess cortisol production. There are 3 tests that can confirm the presence of excess cortisol:

- 24-h urine free cortisol
- Midnight salivary cortisol measurement
- Overnight low-dose dexamethasone suppression

If one test is abnormal, it is recommended that a second test be performed to confirm the diagnosis.

This patient has an abnormal result on all 3 tests, which confirm the diagnosis of Cushing's. The next step is to measure plasma ACTH levels, which will differentiate ACTH-dependent hypercortisolism from ACTH-*independent* hypercortisolism.

- If ACTH is elevated as it is here, do an MRI of the sella turcica to confirm the presence on an adenoma. ACTH can also be secreted ectopically (associated with small cell carcinoma of the lung; paraneoplastic syndrome).
- If ACTH is decreased, that would indicate a possible adenoma in the adrenal gland itself, which directly produces cortisol.

**CLINICAL PEARL**

Cushing's syndrome refers to a state of hypercortisolism. However, if a pituitary microadenoma is the cause of the hypercortisolism, the diagnosis is referred to as Cushing's disease.

The electrolyte abnormalities seen in Cushing's syndrome are secondary to increased mineralocorticoid activity that acts to increase the secretion of potassium and H+ in the kidney. This results in hypokalemia and a metabolic alkalosis.

It is important to rule out other causes for the patient's symptoms such as hypothyroidism by measuring a TSH level. Additionally, it is not unreasonable to check a CBC if the patient presents with easy bruising. These test results were normal in the current scenario.

### Basic Science Correlate

The clinical features of Cushing's syndrome are due to excess cortisol. ACTH stimulates the adrenal gland (mostly in the zona fasciculata) to convert cholesterol into cortisol via a series of enzymatic reactions. Cortisol enhances hepatic gluconeogenesis, which produces hyperglycemia. In turn, increased serum glucose causes insulin secretion from the pancreas. Insulin acts to increase the storage of fat in the adipose tissue causing weight gain and obesity.

- The muscle weakness seen in this patient is due to muscle breakdown via cortisol. Amino acids that are derived from the breakdown of muscle are used to supply the liver with the substrates for gluconeogenesis. The muscle breakdown also thins the extremities in these patients.
- Another key sign of excess cortisol production is hypertension, due to increased activation of mineralocorticoids. Mineralocorticoids retain sodium in the kidney, and thus passive reabsorption of water, which acts to increase the effective circulating blood volume and thus increase BP. Additionally, mineralocorticoids act in the kidney to enhance potassium and H+ secretion causing the classic electrolyte abnormalities that are often observed. Of note, aldosterone production requires angiotensin II activity, which is not affected by increased ACTH. Therefore, aldosterone itself is not increased.
- Cortisol secretion normally exhibits a diurnal rhythm. This means that there is a peak and trough of serum cortisol levels every 24 hrs. Typically, cortisol levels reach their peak early in the morning and a trough late at night. In Cushing's there is no diurnal rhythm because cortisol levels are persistently high. Salivary cortisol is in equilibrium with free cortisol levels; therefore, a late night salivary cortisol level will be elevated in Cushing's and can be diagnostically useful.

### Further Diagnostic Plan/Results

| | | |
|---|---|---|
| 1 | Serum ACTH level | Elevated |
| 2 | High-dose dexamethasone | 4 µg/dL (suppressed) |
| 3 | MRI of the pituitary | Positive for microadenoma |

## Further Management Plan

The management for Cushing's disease should include an endocrinology consult.

- Treatment for an ACTH-secreting adenoma is surgical excision. The surgery may be performed transsphenoidally. After surgery, patients are often deficient in ACTH. Therefore, they may require glucocorticoid replacement for up to a year after the removal of the tumor. Patients may also experience residual disease if the tumor was not completely excised. In this case, stereotactic radiosurgery might be indicated.
- Secondary DM and hypertension usually resolve once the underlying cause of the Cushing's syndrome is treated, though a short course of treatment may be necessary to control excessively high BP or glucose levels.

### CCS NOTE

Normal values for diagnostic results are provided in the case simulations. You do not need to memorize them.

## Discussion

The patient in this case presents with signs and symptoms of Cushing's syndrome. The most common cause of Cushing's syndrome is a pituitary adenoma, which overproduces ACTH (Cushing's disease). Resultant excess cortisol production produces a wide variety of clinical symptoms. Importantly, Cushing's syndrome is a cause of both secondary DM and hypertension.

Diagnosis of Cushing's syndrome should begin with tests to identify excess cortisol levels. If any of the 3 initial tests are abnormal, a second confirmatory test should be performed. Once hypercortisolism is established, a search for the underlying cause is conducted.

In this case, the patient was noted to have a pituitary adenoma on MRI. The appropriate treatment will be surgical resection. In cases where a pituitary adenoma is not the cause of excess cortisol production, one must conduct a search for either ectopic ACTH production or a cortisol-producing adrenal adenoma. If ACTH levels are low, perform a CT scan of the adrenal glands to identify a cortisol-producing adenoma. Small cell carcinoma of the lung can produce a paraneoplastic syndrome in which ectopic ACTH is produced.

## Follow-up Management and Prevention

After the underlying cause of the Cushing's syndrome is treated, the patient should continue to be monitored. The patient should have regular BP checks and follow-up labs (hemoglobin A1c, electrolytes, glucose levels). A lipid profile should also be monitored. Temporary pharmacologic treatment of BP and diabetes may be necessary. Additionally, even though the DM in this patient was secondary to another condition, there is still risk for the macrovascular and microvascular complications of DM. Patients also need assessment for osteopenia/osteoporosis with a bone density scan.

## Final Diagnosis

Cushing's disease

# CASE 7

## Chief Complaint

Headache and palpitations

## History and Physical Examination

A 33-year-old woman comes to the office for evaluation of several hours of severe headache, flushing, and palpitations. She recalls several similar episodes in the past, but her symptoms were less severe and of shorter duration. Each of these episodes occurred after going to the bathroom. Her past medical history is significant only for a long history of migraine headaches, which are difficult to control.

She is diaphoretic and anxious-appearing. Her T is 37.0 C (98.6 F), BP is 195/110 mm Hg, respirations are 20/min, and pulse is 138/min. Orthostasis is elicited. Her head, eyes, ears, nose, and throat are unremarkable. Her heart is tachycardiac with normal heart sounds. Her lungs are clear to auscultation, abdomen is benign, and extremities are unremarkable.

## Differential Diagnosis

1. Pheochromocytoma
2. Primary aldosteronism
3. Renal artery stenosis
4. Essential hypertension

**CCS NOTE**

This patient has severe hypertension and symptoms (headache). Therapy to lower BP should be ordered before the results of all specific diagnostic tests are obtained. Phenoxybenzamine is a good choice for pheochromocytoma.

## Initial Management

**Setting**: outpatient or (rarely) emergency department

## Diagnostic/Therapeutic Plan

- 24-hour urine collection for catecholamines
- Plasma free metanephrines

## Test Results

- Increased urine catecholamines
- Increased plasma metanephrines

## Assessment

The clinical presentation of paroxysms of headache, sweating, palpitations, and anxiety attacks in association with labile hypertension is classic for pheochromocytoma. Patients most commonly seek attention in the setting of a hypertensive crisis.

Patients with pheochromocytoma also present with paroxysmal hypertension or sustained hypertension. Signs and symptoms of an increased metabolic rate may include profuse sweating, tachycardia, and weight loss. Supraventricular arrhythmias are commonly seen.

Measurement of 24-hour urine vanillylmandelic acid levels is diagnostic in 95% of cases of pheochromocytoma. CT scan is used to try to identify the exact location of the tumor.

### Further Management Plan/Results

| Abdominal CT scan | Left adrenal mass present |
|---|---|
| Metaiodobenzylguanidine (MIBG) scan to identify extra-adrenal tumors | No evidence of metastatic disease |

### Treatment Plan

1. Alpha-adrenergic antagonist (phentolamine or phenoxybenzamine) until BP is well controlled (besides an alpha-blocker, no other antihypertensives should be used in the initial management to control symptoms (tachycardia, etc.); use a beta-blocker only after BP is stable)
2. Fluid replacement
3. Surgical consultation for resection of the tumor

### Discussion

Fewer than 0.1% of patients with hypertension have an underlying pheochromocytoma. However, in the appropriate clinical setting, this diagnosis should be aggressively pursued because it is a potentially reversible cause of hypertension. Approximately:

- 90% of lesions are unilateral and localized to the adrenals
- 10% are bilateral
- 10% occur extra-adrenally
- 5% are associated with the familial multiple endocrine neoplasia (MEN) 2 and 3 syndromes

Once the diagnosis is established, surgical excision is the treatment of choice. Preoperative management focuses on establishing alpha-adrenergic blockade. Beta-blockers should be given only once alpha-blockade is achieved. Beta-blockers are used in patients with tachycardia only after alpha-blockers are used. Once the pheochromocytoma is removed, flow cytometry is done to detect abnormal DNA in order to predict malignant tumors.

Ambulatory BP monitoring to detect paroxysm of hypertension is necessary only when its diagnosis is not obvious. It is not necessary in this particular case.

### Final Diagnosis

Pheochromocytoma

**CLINICAL PEARL**

- 10% of pheochromocytomas are extra-adrenal
- 10% are malignant
- 10% are seen in children
- 10% are bilateral
- 10% are multiple
- 10% are familial
- Pheochromocytoma also occurs in MEN2

# CASE 8

## Chief Complaint

Follow-up of uncontrolled diabetes

## History and Physical Examination

A 52-year-old man with an 8-year history of type 2 diabetes mellitus is evaluated in your office for poorly controlled diabetes. He has taken glipizide 10 mg daily for the past few years and reports fasting home glucose measurements >180 mg/dL and postprandial measurements 220–260 mg/dL. He reports no hypoglycemic events. His Hb A1C increased from 7.2% to 8.7%. A recent ophthalmic evaluation showed no retinopathy.

He is obese (BMI 30 kg/m$^2$). His BP is 152/90 mm Hg, pulse 72/min and regular, and respirations 12/min. Physical exam shows a normal cardiac and lung exam. Abdominal exam is benign without evidence of hepatosplenomegaly. Foot exam shows normal sensation (assessed by monofilament), normal skin, and normal pulses. The patient asks about his risk of microvascular disease and for ways to better improve glycemic control.

## Differential Diagnosis

1. No specific differential diagnosis here, since we know the patient has diabetes (type 2 diabetes, given the age group and use of oral agents)
2. Issue surrounding a diabetic with worsening glycemic control is whether the patient is non-adherent to the medication or whether it is a failure of the treatment plan

## Initial Management

**Setting**: outpatient

## Diagnostic/Therapeutic Plan

- Add metformin and determine effectiveness of regimen by monitoring A1C (Hb A1C should fall to ≤7.5% over the next 3 months if treatment is effective; eventually the goal of therapy should be an ideal Hb A1C level <6.5–7%) and home glucose monitoring (fasting glucose should be <126 mg/dL).
- If A1C levels do not fall, the patient should be encouraged to start insulin or add a glitazone to metformin and sulfonylureas (this last option is less effective and predisposes the patient to side effects). Adequate glycemic control reduces the risk for microvascular complication (neuropathy, nephropathy, retinopathy).

## Test Results

- Home-glucose monitoring of fasting glucose 100–120 mg/dL; patient reports no hypoglycemic events

### Assessment

Outpatient management of diabetic patients is one of the most common problems faced by primary care and family practice physicians.

In type 2 diabetes, studies have documented that response to monotherapy is limited (in this case, the patient is taking only sulfonylurea) with rates of failure to sulfonylureas of up to 10% per year. So it is expected that this patient will eventually fail sulfonylurea treatment. Some studies have shown that almost 80–90% of patients who have had diabetes for 10 yrs will benefit from insulin (either as monotherapy or added to oral hypoglycemic agents).

In this case, we have a few options: add metformin, add insulin, or add glitazone.

- Metformin works by inhibiting hepatic neoglucogenesis and provides an effective addition to sulfonylureas. It causes no significant weight gain and hypoglycemia is uncommon. It is contraindicated in patients with renal failure since it may cause lactic acidosis.
- Insulin (NPH or glargine) can be used alone or in combination with oral hypoglycemic agents. It may be the most effective treatment in terms of glycemic control, but it causes significant weight gain.
- Thiazolidinediones and glitazones (pioglitazone) are effective as combination therapy with other oral hypoglycemic agents. They cause edema and weight gain (though not as much as insulin and sulfonylureas). Glitazones lower glucose by sensitizing cells to insulin, and they lower triglycerides in the serum (but increase LDL and HDL cholesterol by 10%).
- A GLP-1 agonist or SGLT-2 inhibitor is recommended for all patients with DM and atherosclerotic cardiovascular disease, kidney disease, or heart failure.

There is no 'single best answer,' but given the patient's obesity, metformin may be the best option since insulin will cause weight gain and predispose the patient to hypoglycemic events.

### Further Diagnostic Plan/Results

- Check A1C at 2 mos after adjustment of medication: 7.0%

### Treatment Plan

Continue metformin and sulfonylureas, and monitor A1C and fasting glucose at home.

### Discussion

This patient has a systolic BP of 152 mm Hg and is considered to be hypertensive since he has diabetes. An ACE inhibitor (ACEI) should be initiated to reduce the risk of nephropathy and renal failure.

Increased urinary protein is the earliest marker for diabetic nephropathy and so a specific test for microalbuminuria should be done frequently to assess for early nephropathy (the urine dipstick is insensitive since it becomes positive with proteinuria >300 mg/day). Consistent microalbuminuria >30 mg/d usually indicates early nephropathy, which should be a consideration for an ACEI. ACEIs have been shown to slow the progression to overt proteinuria, as well as slow the increase in creatinine.

**When should an ACEI be started in patients with diabetes?** With either hypertension or microalbuminuria, or both.

Diabetic patients who develop proliferative retinopathy are at increased risk for blindness. Proliferative retinopathy is characterized by the development of new blood vessels on the retinal surface. These new vessels cause traction as they form and may lead to vitreous hemorrhages and retinal detachment. Diabetic retinopathy may be prevented with adequate glycemic control, but once proliferative changes occur, laser photocoagulation is the only way to stabilize the vessels and prevent blindness. Diabetics are also at risk for cataracts and glaucoma, which are also causes of blindness. Screen type 2 diabetic patients for retinopathy once a year from the onset of diabetes!

**When should we refer a new-onset type 2 diabetic patient to the ophthalmologist?** Immediately and then (at least) 1× a year.

Peripheral neuropathy is the most common form of neuropathy seen in diabetics (mononeuropathy and autonomic neuropathy are the other forms). It sometimes manifests as 'pins and needles' and 'numbness' in areas typically covered by gloves and stockings. Early neuropathy may be asymptomatic but can be picked up on microfilament testing by evidence of decreased sensation. Patients with decreased sensation are at risk for limb-threatening infections as well as ischemia.

Nearly 50% of the amputations caused by neuropathy and poor circulation could have been prevented by careful foot care. Do monofilament testing once a year and teach the patient adequate foot care (inspect feet and toes every day for erythema, swelling, calluses, fungal infections; wear shoes or slippers to protect feet from injuries; wear shoes that fit well, etc.). The pain caused by diabetic peripheral neuropathy is treated with amitriptyline and gabapentin.

### CLINICAL PEARL

Outpatient management for type 2 diabetes is as follows:

- Metformin (**first-line treatment**) alone or with sulfonylureas (both contraindicated in those with renal failure)
- Insulin, if oral hypoglycemic agents ineffective
- Monitor effectiveness with A1C and fasting glucose

## Final Diagnosis

Uncontrolled type 2 diabetes

# CASE 9

## Chief Complaint

Galactorrhea

## History and Physical Examination

A 28-year-old woman comes in for the evaluation of milk-like discharge from both breasts for 3 months. She also reports gradual cessation of menses over the past 4–5 months. Until recently, she has had regular menses; her weight and height have been stable. She reports no fatigue and takes no medications or recreational drugs. She has not noticed acne or striae. She reports no headaches or visual disturbances. Other than 2 episodes of UTI a few years ago which were treated effectively with ciprofloxacin, she has no prior history.

Her family history is significant for hypertension and dyslipidemia. Her BP is 110/70 mm Hg, pulse 74/min, and respirations 14/min. Physical examination reveals no visual field defects. Heart and lung exam are normal. There is expressible milk from both breasts but the rest of the breast exam is unremarkable. Thyroid exam is normal, and abdominal exam is normal. Formal visual field exam shows no evidence of hemianopsia. An office test for pregnancy is negative.

## Differential Diagnosis

1. Prolactinoma
2. Hypothyroidism
3. Pregnancy

## Initial Management

**Setting**: outpatient

## Diagnostic/Therapeutic Plan

- Prolactin level
- TSH
- Repeat pregnancy test

## Test Results

- Prolactin level: 260 ng/mL
- TSH: normal
- Repeat pregnancy test: negative

## Assessment

Prolactinomas are the most common active (secretory) adenomas of the pituitary. The most common symptoms of small prolactinomas are amenorrhea, infertility, and galactorrhea. There are causes of galactorrhea and hyperprolactinemia that are not associated with pituitary adenomas (secondary hyperprolactinemia).

Causes of secondary hyperprolactinemia are the following:

1. Primary hypothyroidism: Due to activation of TRH, the hypothalamic hormone that activates TSH and prolactin.
2. Dopamine-inhibiting drugs (haloperidol, metoclopramide, trifluoperazine): Since prolactin is under constant inhibition from dopamine drugs that inhibit, dopamine will increase serum prolactin levels. A drug history is very important in this case!
3. Pregnancy: This must be excluded first in all patients with new-onset galactorrhea.

In this patient with galactorrhea in the setting of an initial negative pregnancy test and no history of drug/medication use, the likely diagnosis is a prolactinoma or hypothyroidism. In secondary hyperprolactinemia, prolactin <200 ng/mL.

### Further Management Plan/Results

- MRI of brain: pituitary microadenoma

### Treatment Plan

- Trial of dopamine agonists: cabergoline or bromocriptine (cabergoline preferred due to better side-effect profile)
- Monitor prolactin levels

### Discussion

Prolactinomas in women cause galactorrhea, oligomenorrhea, amenorrhea, and infertility. Hypogonadism is thought to result from suppression of GnRH by the elevated prolactin levels. Large prolactinomas, commonly seen in men, present with bitemporal hemianopsia, headaches, and blurry vision. Serum prolactin in prolactinomas is almost always >200 ng/mL.

Pituitary MRI is the most sensitive test for detecting pituitary tumors and determining their size; it may be repeated periodically to assess tumor progression and the effects of therapy. CT scan can also visualize the pituitary but is less sensitive than the MRI.

The goal of treatment in prolactinomas is to reduce prolactin secretion, reduce tumor size, and correct any visual field defects. In the case of very large tumors, only partial achievement of this goal is possible. Because dopamine normally inhibits prolactin secretion, treatment with dopamine agonists like bromocriptine or cabergoline is effective and usually the first step in the management. These drugs also shrink the tumor and return prolactin levels to normal in approximately 80% of cases.

#### CLINICAL PEARL

In patients with galactorrhea, exclude primary hypothyroidism and pregnancy, and then confirm that patient is not using dopamine-depleting drugs. Prolactinomas cause significantly elevated prolactin (>200 ng/mL).

Bromocriptine is associated with side effects such as nausea and dizziness. Cabergoline is associated with the same side effects, but these seem to be less common and less severe than with bromocriptine. Surgery should be considered if medical therapy cannot be tolerated or if it fails to reduce prolactin levels and reduce tumor size. Normalization of prolactin levels always results in restoration of fertility and gonadal function.

Men with prolactinoma will not have galactorrhea; they will have hypogonadism. In a man with ED, low libido, and low energy, check an 8 AM total testosterone level and if it is low, repeat it. After 2 low total T levels, the next step is to check LH. High LH means it is a primary (testicular) source, while low or normal LH means it is a secondary or pituitary source. Because of negative feedback inhibition, low testosterone should cause high LH. Normal LH in the setting of low testosterone is abnormal and it means the pituitary gland is the source.

Once you confirm it is secondary hypogonadism, check the prolactin level. If it is high, the patient has a prolactinoma.

### Final Diagnosis

Prolactinoma

# CASE 10

## Chief Complaint

Weight loss, weakness, and dizziness

## History and Physical Examination

A 42-year-old woman presents with a 2-month history of weight loss (22 lb), generalized weakness, and dizziness when standing. Her medical history is negative except for hypothyroidism, which was diagnosed 4 years ago and is treated with levothyroxine 125 mcg daily. She has had no recent travel. A recent PPD and chest x-ray done while starting a new job in a hospital were both negative. She takes no medication or recreational drugs.

On physical examination the patient weighs 106 lb. Her blood pressure is 98/68 mm Hg with evidence of orthostasis when sitting up. The nails and palms have increased pigment. Cardiac exam shows evidence of tachycardia at 102/min. Lung and abdominal exams are unremarkable. Laboratory studies completed at another institution include Na 129 mEq/L, K 5.2 mEq/L, and glucose 58 mg/dL. CBC is normal except for an increase in peripheral eosinophils.

## Differential Diagnosis

1. Primary adrenal insufficiency
2. Small-cell lung cancer secreting ACTH (Cushing's syndrome)
3. Chronic infectious diseases (tuberculosis, HIV)
4. Malabsorption syndrome (celiac sprue, IBD)

## Initial Management

**Setting**: outpatient

## Diagnostic/Therapeutic Plan

- Cosyntropin stimulation test
- HIV test

## Test Results

- Cosyntropin stimulation test: minimal increase in cortisol levels after ACTH stimulation
- HIV test negative

## Assessment

This patient has the classic features of primary adrenal insufficiency (Addison's disease): weakness, orthostasis, hyperpigmentation, electrolyte abnormalities (hyperkalemia and hyponatremia), and peripheral eosinophilia.

Other diseases that should be considered are paraneoplastic syndrome (small-cell lung cancer) causing Cushing's syndrome (less likely with negative smoking history and recent normal chest x-ray); malabsorption syndromes such as sprue and IBD (less likely given absence of diarrhea); and TB and HIV, which should always be excluded (though this patient had a recent PPD that was negative).

### Further Management Plan/Results

| CT scan of the adrenals | Evidence of adrenal atrophy; no evidence of scarring or granulomas |
|---|---|

### Treatment Plan

1. Start hydrocortisone and fludrocortisone

### Discussion

Adrenal insufficiency or Addison's disease is characterized by weakness, weight loss, low BP, and orthostasis, as well as hyperpigmentation. The symptoms can be non specific and the disease sometimes eludes diagnosis. It can occur after recent steroid use (prednisone), but this should be evident from the history.

In the United States, most cases of adrenal insufficiency are due to autoimmune disorders. Sometimes it can be part of polyendocrine deficiency syndrome, where adrenal insufficiency is accompanied by other gland failure (pernicious anemia, hypothyroidism, vitiligo, etc.). In the developing countries, about 20% of adrenal insufficiency cases are due to TB.

The most specific test to diagnose adrenal insufficiency is the ACTH stimulation test (cosyntropin test). (An 8 AM cortisol test <3 mcg/dL is diagnostic of adrenal insufficiency, and thus ACTH stimulation test is not needed.) The test will identify both primary adrenal insufficiency as well as chronic adrenal insufficiency (the adrenal glands atrophy in the absence of ACTH). Patients with adrenal insufficiency typically fail to respond to an ACTH injection with increased cortisol. ACTH level should be checked next to determine if it is primary or secondary (high, primary, low, or inappropriately normal is secondary).

Once the diagnosis of adrenal insufficiency is made, additional imaging of the adrenals with CT scan or MRI is needed. Scarring and calcification of the adrenals may indicate TB, and thus further evaluation may be warranted. Treatment involves replacing the missing hormones. Hydrocortisone is given to replace cortisol; if aldosterone is missing, fludrocortisone should be added.

### Final Diagnosis

Primary adrenal insufficiency associated with polyendocrine deficiency syndrome

**CLINICAL PEARL**

Primary adrenal insufficiency (Addison's disease):

- Hyperpigmentation (not evident in secondary adrenal insufficiency)
- Hypotension
- Hyperkalemia
- Eosinophilia
- Treat with hydrocortisone +/− fludrocortisone

Secondary adrenal insufficiency (occurs with Sheehan's syndrome, hemochromatosis, pituitary apoplexy)

- Other hormones are deficient: LH, FSH, GH, TSH
- No evidence of hyperpigmentation
- Hypotension and hyperkalemia uncommon
- Treat with hydrocortisone

# CASE 11

## Chief Complaint

Headache and blurry vision

## History and Physical Examination

A 52-year-old man with past medical history of pituitary adenoma presents to the emergency medicine department with a few hours of left eye diplopia, blurry vision, and ptosis. Prior to this presentation he reported 1 week of constant excruciating occipital headaches not alleviated by naproxen. The patient denies any focal weakness, sensory changes, fevers, and vomiting. There is also no report of weight loss, skin changes, recent travel, or head injury.

On initial presentation his blood pressure is 82/44 mm Hg and he is afebrile. On examination he has mild neck stiffness. He exhibits left eye ptosis with a left pupil 6 mm dilated but minimally reactive. The right pupil is 3 mm and strongly reactive to light. Visual acuity is 20/70 on the right and 20/100 on the left. Extra-ocular movements are intact on the right but the patient cannot adduct or look superiorly or inferiorly on the left. Other cranial nerves are intact. The rest of the neurologic and physical exam is normal. Routine laboratory studies show normal CBC and normal basic metabolic panel and urine studies.

## Differential Diagnosis

1. Pituitary apoplexy, given history of prior adenoma
2. Subarachnoid bleed (SAB)
3. Meningitis

**CLINICAL PEARL**

Always consider subarachnoid bleed and pituitary apoplexy in patients presenting with acute-onset neck stiffness. Bacterial and viral meningitis typically are associated with fever and evolve over days.

## Initial Management

**Setting:** emergency department

## Diagnostic/Therapeutic Plan

- Emergency CT scan of head without contrast

## Test Results

- Hyperdense mass with bleeding in area of pituitary gland and optic chiasm

**CLINICAL PEARL**

In patients with neck stiffness, CT scan should be done before lumbar puncture, if the patient has focal neurologic signs (in this case, ophthalmoplegia), papilledema, or immunodeficiency.

## Assessment

This patient has the typical features of pituitary apoplexy. The lack of fever and the acute onset make meningitis less likely. SAB needs to be considered as a possibility, but the existence of prior adenoma makes apoplexy more likely. In any event, CT without contrast will help to differentiate the two.

### Further Management Plan/Results

- **Pituitary MRI:** confirms existence of pituitary macroadenoma with acute hemorrhage; MRI findings also show that the tumor was displacing the optic chiasm, explaining the acute visual field changes
- Cortisol level: low
- TSH level: low
- FSH and LH: low

### Initial Management

The ICU setting is required, since pituitary apoplexy is considered an endocrinologic emergency.

- Initiate hormone replacement with hydrocortisone and levothyroxine
- Start IV fluids to stabilize BP
- Initiate neurosurgery consult if surgical intervention needed

In patients with acute visual loss, neurosurgeons sometimes perform an emergency transsphenoidal resection.

### Discussion

Pituitary apoplexy is an emergency that causes acute hypopituitarism. It is typically due to bleeding into or impaired blood supply of the pituitary. It occurs in the presence of a pituitary adenoma (or another pituitary tumor, <30% of cases).

The most common initial symptom (>90%) is sudden headache, often associated with blurry vision and worsening visual field defects. This is caused by compression of the nerves around the optic chiasm. The oculomotor nerve is predominantly affected as it lies closest to the pituitary. It is also commonly associated with nausea and vomiting. In 25% of cases, the presence of blood irritates the meninges, which may cause neck stiffness and photophobia.

This initial stage is then followed by hormonal defects. Especially important is adrenal insufficiency (70% of cases), which is due to a decrease in production of ACTH. The sudden decrease in cortisol production causes an adrenal crisis (Addisonian crisis). This may cause hypotension (as noted in our patient) and hypoglycemia. The hypotension and hypoglycemia can be life-threatening and require immediate intervention.

Hyponatremia may occur and can be profound. It is thought to be due to the low cortisol or elevated levels of ADH (inappropriate secretion). Several other hormonal deficiencies may develop in the subacute phase including deficiency in TSH, LH, and FSH. This leads to hypothyroidism, and in women amenorrhea and infertility.

Diagnosis is confirmed by MRI scan of the pituitary, which may demonstrate hemorrhage or infarction (due to reduced blood supply). Note: It makes sense to start with CT scan without contrast in the ED, in order to rule out SAB. The hormonal dysregulation is confirmed by showing low levels of ACTH (and cortisol), TSH, FSH, and LH.

Treatment is timely correction of hormone deficiencies and in some cases, surgical decompression (neurosurgery consult). The decision on whether to neurosurgically decompress the pituitary gland will depend on the severity of visual loss and visual field defects. Most patients will need long-term hormonal supplementation so they will require long-term follow-up by an endocrinologist.

In the acute phase, the first priority is to stabilize the BP. Cortisol deficiency can cause severe hypotension.

Treatment requires IV fluids (normal saline or dextrose if patient is hypoglycemic) and IV hydrocortisone (or dexamethasone if there is significant swelling in the brain).

### Final Diagnosis

Pituitary apoplexy

# Gastroenterology 9

## CASE 1

### Chief Complaint

"My belly is swollen and it hurts."

### History and Physical Examination

A 58-year-old woman comes to the emergency department with fever, abdominal pain, and abdominal distention. In the last several months, she has developed ascites, anorexia, and progressive wasting. She also complains of severe itching. She is on no medications. She is a former IV drug user who was discharged several months ago from an alcohol-detoxification unit.

She is disheveled-appearing and cachectic with a grossly distended abdomen. Her T is 38.3 C (101.0 F), BP 110/70 mm Hg, pulse 107/min, and respirations 22/min. Physical examination shows poor dentition, parotid gland enlargement, and scleral icterus. Her lungs are clear and the heart has an RRR. The abdomen is distended, tympanitic, tender, and with shifting dullness. A liver edge is not palpable, but the spleen is palpable 3 cm below the left costal margin. Bilateral palmar erythema is noted. Multiple spider angiomata and excoriations are also present. A flapping tremor is noted when the patient is asked to extend her wrists while her arms are outstretched.

### Differential Diagnosis

1. Alcoholic cirrhosis
   - More likely, as patient has signs of chronic liver disease and was recently discharged from alcoholic detoxification center
2. Chronic viral hepatitis or acute hepatitis
   - Could be a possible diagnosis, given that the most common cause of cirrhosis in the United States is hepatitis C (especially since patient is prior IV drug user and in an age group with high rates of infectivity, i.e., baby boomer generation)
3. Spontaneous bacterial peritonitis
   - Must be ruled out in all patients who present with fever and ascites, with or without fever or abdominal pain
4. Peritoneal carcinomatosis secondary to ovarian cancer
   - Must be considered as an alternative source of ascites in a female patient

### Initial Management

**Setting:** emergency department

### Diagnostic/Therapeutic Plan

- PT, PTT, INR
- CBC, peripheral smear
- BUN/creatinine
- Aspartate aminotransferase (AST)
- Alanine aminotransferase (ALT)
- Alkaline phosphatase
- Total and fractionated bilirubin
- Albumin
- Total protein

### Test Results

- PT 16 sec (normal <13 sec), PTT 38 sec, INR 1.4
- WBCs 4,800/mm$^3$, hemoglobin 11 mg/dL, platelets 120,000/mm$^3$, MCV 102 mm$^3$; acanthocytosis on peripheral smear
- BUN/creatinine 30 mg/dL, 1.0 mg/dL
- AST 200 U/L
- ALT 100 U/L (normal: 8–20 U/L)
- Alkaline phosphatase 150 U/L (normal: 20–70 U/L)
- Total bilirubin 3.4 mg/dL (normal: 0.1–1.0 mg/dL)
- Albumin 2.8 g/dL (normal: 3.5–5.5 g/dL)
- Total protein 6.5 g/dL (normal: 6–7.8 g/dL)

### Assessment

This patient has stigmata of chronic liver disease or cirrhosis. Signs of chronic liver disease on physical examination include ascites, spider angiomata, caput medusa, splenomegaly, palmar erythema, and asterixis (a flapping tremor when the wrists are extended), which this patient has.

The patient's lethargy is indicative of hepatic encephalopathy, but the neurologic findings can range from confusion and irritability to obtundance and personality change. Also common in hepatic encephalopathy is a **reversal of the sleep-wake cycle**.

**CLINICAL PEARL**

Elevated arterial or free venous serum ammonia is the classic lab abnormality for hepatic encephalopathy. Ammonia level does not, however, correlate with the degree of hepatic encephalopathy.

In liver disease, the **Child-Pugh score** helps to delineate prognosis.

| Parameter | 1 point | 2 points | 3 points |
|---|---|---|---|
| Total bilirubin, µmol/l (mg/dL) | <2 | 2–3 | >3 |
| Serum albumin, g/dL | >3.5 | 2.8–3.5 | <2.8 |
| PT INR | <1.7 | 1.71–2.30 | >2.30 |
| Ascites | None | Mild | Moderate to severe |
| Hepatic encephalopathy | None | Grade I–II (or suppressed with medication) | |

| Points | Class | 1-yr survival |
|---|---|---|
| 5–6 | A | 99% |
| 7–9 | B | 81% |
| 10–15 | C | 45% |

### Basic Science Correlate

- In portal hypertension, portosystemic shunting allows thiols, dimethyl sulfide, and trimethylamine to pass into the lungs and be breathed out. These compounds lead to the odor of fetor hepaticus (sweet, feces).
- Spider angiomata are vascular lesions with a central arteriole surrounded by smaller vessels and occur due to a rise in estradiol. The liver normally clears estradiol.
- Palmar erythema is due to vasodilation due to increased estrogen.
- Gynecomastia also occurs from an increase in free estradiol.
- Caput medusa occurs when blood from the portal venous system is shunted through the periumbilical veins and ultimately to the abdominal wall veins. This can lead to a Cruveilhier-Baumgarten murmur.
- PT and PTT elevations are due to a lack of clotting factor production (clotting factors made in the liver).
- The only clotting factors not made in the liver are von Willebrand's factor and factor VIII.

This patient has a history of alcoholism, and the increase in AST when compared with ALT points to alcohol-related liver disease. Chronic viral hepatitis should be ruled out given the history of IV drug use. Serologies for hepatitis B and C should be performed. Hepatitis A does not cause chronic liver disease, but an acute infection can be particularly severe when there is underlying chronic hepatitis, and may lead to fulminant failure.

In a patient with or without a history of alcohol abuse who has ascites, always consider cancer and tuberculosis as a potential etiology of the ascites. Vascular causes of ascites are less likely in this case but may be ruled out through the use of Doppler U/S or CT of the abdomen with contrast.

Other improbable causes of cirrhosis are primary biliary cirrhosis, hemochromatosis, Wilson disease, and alpha 1-antitrypsin deficiency. These diseases should be ruled out in this patient, given that they may be reversible. A thorough history should be obtained to rule out drug-related hepatotoxicity secondary to isoniazid, methotrexate, or acetaminophen.

#### CLINICAL PEARL

Beware of the female patient who has a history of significant alcohol abuse and presents with new ascites. She may have alcoholic liver cirrhosis, but you should also consider ovarian cancer with peritoneal carcinomatosis. Ovarian cancer causing ascites will have a low albumin gradient, indicating no evidence of portal hypertension.

#### CLINICAL PEARL

The most common cause of cirrhosis in the United States is hepatitis C, followed by alcoholic liver disease.

### CLINICAL PEARL

Paracentesis should **always** be attempted, even if an obvious cause of liver disease is assumed. The most important tests to do with the paracentesis fluid are SAAG and WBC. A patient with cirrhosis and ascites is at high risk for the development of spontaneous bacterial peritonitis. In a febrile patient with ascites, perform a diagnostic paracentesis to exclude this. Peritoneal fluid with absolute polymorphonuclear leukocytes >250/mm$^3$ (or total WBC 500/mm$^3$) suggests the presence of infection.

### CLINICAL PEARL

When sudden worsening of ascites occurs in a patient with cirrhosis, you have to consider hepatoma, spontaneous bacterial peritonitis, and viral hepatitis. A repeat paracentesis is mandatory to exclude spontaneous bacterial peritonitis.

Hepatoma can be evaluated through diagnostic imaging such as ultrasonography or CT scan, as well as serum alpha-fetoprotein (which is elevated with hepatoma).

Liver-generated ascites is a sign of advanced disease and usually results from portal hypertension, which leads to vasodilatation. The vasodilatation that occurs triggers renal sodium retention and results in high intravascular volume and ascites formation. The volume/pressure sensors in the cirrhotic patient are limited in the face of volume overload. Consequently, these volume/pressure sensors sense volume depletion in the face of volume overload and paradoxically stimulate release of renin/aldosterone, which leads to more increased sodium retention and increased fluid volume.

Other causes of progressive ascites include malignant ascites (e.g., ovarian carcinoma), right-sided heart failure, and vascular obstruction due to hepatic vein thrombosis (Budd-Chiari) or inferior vena cava thrombosis.

The etiology of ascites can be distinguished by obtaining a serum ascites-albumin gradient (SAAG). This is a gradient obtained by taking the difference between the serum albumin and the albumin in the ascitic fluid.

A serum ascites-albumin difference of >1.1 g/dL is indicative of portal hypertension and is seen in cirrhosis, cardiovascular ascites (congestive heart failure), or hepatic/portal vein thrombosis syndromes. If the serum ascites albumin gradient (SAAG) is <1.1, portal hypertension is absent; this can be seen in peritoneal carcinomatosis, peritonitis in the absence of cirrhosis (i.e., tuberculosis), nephrotic syndrome, or pancreatic or biliary ascites. Basically, if the ascitic fluid albumin level is much lower than the serum albumin level, it is from a hydrostatic problem like portal hypertension.

| | |
|---|---|
| **SAAG (gm/dL) <1.1** | • Ascitic total protein >2.5 gm/dL is consistent with carcinomatosis, tuberculosis, pancreatitis, or serositis<br>• Ascitic total protein <2.5 gm/dL is consistent with nephrotic syndrome |
| **SAAG (gm/dL) ≥1.1** | • Ascitic total protein <2.5 gm/dL is consistent with portal hypertension<br>• Ascitic total protein >2.5 mg/dL is consistent with CHF or Budd-Chiari syndrome |

The liver has a large role in synthesis of albumin and proteins involved in coagulation. Laboratory abnormalities of cirrhosis include evidence of poor synthetic function demonstrated by low serum albumin levels and elevated PT and PTT. Elevation of the PT and PTT is caused by deficient production of clotting factors, which results from loss of liver parenchymal cell function. Vitamin K serves as a cofactor used by liver parenchymal cells in the production of these clotting factors. Other hematologic abnormalities seen in cirrhosis include anemia and thrombocytopenia from hypersplenism, marrow suppression, or the anemia of chronic disease.

Liver failure is often associated with an elevation in the direct bilirubin, transaminases, lactate dehydrogenase, and alkaline phosphatase. However, patients with a cirrhotic liver that becomes progressively more fibrotic may lose their ability to produce these enzymes, and, consequently, their levels can be normal.

### Further Tests/Results

| | |
|---|---|
| Hepatitis B and C serologies | Negative |
| Paracentesis | WBCs 50 mm$^3$; Gram stain and culture negative; albumin 1.2 |
| Fe (iron) studies | Normal |
| Ceruloplasmin levels | Normal |
| Alpha-1 antitrypsin levels | Normal |
| Antimitochondrial antibodies | Negative |
| Liver U/S mass | Shrunken nodular fatty liver; normal bile ducts; no evidence of mass |

### Further Management

- Salt restriction, diuretics (spironolactone and furosemide)
- Balanced diet with adequate protein ingestion, diet-enriched branched chain amino acids to protect against development of hepatic encephalopathy
- Counseling against further alcohol ingestion/recommend enrollment in alcohol treatment
- Follow patient closely and watch for signs of GI bleed and encephalopathy
- Upper endoscopy to exclude esophageal varices (given patient's portal hypertension and ascites)
- Lactulose and rifaximin (given patient's hepatic encephalopathy)
- If patient has SBP, you must cover gram negatives and *Streptococcus pneumoniae*: ceftriaxone or cefotaxime (metronidazole not needed); add albumin infusions on day 1 and 3 to prevent HRS

#### Basic Science Correlate

- Spironolactone, a direct aldosterone antagonist, can lead to gynecomastia and hyperkalemia.
- Furosemide, a loop diuretic, inhibits Na-K-2Cl symporter in the thick ascending limb of the loop of Henle and can lead to hypokalemia.
- Lactulose is a non digestible disaccharide that reduces the ammonia levels through increased bowel movements. It is titrated until the patient has 2–3 bowel movements per day. Dehydration is a common side effect.
- Rifaximin interferes with transcription by binding to the γ-subunit of bacterial RNA polymerase. This reduces relapse of hepatic encephalopathy and improves quality of life.

#### CLINICAL PEARL

Fever + abdominal + cirrhosis = SBP must be ruled out.

#### NOTE

Hepatorenal syndrome is diagnosed by the following:

- Increase in creatinine by 0.3 mg/dL or ≥50% in 48 hours
- Bland urinalysis (not RBCs or protein or cast)
- Normal ultrasound
- Not in sepsis
- No improvement in kidney function after 48 hours of holding diuretics and IV albumin

## Discussion

This patient presents with several classic findings of cirrhosis secondary to alcoholic liver disease. The other disease entities in the differential have been ruled out by negative testing.

Alcoholic hepatitis may present with acute symptoms of fever, hepatosplenomegaly, and elevated transaminases. In alcoholic cirrhosis, patients usually present with anorexia, loss of muscle mass, and fatigue. The liver may be enlarged and fatty, but as the disease progresses, cirrhosis develops and the liver becomes hard, nodular, shrunken, and scarred. Fibrous bands connecting portal triads and central veins, as well as regenerative parenchyma-forming micronodules, characterize liver histology in cirrhosis.

Men often present with gynecomastia and testicular atrophy caused by decreased hepatic clearance of androstenedione that is converted to estrogen and leads to increased estrogen levels. Patients with alcoholic cirrhosis usually have signs of portal hypertension, which include ascites, hemorrhoids, splenomegaly, and esophageal varices.

In alcoholic liver disease, transaminase elevations are usually mild and do not exceed 500 U/L. The transaminase elevation is characterized by an AST that is approximately 2 to 3x ALT, as is seen here. Bilirubin elevations are often modest but progress as the disease worsens. Patients have decreased albumin levels and oncotic pressure, which increase the risk of ascites formation. Splenomegaly can be associated with pancytopenia. Coagulopathy is another sign of liver dysfunction. Hepatic encephalopathy is seen in end-stage disease (to be discussed in a later case).

Patients with alcoholic fatty liver have a good prognosis, and the problem may resolve after cessation of drinking. Patients with alcoholic hepatitis who stop drinking rarely develop cirrhosis. Of those who continue drinking, the incidence of cirrhosis is 45–80%. Hyperbilirubinemia, prolongation of clotting times, ascites, and encephalopathy are associated with a mortality, which may exceed 50%. Prognosis is largely determined by whether the patient continues to drink. In a large study from Copenhagen, the 5-year survival for nondrinkers without jaundice was 85%, whereas it was only 60% for those who drank. Once jaundice occurs, survival falls to 50% in nondrinkers and 30% in drinkers. GI bleed carries the worst prognosis.

Treatment is largely supportive. Corticosteroids may be used in treatment of acute alcoholic hepatitis in patients who are very coagulopathic, but corticosteroids play no role in treatment once cirrhosis occurs. Advanced disease can be treated with liver transplantation if the patient discontinues drinking.

## Follow-up Management and Prevention

- Surveillance for varices every 2 years if initial scope was negative
- Nonselective beta blocker (propranolol or nadolol) for prevention of variceal bleeds
- Surveillance for HCC with ultrasonography every 6 mos for patients with cirrhosis
- Band ligation (most appropriate therapy) if varices are present
- If patient had SBP, subsequent antibiotic prophylaxis with norfloxacin

## Final Diagnosis

Cirrhosis

# CASE 2

## Chief Complaint

"I'm vomiting blood."

## History and Physical Examination

A 72-year-old man comes to the emergency department vomiting blood. The patient has a known history of ethanol abuse and has had a couple of upper GI bleeds in the past. He was on a drinking binge earlier today, and an hour ago he was found by the emergency workers in a pool of blood on the sidewalk. He denies any pain at this time.

He is afebrile. His BP is 80 mm Hg/palpation and pulse 125/min. He is stuporous and smells of alcohol. Physical examination shows scleral icterus, gynecomastia, and spider angiomata. Cardiovascular examination is normal except for tachycardia. The chest is clear to auscultation. The abdomen is soft, non-tender, and nondistended; splenomegaly is evident. Rectal exam is significant for melena.

## Differential Diagnosis

1. Bleeding esophageal varices
    - The most likely diagnosis of upper GI bleed in patients with known cirrhosis or who have stigmata of chronic liver disease
2. Mallory-Weiss tear
    - Occurs most commonly in patients with a history of retching and vomiting; although this patient did have an alcoholic binge earlier, there is no mention of vomiting or retching
3. Erosive gastritis
    - A common finding in patients with alcoholism; however, less likely to cause severe upper GI bleed and more likely to cause melena
4. Peptic ulcer bleeding
    - Caused by NSAIDs or *H. pylori*, which can cause upper GI bleed; however, in the setting of chronic liver disease, the more likely cause is varices due to portal hypertension

## Initial Management

**Setting:** emergency department

## Diagnostic/Therapeutic Plan

In the case of upper GI bleed, the initial management plan is the same whatever the cause. It always focuses on stabilizing the patient.

- Insert 2 large-bore IV lines and start fluids (normal saline or crystalloid)
    - Continue saline infusion until systolic BP is >90 mm Hg, HR decreases <90/min, or urine output (if affected) increases
- Obtain a CBC, biochemical profile, and PT/PTT
- Give transfusions of packed RBC as needed
    - Fresh frozen plasma in patients with coagulopathy
- May require urgent upper endoscopy and therapeutic intervention
- Insert a nasogastric tube to determine if there is ongoing, active bleeding

**CLINICAL PEARL**

Upper GI bleed can manifest as hematemesis, melena, hematochezia, or hemodynamic changes (dizziness).

## Test Results

- Hemoglobin 10 mg/dL (normal 13–16 mg/dL)
- Platelets 80,000/mm$^3$ (normal 140,000–340,000/mm$^3$)
- Sodium 150 mEq/L (normal 135–150 mEq/L), BUN 30 mg/dL (normal: 8–18 mg/dL), creatinine 1.4 mg/dL (normal: 0.6–1.3 mg/dL)
- Bilirubin 3.5 mg/dL (normal: 0.1–1.0 mg/dL), AST 240 U/L, ALT 80 U/L (normal: 8–20 U/L), alkaline phosphatase 160 U/L, PT/PTT: 17 sec/45 sec (elevated)

## Assessment

The patient presents with evidence of vomiting bright red blood and with melena in the rectal vault. The presence of melena suggests a bleed greater than 100 mL, originating from a source proximal to the ligament of Treitz.

**CLINICAL PEARL**

Because there is significant mortality and morbidity associated with upper GI bleed, an upper endoscopy should be performed before discharge from the hospital. However, nasogastric lavage showing bright blood (especially if the patient is hemodynamically unstable) mandates an emergent consult with gastroenterology and endoscopy.

Upper GI bleed in an alcoholic patient has several possible etiologies. Massive blood loss is often caused by esophageal varices resulting from progressive portal hypertension. However, even alcoholics with known esophageal varices often suffer upper GI bleed from other causes. Other possibilities include peptic ulcer disease or severe gastritis. Recurrent retching can result in a Mallory-Weiss tear and subsequent bleeding.

This patient also has evidence of cirrhosis and alcoholic liver disease on physical examination (gynecomastia, spider angiomatas, icteric sclera) and lab findings (elevated bilirubin, elevated AST/ALT ratio 3:1, elevated PT/PTT, low albumin).

In assessing this patient, primary attention is given to determining the extent of blood loss and stabilizing intravascular volume with crystalloids and packed RBC transfusions. Given the history of alcoholism, evidence for an underlying coagulation defect should also be explored and corrected. Emergent endoscopy should be performed to determine the source of bleeding once the patient is stabilized.

### Further Management Plan/Results

| | |
|---|---|
| Emergent upper endoscopy once patient is stabilized | Esophageal varices with cherry red spots and a varix with a clot but no active bleeding; normal gastric mucosae with no evidence of peptic ulcers |
| Banding of the esophageal varices to control the bleeding | |

**CLINICAL PEARL**

Nonselective beta-blockers (propranolol, nadolol) are the only effective treatment for esophageal varices for first-time, as well as recurrent, bleeding.

### Follow-up Management

1. Admission to ICU for continued observation and blood transfusion as appropriate
2. Fluid resuscitation (important in any GIB); keep SBP >100 mm Hg and HR <100/min
3. IV somatostatin/octreotide
4. Monitor for signs of recurrent bleeding
5. Propranolol once BP is stable
6. Monitor for signs of delirium tremens
7. Fresh frozen plasma if increased PT
8. Ciprofloxacin or ceftriaxone (prophylaxis against SBP)

### Discussion

This patient has bleeding esophageal varices as a result of portal hypertension secondary to alcohol-induced cirrhosis. Varices are portosystemic collaterals that can develop in the esophagus, stomach, or rectum in patients with portal hypertension. Varices in the esophagus and stomach can be seen in up to 60% of cirrhotic patients and have a 30% chance of bleeding. Factors which increase the likelihood of variceal bleeding include size and presence of cherry red spots or red streaks on varices. This patient had cherry red spots as well as a clot on a varix that had recently bled.

About 60% of upper GI bleed in cirrhotics is caused by esophageal varices, while 7% is caused by gastric varices. Variceal bleeding carries a high mortality rate of up to 70%.

**NOTE**

Giving antibiotics for SBP prophylaxis is very important and very commonly tested on the exam.

Upper endoscopy is the mainstay of both diagnosis and treatment of varices. Octreotide should be used immediately in all patients with variceal bleeding. The somatostatin analog inhibits the release of vasodilator hormones such as glucagon, indirectly causing splanchnic vasoconstriction and decreased portal inflow. Variceal rubber band ligation and sclerotherapy are treatment options to control bleeding, but they do not treat portal hypertension. Banding is used in patients with bleeding to prevent recurrent bleeding. Band ligation is superior. Sclerotherapy has more complications, such as stricture formation and scarring. It is important to stabilize the patient before any procedure and to try to correct coagulopathy as well. The risk of recurrent bleeding from varices is very high and ranges from 40–80%. Risk of recurrent variceal bleeding can be reduced with the use of nonselective beta-blockers (e.g., propranolol) once the patient is stable.

If bleeding cannot be controlled with banding, the next line of treatment includes TIPS, or transjugular intrahepatic portosystemic shunting. Somatostatin/octreotide causes splanchnic vasoconstriction and should be used as adjuncts to endoscopic therapy to control bleeding and prevent further bleeding. If the above measures fail, shunt operations can be considered to decrease portal hypertension. A Blakemore tube is rarely used and only as a bridge to surgery.

**NOTE**

Factor VIII is generally increased or normal in liver disease. The reason is because factor VIII is produced in hepatic and non-hepatic endothelial cells, so with chronic liver disease a significant proportion of factor VIII production is unaffected.

On the other hand, in DIC, consumption of factor VIII causes a decrease in its level.

Platelet transfusions are used as needed if the platelet count <50,000. Cryoprecipitate (preferred over fresh frozen plasma [FFP] because it has fibrinogen and less volume) is used to correct the elevation. This elevation is common in alcoholics and can be secondary to nutritional deficiency or liver disease with poor synthetic function. Give PRBCs to keep the hemoglobin >7 g/dL (over-transfusing can increase portal pressures).

Given the history of recent alcohol use and severe bleeding, this patient should also be monitored in an intensive care setting for signs of delirium tremens. Gastric varices can regress in alcoholic patients who abstain from alcohol. Once this patient recovers, he should be advised to stop alcohol consumption and seek professional treatment regarding this.

Vasopressin is no longer used with variceal bleeding. It has no additional efficacy when compared with octreotide and has more potential cardiac adverse effects.

### Follow-up Management and Prevention

- Surveillance for varices every 2 years after initial presentation
- If varices are present on subsequent endoscopies, band ligation is the most appropriate therapy
- To prevent further variceal bleeds, use a nonselective beta blocker (propranolol or nadolol) after the bleed is stabilized

### Final Diagnosis

Bleeding esophageal varices

# CASE 3

## Chief Complaint

"My gut hurts, but it feels better after I eat."

## History and Physical Examination

A 52-year-old man presents with a 2-month history of epigastric pain. The pain wakes him up from his sleep. Eating and over-the-counter antacids relieve it. He has no significant weight loss and no nausea or vomiting. He has no known history of pancreatic or ulcer disease. He does not drink alcohol. He occasionally smokes and takes aspirin for back pain.

He is a healthy-appearing man in very mild distress. His vital signs are stable. Examination of his heart and lungs is WNL. His abdomen is soft, nontender, nondistended, and there are no palpable masses. Rectal examination is without any masses and is guaiac-negative.

## Differential Diagnosis

1. Duodenal ulcer
   - Epigastric pain that is long-standing and awakens someone from sleep can be gastric or duodenal, but classically pain that is better with eating is duodenal in nature
2. Gastric ulcer
   - More common when patient has pain that is worsened with eating
3. Esophagitis
   - Commonly found in patients with GERD; would have complaints of chest pain
4. Gastric cancer
   - Does have dull epigastric pain that is unrelated to eating; would be associated with early satiety
5. Cholelithiasis
   - Would have postprandial pain; would localize to right upper quadrant

## Initial Management

**Setting**: outpatient

## Diagnostic/Therapeutic Plan

- CBC
- Liver function tests
- U/S of the gallbladder
- Amylase/lipase

### Test Results

- CBC: normal
- LFTs: normal
- U/S: negative for cholelithiasis
- Amylase/lipase: normal

### Assessment

The patient presents with epigastric pain relieved partially with antacids. This is suggestive of peptic ulcer disease, specifically duodenal ulceration. Pain is classically described as burning or gnawing and is most severe in early morning and 2–3 hrs after eating. Gastric ulceration can be associated with a worsening pain on eating. Complications of peptic ulcer disease include bleeding, perforation, and gastric outlet obstruction, which may present as protracted vomiting immediately after eating.

Cholelithiasis may also present with postprandial epigastric pain and may be excluded with U/S of the gallbladder. Initial diagnostic assessment should exclude evidence of chronic blood loss. A young patient with classic presentation for peptic ulcer disease can be treated empirically with H2 blockers or proton pump inhibitors. If symptoms persist, then an evaluation should be pursued.

If ulcers recur, an underlying disorder such as Zollinger-Ellison syndrome should be excluded. A patient age >50 is at greater risk for a malignant ulcer and should be evaluated initially with endoscopy.

**NOTE**

Around 10% of upper GI bleeds present with bright red blood per rectum. Patients will be hypotensive due to rapid bleeding. In patients with bright blood per rectum and hypotension and high BUN:cr, perform upper endoscopy.

**CLINICAL PEARL**

To test for eradication of *H. pylori* (recommended for all), use urea breath or stool antigen testing. Both are effective but stool testing is more cost-effective. Testing should be done 4–8 weeks after completing the regimen.

Do not order serum antibody testing for *H pylori*.

**CLINICAL PEARL**

If a patient has a duodenal ulcer and is *H. pylori*-negative, the likely cause is NSAID-induced peptic ulcer disease. The chance of getting peptic ulcer disease and bleeding with NSAIDs increases with advanced age, comorbid conditions, and concomitant use of corticosteroids and high-dose NSAIDs.

### Further Management Plan/Results

| | |
|---|---|
| Upper endoscopy with biopsy | • Nondilated stomach with 1-cm ulceration in the first portion of the duodenum; no bleeding or evidence of gastric outlet obstruction<br>• Biopsy with Warthin-Starry stain is positive for *H. pylori*; in actively bleeding ulcers, sensitivity is low so stool antigen or urea breath test should be done |

#### Basic Science Correlate

- *H. pylori* is a microaerophilic helix-shaped gram-negative bacterium
- *H. pylori* produces oxidase, catalase, and urease

### Discussion

This patient has a duodenal ulcer secondary to *H. pylori*. The initial medical management of peptic ulcer disease is antisecretory therapy with proton pump inhibitors (e.g., omeprazole, lansoprazole). There is no difference between the different medications within a class; however, the proton pump inhibitors produce more rapid healing of duodenal ulcers because of their sustained antacid secretory effect compared with H2 blockers.

Antacids are composed of aluminum and magnesium hydroxide and act by neutralizing gastric acid and protecting gastric mucosa. Antacids at high doses also demonstrate healing rates comparable with H2 blockers, but the ulcers will recur without eradicating *H. pylori.*

*H. pylori* infection is associated with 90% of duodenal ulcers and 70% of gastric ulcers. Therapy for *H. pylori* dramatically reduces the recurrence of ulcer disease (75–90% reduction in peptic ulcer). Almost 50–60% of patients will have a recurrence after treatment with H2 blockers or PPIs alone if *H. pylori* is not eradicated with antibiotics. When testing for *H. pylori,* patient should be off antibiotics for 4–8 weeks and off PPIs for 2 weeks.

Triple therapy with clarithromycin, amoxicillin, and a PPI is commonly used; however, if there was recent treatment with a macrolide, local resistance to clarithromycin is >15% so use quadruple therapy or replace clarithromycin with levofloxacin. Quadruple therapy is tetracycline, metronidazole, bismuth, and a PPI.

**NOTE**

Aspirin for secondary prophylaxis and anticoagulation in A-fib should be restarted within 24 hours.

### Follow-up Management and Prevention

- *H. pylori* therapy for 2 wks with an oral PPI (such as omeprazole, pantoprazole, or rabeprazole), combined with amoxicillin/clarithromycin or metronidazole/clarithromycin. Alternatives include tetracycline/metronidazole/bismuth subsalicylate or tetracycline/clarithromycin/bismuth subsalicylate. Any PPI with amoxicillin/clarithromycin is the single best answer.
- Surgery for severe complications such as severe bleeding not responsive to local therapy, perforation, or obstruction; although duodenal ulcers are not associated with malignancy, refractory cases may rarely require surgery.
- Counseling of patients:
  - Avoid excess use of NSAIDs (if must use, give COX-2 inhibitor and a PPI)
  - Smoking and alcohol use prevent the healing of ulcers but do not cause them
  - Bland (nonspicy) diets do not help, nor does removing spicy food from diets

**CLINICAL PEARL**

*H. pylori* is not associated with GERD.

### Final Diagnosis

Duodenal ulcer

# CASE 4

## Chief Complaint

Confusion

## History and Physical Examination

A 45-year-old man was admitted 2 days ago for an acute upper GI bleed. The patient is an alcoholic with a long history of alcoholic liver disease. He underwent endoscopy on admission and was found to have a bleeding duodenal ulcer that responded to treatment with omeprazole. The patient appeared to be stabilizing. This morning, however, the nurse noted that the patient was becoming increasingly confused. He appeared agitated and was oriented to his name, but thought the current year was 1972 and that Nixon was president. The patient has become increasingly lethargic over the last few hours. He has been on thiamine since admission.

He is afebrile, BP is 130/80 mm Hg, pulse 80/min, and respirations 16/min. The neck is supple, lungs are clear, and heart has RRR. His abdomen is soft, nontender, liver edge not palpated, splenic tip 3 cm below the left costal margin. He is lethargic and uncooperative, withdraws to pain, and is hyperreflexic bilaterally. Asterixis is present, while nystagmus is not. Cranial nerve examination reveals no overt ophthalmoplegia.

## Differential Diagnosis

1. Hepatic encephalopathy
   - Confusion in liver disease is highly suspicious for hepatic encephalopathy, compounded by the fact that the patient recently had an upper GI bleed (a known trigger for worsening hepatic encephalopathy).
2. Alcohol withdrawal/delirium tremens
   - Liver disease can be secondary to alcoholism and so a concurrent syndrome could be seen. However the finding of asterixis and normal vital signs make it less likely.
3. Infection: meningitis, bacterial peritonitis if patient has ascites
   - Any infection has the potential to cause sepsis and lead to end-organ damage (AMS, confusion, low urine output, etc.).

### Initial Management

**Setting:** emergency department

### Diagnostic/Therapeutic Plan

- CBC
- BUN/creatinine
- AST/ALT
- Lactate dehydrogenase
- Bilirubin
- Glucose
- Ammonia

### Test Results

- WBC 5,000/mm$^3$ (normal 4,000–11,000/mm$^3$), hemoglobin 10 mg/dL (normal 13–17mg/dL), platelets 110,000/mm$^3$ (normal 150,000–350,000/mm$^3$), MCV 92 μm$^3$
- BUN 20 mg/dL, creatinine 1.1 mg/dL
- AST 60 U/L (normal 8–30 U/L), ALT 48 U/L (normal 8–30 U/L)
- Lactate dehydrogenase 250 U/L (normal 100–300 U/L)
- Bilirubin 1.5 mg/dL (normal 0.1–1.0 mg/dL)
- Glucose 110 mg/dL (normal 80–120 mg/dL)
- Ammonia 180 (normal 47–65)

### Assessment

A stressor such as GI bleed or infection often precipitates hepatic encephalopathy. An elevated ammonia level roughly correlates with this diagnosis. Ammonia levels by themselves do not adequately diagnose hepatic encephalopathy. Confusion and agitation several days into hospitalization are suggestive of delirium tremens, but this patient appears more confused than agitated and does not appear to be in a hypersympathetic state.

Wernicke encephalopathy is possible, particularly in a patient receiving IV glucose solution who has underlying thiamine depletion, but this patient has been on thiamine replacement.

### Further Management Plan

1. Correct precipitating factors (GI bleed or infections)
2. Airway protection including intubation if necessary
3. Lactulose to prevent ammonia absorption and facilitate excretion; the dose of lactulose should be titrated to produce 2–4 stools a day
4. Rifaximin (antibiotic with poor oral bioavailability) for reducing nitrogenous production in the gut and helping to prevent relapse of hepatic encephalopathy episodes

#### CLINICAL PEARL

The most common predisposing factor for hepatic encephalopathy is GI bleed (increased absorption of nitrogenous substances). Patients with cirrhosis are especially prone to upper GI bleed because of portal hypertension-induced varices. Hepatic encephalopathy is associated with increased nitrogenous substances generated by colonic bacteria. Aggressive use of diuretics and associated electrolyte disturbances may also precipitate an event. Dehydration from overdiuresis is associated with a contraction alkalosis, which increases the proportion of circulating uncharged ammonia that can penetrate the blood-brain barrier.

## Discussion

This patient has hepatic encephalopathy precipitated by recent GI bleed. Hepatic encephalopathy is a reversible change or decrease in neurologic status that is secondary to liver disease.

The etiology of hepatic encephalopathy is not fully understood. It is associated with severe hepatocellular dysfunction, portal hypertension, shunting of blood away from portal circulation, and ingestion of high-protein meals. Toxic nitrogenous by-products of proteins absorbed from the intestine are not detoxified by the liver and gain access to the systemic circulation, leading to encephalopathy.

**NOTE**

Ammonia level is not correlated with the degree of encephalopathy and should not be checked.

Patients with hepatic encephalopathy usually present with progressive confusion that may lead to stupor and coma. Focal signs may transiently develop. Hyperreflexia, rigidity, and asterixis are present. Fetor hepaticus refers to a musty smell associated with encephalopathy; it is related to the presence of mercaptans in the blood. Cerebral edema may be present. The diagnosis of hepatic encephalopathy is one of exclusion.

Treatment of encephalopathy is identification and elimination of the precipitating causes, such as protein sources in the gut (e.g., blood or food).

- Assess patients for GI bleed
- Eliminate sedatives or tranquilizers
- Check paracentesis to look for SBP. Hypokalemia can also lead to hepatic encephalopathy.
- Initiate ammonia-lowering therapy with lactulose (an osmotic diuretic that acidifies colonic contents, which trap ammonia in the lumen and prevent its absorption)
  - Lactulose also reduces ammonia production by colonic bacteria
  - Antibiotics such as rifaximin reduces ammonia level by killing urease-producing colonic bacteria

**CLINICAL PEARL**

Beware of the alcohol liver disease patient whom you elect to treat with sedatives (benzodiazepines) for presumed delirium tremens. Benzodiazepines are also common precipitants of hepatic encephalopathy.

## Final Diagnosis

Hepatic encephalopathy

# CASE 5

## Chief Complaint

"I've had diarrhea, weight loss, and abdominal distension."

## History and Physical Examination

A 27-year-old woman comes to the office with 8 months of diarrhea, weight loss, and a pruritic skin rash. There is no blood or mucus in the diarrhea. She is a very anxious person and has recently been more depressed. She is frustrated because she cannot identify a cause of the diarrhea and has become obsessive about eating food she is sure cannot be contaminated with any type of food poisoning. She denies fevers, abdominal pain, or bleeding, and her appetite is excellent.

Her T is 37.0 C (98.6 F), BP 130/80 mm Hg, pulse 70/min, and respirations 14/min. Examination of the eyes, ears, nose, throat, and neck is normal. The abdomen is soft, nontender, and somewhat distended with hyperactive bowel sounds. Rectal examination shows guaiac-negative, brown stool. She has a diffuse, papulovesicular rash over her elbows, knees, buttocks, and back.

## Differential Diagnosis

1. Celiac disease: the likely diagnosis given the diarrhea and weight loss, which indicate malabsorption; the pruritic vesiculated lesions are consistent with dermatitis herpetiformis
2. Inflammatory bowel disease: seen in young patients with diarrhea but lack of blood in stool makes it unlikely; family history is common; pruritic skin lesions are not a characteristic extra-intestinal manifestation
3. Lactose intolerance: diarrhea is commonly seen in lactose intolerance but would be accompanied with gas, bloating, and worsening after eating dairy; typically not associated with malabsorption
4. Tropical sprue: produces malabsorption but would need travel history to endemic regions
5. Irritable bowel syndrome
    - Diarrhea is seen but there is predominately abdominal pain and possible constipation (diarrhea would alternate with constipation in a patient who is under stress/emotional distress)
    - Anyone with irritable bowel syndrome plus diarrhea should be tested for celiac sprue
6. Whipple disease: produces malabsorption but additionally has arthritis and neurologic symptoms and signs

7. Microscopic colitis
    - Chronic watery diarrhea in post-menopausal women
    - Colonoscopy shows normal mucosa
    - Biopsy shows lymphocytic or collagenous colitis
    - Can be caused by certain drugs: NSAIDs, PPIs, SSRIs (stop them right away)
    - Treatment: loperamide or bismuth (for mild disease); budesonide (severe disease)
8. Small intestinal bacterial overgrowth
    - Nocturnal diarrhea and history of gastric bypass surgery, diabetic neuropathy, or scleroderma
    - Caused by decreased peristalsis of the small intestines
    - Check glucose with hydrogen breath test or treat with empiric antibiotics
    - Treatment: rifaximin

### Initial Management

**Setting**: outpatient

### Diagnostic/Therapeutic Plan

- CBC, serum iron, calcium, B12, folate
- Stool culture
- Stool examination for ova and parasites
- Smear for fecal leukocytes
- Stool for fat determination (Sudan stain)
- D-xylose absorption test

**CLINICAL PEARL**

The organisms that most commonly cause fecal leukocytes are *Shigella*, *C. jejuni*, *E. coli* 0157:H7, enteroinvasive *E. coli*, *C. diff*, and *Salmonella*.

### Test Results

- Mild macrocytic anemia; B12, folate, serum iron, calcium, and magnesium all mildly decreased
- Stool culture negative for enteric pathogens
- Stool exam negative
- Smear negative for fecal leukocytes
- Stool for fat determination: multiple fat globules seen
- D-xylose absorption test abnormal

### Assessment

The differential diagnosis of chronic diarrhea includes infectious etiologies, inflammatory bowel disease, and malabsorption syndromes. Infectious causes are less likely since bacterial gastroenteritis would present acutely and often resolves spontaneously over several days. *Giardia* may cause a chronic diarrheal syndrome associated with bloating and dyspepsia. In immunocompromised patients (e.g., AIDS patients), cryptosporidia, microsporidia, *Giardia*, and *Mycobacterium avium* intracellulare are common causes of chronic diarrhea.

Malabsorption syndromes are characterized by steatorrhea and weight loss. Pancreatic insufficiency-induced malabsorption is caused by chronic pancreatitis or cystic fibrosis. Injury to the small bowel surface is seen with celiac sprue, Whipple disease, or tropical sprue. If in doubt, use D-xylose to differentiate, despite patient's history.

Finally, lactase deficiency results in bloating and diarrhea after ingesting milk products. It is documented by history and the impact of cessation of milk products in the diet.

An association between IgA deficiency and celiac disease can cause a false-negative IgA based test. Check assays for IgG.

### Further Management Plan/Results

| | |
|---|---|
| • Antiendomysial, anti-tissue transglutaminase antibodies | Positive |
| • Small bowel biopsy | • Abnormal, with total villous atrophy<br>• Mosaic pattern appearing mucosa "cracked mud" and villous atrophy seen |

#### Basic Science Correlate

Patients with celiac disease may have a variant HLA-DQ2 (most common) allele or the HLA-DQ8 allele.

#### Basic Science Correlate

Gluten activates an immune-mediated reaction, which involves the innate and the adaptive immune systems.

- Tissue transglutaminase, an enzyme present in the lamina propria, deamidates glutamine residues in gluten to form glutamic acid.
- Glutamic acid is a negatively charged molecule that is recognized by the antigen-precipitating cells, which express the HLA DQ2/DQ8 receptors for T lymphocytes.
- T lymphocytes become activated and then begin to divide rapidly and secrete several immunomodulators such as immunoglobulins, cytokines, interferons, tumor necrosis factor, and interleukin 15 and 17.
- These attack and cause damage to villous atrophy.
- The various antibodies seen in celiac disease are:
  - IgA endomysial antibody
  - IgA tissue transglutaminase antibody
  - IgG tissue transglutaminase antibody
  - IgA deamidated gliadin peptide
  - IgG deamidated gliadin peptide

#### CLINICAL PEARL

Anti-tissue transglutaminase antibody (IgA) is the most sensitive and specific.

#### CLINICAL PEARL

A diagnosis of celiac sprue requires histologic confirmation. Also know the recent serologic studies used for diagnosis (transglutaminase antibodies and antiendomysial antibodies). These antibodies should disappear following the institution of a gluten-free diet. The most common cause of persistent symptoms with celiac sprue is nonadherence to a gluten-free diet.

Patients with celiac disease present with diarrhea, weight loss, abdominal distention, fatigue, and skin lesions. The skin lesions are characteristically vesiculopapular and intensely pruritic and are known as dermatitis herpetiformis. Treatment is dapsone.

### Discussion

Celiac sprue is suggested here, given laboratory and endoscopic findings. Celiac disease or gluten-sensitive enteropathy results from damage to the mucosa of the proximal small intestine from an unknown mechanism. There seems to be an immunologic reaction that causes the development of an immune response against the intestinal mucosa that is stimulated by digestion of gluten (a protein contained in grains). The disease seems to be somewhat genetically predisposed, because there are certain HLA haplotypes that are more common in these patients and their relatives.

**CLINICAL PEARL**

Shortness of breath after treatment with dapsone is most commonly due to methemoglobinemia.

In some patients, celiac disease can first present in childhood and resolve spontaneously, only to recur as an adult in decades 4 or 5. Other patients may not manifest symptoms until middle- or old-age. Patients may have asymptotic disease in childhood or may develop the disease in adulthood, as may be the case here.

The 3 features of celiac sprue that establish diagnosis include:

1. Evidence of malabsorption
2. Characteristic duodenal mucosal changes seen on biopsy
3. Symptomatic improvement on gluten-free diet

Diarrhea occurs secondary to malabsorption, and hence steatorrhea occurs. Serum iron, vitamin B12, zinc, magnesium, and calcium can also be decreased because of the malabsorption, given that these elements are absorbed in the small intestine. Osteoporosis is common but iron deficiency anemia is most common due to impaired absorption in the duodenum. Liver enzymes can also be increased.

The major method of establishing a diagnosis of celiac disease is with antigliadin, antiendomysial, and antitransglutaminase antibodies. The single most important test is small bowel biopsy.

#### Basic Science Correlate

The D-xylose test helps to differentiate malabsorption from pancreatic insufficiency from sprue because sprue is caused by an intestinal mucosal defect and not an enzyme secretory defect. D-xylose is a 5-carbon sugar that should be absorbed in the proximal small intestine and excreted in the urine easily as long as the small bowel mucosa is intact. Because metabolism of the sugar is not necessary for absorption, pancreatic and other enzyme deficiencies do not affect it. In this patient, the D-xylose level in the urine was low, indicating that the defect lies at the level of the intestinal mucosa and that D-xylose was not absorbed.

**NOTE**

Type 1 diabetes and thyroid disease are common in celiac patients. Consider celiac in those with poorly controlled hypothyroidism because they cannot absorb the thyroid hormone.

The small bowel duodenal biopsy is essential in the diagnosis of this disease because it identifies the total villous atrophy that is seen in 80% of patients and mononuclear infiltrate in the lamina propria. Celiac sprue patients should respond to the gluten-free diet. Diagnosis can be confirmed with resolution of symptoms while on a gluten-free diet. Antibody tests, including antiendomysial antibody and antigliadin, can also assist in diagnosis. Antiendomysial antibody is more useful with a specificity and sensitivity of 90%.

Lymphoma (enteropathy-associated T-cell lymphoma) can occur in 10–15% of cases of celiac disease. It is unclear whether therapy with a gluten-free diet decreases the incidence of lymphoma. Patients with celiac disease are also at risk for adenocarcinoma of the intestine.

The mainstay of therapy is a gluten-free diet (free of wheat, rye, and barley gluten). Over time, the small intestinal mucosa will normalize. Patients with anemia and electrolyte abnormalities may require supplemental therapy.

### Follow-up Management and Prevention

- Gluten-free diet (no wheat, rye, oats, bran)
- Use of rice and corn-containing products
- Folate and iron supplementation as needed
- If symptoms persist after 3 mos of dietary modification, non adherence to diet is most likely cause but also consider lymphoma (especially if patient has fevers)
- If patient develops abdominal pain several months/yrs after being stable and without symptoms, the most common cause is lymphoma (bone mineral density should be done)

### Final Diagnosis

Celiac sprue

# CASE 6

## Chief Complaint

Left-sided abdominal pain

## History and Physical Examination

A 78-year-old woman comes to an unscheduled office visit complaining of left-sided abdominal pain for the past 24 hours. She had a similar episode 3 months ago, but that went away on its own. Yesterday she noted some mild abdominal pain on the left lower abdomen, which has steadily worsened over the course of the day in association with low-grade fever. She denies nausea or vomiting. She denies a change in bowel habits and blood per rectum. She denies any change in urinary habits or weight. Her appetite is good.

Her T is 38.3 C (101.0 F), BP 130/80 mm Hg, pulse 90/min, and respirations 18/min. Examination of the heart and lungs is normal. The abdomen is soft, nondistended, and mild rebound is noted in the left lower quadrant. There is no evidence of diffuse peritonitis or costovertebral angle tenderness. Rectal examination shows guaiac-negative stool with no masses.

## Differential Diagnosis

1. Diverticulitis
    - Most common cause of LLQ pain with fever in an older adult patient; the lack of blood also fits the description
2. Pyelonephritis
    - Seen in patients who have dysuria and flank pain with positive costovertebral angle tenderness
3. Appendicitis
    - Causes abdominal pain and fevers but in right lower quadrant
4. Colon cancer
    - Does not present with pain but causes change in stool caliber and often guaiac-positive stool

## Initial Management

**Setting**: outpatient or emergency department

## Diagnostic/Therapeutic Plan

- CBC
- Biochemical profile
- Chest x-ray
- Abdominal x-ray
- Urinalysis

### Test Results

- WBC count 15,000/mm$^3$ (normal 4,000–11,000/mm$^3$), normal hemoglobin
- Biochemical profile normal
- Chest x-ray normal
- Abdominal x-ray: air-filled small bowel in lower pelvis; no evidence of intestinal obstruction; no free air
- Urinalysis: no pyuria or blood

### Assessment

Fever and lower abdominal pain are worrisome findings that could be consistent with appendicitis. Pain and tenderness exclusively on the left is inconsistent with appendicitis. A good appetite and the absence of tenderness on rectal examination are also inconsistent with appendicitis. Colitis is unlikely without diarrhea or blood in the stool.

### Further Management Plan/Results

| | |
|---|---|
| CT scan of abdomen and pelvis | • Shows localized inflammatory changes along sigmoid colon with no evidence of free air or abscess<br>• Bowel loops and diverticula are visible |

### Further Management

- Nothing by mouth
- IV hydration
- IV antibiotic such as ciprofloxacin or metronidazole; any fluoroquinolone in combination with metronidazole is also effective; cephalosporins such as cefoxitin are also effective
- Surgical exploration if patient worsens

### Discussion

This patient has findings consistent with diverticulitis. Diverticulitis results from inflammation and microperforation of colonic diverticulum. The microperforation is thought to occur secondary to a fecalith, which becomes trapped in the diverticulum and causes inflammation. Diverticulitis is seen in up to 25% of patients with diverticula. It most commonly occurs on the left side of the colon. Patients commonly present with fever, leukocytosis, and left lower quadrant abdominal pain.

#### Basic Science Correlate

A true diverticulum includes all 3 layers of the gut; the lining mucosa, the muscularis, and the outer serosa. Colonic or false diverticula are missing the muscularis and are therefore very thin-walled.

**CLINICAL PEARL**

Consider surgical therapy for diverticulitis in those:

- With recurrent cases
- Who do not promptly improve with medical treatment
- With complicated diverticular disease (i.e., abscess)
- Who are young (age <40) because disease tends to be aggressive

Complications of diverticulitis include abscess formation, colovesical fistula formation (causing recurrent urinary tract infections or pneumaturia), or perforation leading to peritonitis. Occasionally, an inflammatory phlegmonous mass can be felt on palpation.

Diagnosis can be suspected from the clinical findings listed above. CT scan confirms diagnosis and often reveals a thickened (inflamed) colon with a possible abscess or fistula.

Patients with minimal symptoms can be treated as outpatient with an oral antibiotic such as amoxicillin-clavulanate or ciprofloxacin-metronidazole. Patients with more significant signs of inflammation, such as this patient, should be admitted to the hospital and given nothing by mouth, started on IV hydration, and administered broad-spectrum antibiotics to cover gram-negative and anaerobic colonic flora.

If the patient's clinical condition improves and physical findings normalize, slowly start the patient on oral intake and advance the diet as tolerated. Once resolution occurs, give 7–10 days of oral antibiotics. Most patients display symptomatic improvement within 72 hrs.

If the patient's clinical condition worsens while on IV antibiotics or if peritonitis of a more diffuse nature develops, surgical intervention and an exploratory laparotomy are indicated. Resection of the involved area would be necessary, in addition to creating a colostomy. Surgery can also be considered on an elective basis in patients with recurrent episodes of diverticulitis. Abscess drainage and fistula repair may also be needed.

Colonoscopy and barium enemas are contraindicated in active diverticulitis because of the potential for perforation. However, in all patients perform **colonoscopy about 4 weeks after the inflammation resolves to rule out carcinoma.**

## Follow-up Management and Prevention

- Patient should consume adequate fiber and be well hydrated, as constipation is a risk factor for the development of diverticulitis.
- Avoiding nuts and seeds is a myth; do not counsel patients to remove them from the diet.

## Final Diagnosis

Diverticulitis

# CASE 7

## Chief Complaint

"I'm having red blood mixed with loose stools."

## History and Physical Examination

A 17-year-old woman comes to the office because of bright red blood per rectum and loose stools for the past 2 weeks. She associated the rectal bleeding with 5–6 soft/loose stools per day and lower abdominal discomfort. There is no history of antibiotic use, fever, unusual travel, or joint discomfort.

She is afebrile, and vital signs are stable. Cardiovascular and pulmonary examinations are WNL. Her abdomen is non distended, with normal bowel sounds. There is tenderness in the left lower quadrant and painful, tender coin-sized lesion on the left shin. Rectal examination shows bright red blood in rectal ampulla. Nothing abnormal is palpated.

## Differential Diagnosis

1. Infectious enterocolitis
   - Common cause of bloody diarrhea, but usually self-resolves in a few days and does not extend 2 weeks
   - Infectious causes of bloody diarrhea do not cause tender shin lesions.
2. Inflammatory bowel disease (IBD)
   - Most likely diagnosis, as patient fits the age group, presents with several episodes of loose blood BMs, and has a classic extraintestinal manifestation of IBD known as erythema nodosum
3. Hemorrhoidal bleeding
   - Does cause blood in the stool but would be bright red blood and would be associated with constipation. Furthermore, the description would be blood streaking the stool as opposed to diarrhea.

### CLINICAL PEARL

Bloody diarrhea in the young patient usually represents enteroinvasive bacterial infection (e.g., *Campylobacter*) or the first bout of IBD.

## Initial Management

**Setting:** outpatient

## Diagnostic/Therapeutic Plan

- Examine stool for culture
- Examine stool for ova and parasite
- Examine stool for fecal leukocytes
- Abdominal x-ray
- CBC and ESR

### Test Results

- Stool for culture: negative
- Stool for ova: negative
- Stool for fecal leukocytes: positive
- X-ray: normal
- WBC and ESR: elevated

### Assessment

IBD is a good consideration in this case and is divided into ulcerative colitis (UC) and Crohn's disease. The predominant symptom of UC is bloody diarrhea, given rectal involvement in almost 100% of cases. Infection is unlikely, given negative stool studies. Hemorrhoids can occur at any age but should be palpable on examination.

### Further Management Plan/Results

- Colonoscopy: continuous petechial hemorrhage, mild exudate, edema, and hyperemia are seen in rectosigmoid colon extending to sigmoid flexure; a few superficial ulcerations are noted

### Further Management

- Mesalamine for maintenance in UC (not effective for flares)
- Only when mesalamine not effective, use 6MP or azathioprine for long-term immunomodulators and to bridge patient off steroids; needs several months to have an effect (not effective for flares)
- Corticosteroids in severe disease to induce remission
- Supportive antidiarrheal agents
- Total colectomy should be considered in severe cases refractory to steroids
- Biologics such as infliximab, adalimumab, and golimumab when patient has symptoms despite immunomodulators
- Anti-TNF antibodies are approved for inducing and maintaining remission in UC; use when no response to glucocorticoids but first check PPD and hepatitis B
- Ustekinumab or vedolizumab for cases refractory to anti-TNF antibodies

### Discussion

This patient has ulcerative colitis (UC). UC is seen predominantly in young adults but has a second peak of incidence in the older adult. It has a genetic predisposition, with up to 20% of patients having a family member with the disease. The etiology is unknown but is thought to be immune-mediated or related to food allergy or infection.

Patients with UC initially present with bloody diarrhea and abdominal pain for several weeks duration. The disease course can vary from mild proctitis to fulminant pancolitis. There is an increased risk of cancer in UC patients with disease >10 years duration. These patients need to have a colonoscopy with biopsy to rule out dysplasia.

Crohn's disease differs from UC in that it has transmural granulomas, which can cause fistula formation. Crohn's also involves any part of the GI tract from the mouth to the anus but "skips" parts of the bowel, leaving it normal. Fistulas are treated with infliximab and other TNF modifiers. Infliximab use has been associated with reactivating tuberculosis.

Recent research has shown that mesalamine is effective only in limited, mild ileocolonic Crohn's disease. Crohn's is mostly treated with anti-TNF antibodies now. Infliximab, adalimumab and certolizumab are used. They are effective both for Crohn's flares and maintenance. They are also used to treat fistulas.

| Crohn's Disease | Ulcerative Colitis |
|---|---|
| Skip lesions | Curable by surgery |
| Transmural granulomas | Entirely mucosal |
| Fistulas and abscesses | No fistulas, no abscesses |
| Masses and obstruction | No obstruction |
| Perianal disease | No perianal disease |

### Basic Science Correlate

| ANCA and ASCA Results in IBD | | |
|---|---|---|
| **Test** | **Crohn's Disease** | **Ulcerative Colitis** |
| Antineutrophil cytoplasmic antibody (ANCA) | Negative | Positive |
| Anti-Saccharomyces cerevisiae antibody (ASCA) | Positive | Negative |

It is important to rule out infectious cause of diarrhea, which in this condition can present in a similar fashion.

- Stool studies should be checked.
- Sigmoidoscopy is useful in diagnosis and is best performed in an unprepped bowel
- Colonic findings may reveal mucosal inflammation extending from the rectum proximally
  - Inflammation is continuous (unlike CD, which has skip lesions)
- Biopsy sample can assist in diagnosis.
- It is important to rule out toxic megacolon (a complication of UC), with abdominal film.

In an acute flare, patients have elevated CBC and sedimentation rate. If significant blood loss occurs, anemia can be seen. Patients should be given 13-valent pneumococcal conjugate and 23-valent pneumococcal polysaccharide vaccines.

**NOTE**

All patients with IBD flare must have *Clostridiodes difficile* test checked.

Patients with UC and CD may have extra-intestinal manifestations, such as arthritis, erythema nodosum, episcleritis, iritis, and sclerosing cholangitis. If someone is diagnosed with PSC, check colonoscopy to evaluate for IBD. These patients are also at risk for gallbladder cancer (if gallbladder polyps are found, remove the gallbladder).

For initial therapy, use a salicylate such as mesalamine. For severe cases, use corticosteroids. For chronic active disease, immunosuppressive agents (azathioprine and 6MP) can be used where they have a steroid-sparing effect in patients who are steroid-dependent. For proctosigmoiditis, use enemas. For severe UC refractory to steroid therapy, surgery may be needed.

### Follow-up Management and Prevention

Patients with UC should be counseled that use of NSAIDs can cause flares. Cigarette smoking has been shown to be protective in UC.

There is a risk of colorectal cancer in IBD (both UC and Crohn's), associated with duration and extent of disease. In UC, annual surveillance colonoscopy is started 8 years after diagnosis and repeated every 1-2 years.

### Final Diagnosis

Inflammatory bowel disease: ulcerative colitis

# CASE 8

## Chief Complaint

"Severe, dull abdominal pain"

## History and Physical Examination

A 32-year-old man with a history of alcohol abuse comes to the emergency department with a 2-day history of increasing, constant, dull epigastric pain that radiates to the back. He has had 2 episodes of emesis without any blood or coffee grounds. The patient admits to an alcoholic binge yesterday. He denies prior history of similar episodes. He denies any history of trauma and medication use.

His T is 37.7 C (99.9 F). Supine BP is 110/70 mm Hg, pulse 100/min; standing BP 90/60mm Hg, and pulse 120/min. The heart is tachycardic and lungs are WNL. The abdomen has decreased bowel sounds, tenderness to palpation in the epigastric region, but no guarding or rebound tenderness. Rectal examination shows guaiac-negative stool.

## Differential Diagnosis

1. Pancreatitis
   - Most common cause of acute epigastric pain in an alcoholic patient
2. Peptic ulcer disease with possible perforation
   - Commonly seen in patients with long-standing history of peptic ulcer disease

## Initial Management

**Setting:** emergency department

## Diagnostic/Therapeutic Plan

- Stabilize patient
- CBC
- Biochemical profile
- Amylase and lipase
- Abdominal x-ray

## Test Results

- Place large bore catheters and start fluids
- WBC 15,000/mm$^3$ (normal 4,000–11,000 mm$^3$)
- Glucose 204 mg/dL (normal 80–120 mg/dL), calcium 7.2 mg/dL (normal 8.5–10.5 mg/dL)
- Amylase 460 U/L (normal 60–180 U/L); lipase 1,000 U/L (elevated 3x normal)
- X-ray: no evidence of free air

### Basic Science Correlate

Amylase has the highest sensitivity, while lipase has the highest specificity

## Assessment

People with a history of alcohol abuse are at risk for acute pancreatitis, which classically presents with abdominal pain that radiates to the back. There is no rebound tenderness or guarding, arguing against a perforated peptic ulcer. Risk factors for severe pancreatitis are age >55, comorbidities, SIRS, signs of hypovolemia (BUN >20 mg/dL and rising and hematocrit >44%, and elevated serum creatinine.

Patients with pancreatitis can have low-grade fever, increased WBC, and electrolytic abnormalities, especially hypocalcemia. Diagnosis requires at least 2 of the following:

- Acute onset upper abdominal pain
- Serum amylase or lipase increased ≥3 the upper limit of normal (ULN)
- Findings on CT suggestive of pancreatitis

**NOTE**

- Do an abdominal ultrasound on all patients with acute pancreatitis (even alcoholics) to evaluate for biliary stones.
- Do a CT only if severe symptoms persist for more than 48 hours (rebound tenderness, absent bowel sounds, high fever) to look for complications.

## Further Management Plan/Results

- CT scan of abdomen: diffuse pancreatic edema with extension to the pancreatic fat is seen

## Further Management

- Nothing by mouth
- Analgesics, e.g., morphine
- IV hydration
- If CT shows necrosis, administer imipenem and consider surgical evaluation for debridement
- Gallbladder U/S to exclude gallstone pancreatitis

**CLINICAL PEARL**

Causes of pancreatitis:

- Gallstones
- Ethanol
- Trauma
- CF (young people)
- Sulfonamides, didanosine, valproic acid, thiazides, azathioprine/6-MP, pentamidine, estrogen, furosemide
- Autoimmune disease
- Scorpion stings
- Hypertriglyceridemia/hypercalcemia
- ERCP

## Discussion

This patient has alcohol-induced pancreatitis. In acute pancreatitis, there is pancreatic inflammation, and autodigestion occurs within acinar cells by activated pancreatic enzymes. In the United States, alcohol abuse accounts for 30% of cases of acute pancreatitis, followed by gallstones. The exact mechanism of alcoholic injury to the pancreas is unknown.

- Most patients present with abdominal pain in the upper abdomen or epigastric region that usually radiates to the back. The pain is often dull in nature.
- Patients may have nausea and vomiting accompanied by severe abdominal pain.
- On physical examination, upper abdominal tenderness is typically seen.
- Pancreatic enzymes amylase and lipase are elevated at least to 3x their normal limit. Amylase increases first, followed by the lipase, which is more specific for pancreatic injury.
- Increased glucose levels are seen in B-cell dysfunction that results in decreased levels of insulin.
- A decrease in calcium may occur and does not mandate treatment.

Pancreatic inflammation can be seen on CT, as well as phlegmonous changes, pseudocysts formation, and pancreatic necrosis.

Other complications of pancreatitis include phlegmonous changes (early in disease), abscess formation (4–6 weeks), formation of pseudocyst (collection of pancreatic fluid surrounded by fibrous or granulation tissue occurring at 1–4 weeks), necrosis (2 weeks), and acute respiratory distress syndrome. The mortality rate for acute pancreatitis is 10% and is related to the presence and severity of pancreatic necrosis.

The mainstay of treatment for pancreatitis is supportive, and 90% of cases resolve spontaneously. Support consists of putting the pancreas to rest: stop all oral intake and correct all the fluid sequestration by providing IV fluids (250-500 mL/h) and analgesic therapy. Aggressive IVFs are most beneficial in the first 12-24 hours and may be detrimental after that window (**high-yield**).

- Encourage patient to stop alcohol ingestion; monitor for delirium tremens.
- Start on oral intake once abdominal pain resolves and narcotic analgesics are not needed. Normalization of amylase or lipase is not needed to initiate oral intake.
- If pain and nausea persist and patient cannot tolerate PO by 72 hours after admission, start on enteral nutrition.
- Nasogastric or nasojejunal enteral feeding has been shown to promote healthy gut-mucosal barrier and prevent trans location of bacteria. Enteral feeding should be used over total parental nutrition (which is discouraged, due to high infection rates with bacteria and fungi).

There is no evidence that antibiotics help resolve uncomplicated episodes of pancreatitis, but imipenem and cefuroxime may be helpful in some scenarios: severe pancreatitis with infected necrosis, cholangitis, and infected pseudocysts. Surgery may be needed for pseudocyst removal, necrotic debridement, and infected pancreatitis debridement. CT-guided needle biopsy is helpful for determining if the patient has infected necrosis. Most pseudocysts resolve spontaneously and do not need drainage.

### Follow up-Management and Prevention

In patients with gallstone pancreatitis, cholecystectomy is required. In patients who abuse alcohol, addiction counseling for alcohol is required.

### Final Diagnosis

Acute pancreatitis

#### CLINICAL PEARL

Up to 70% of idiopathic cases of pancreatitis are secondary to biliary microlithiasis.

#### CLINICAL PEARL

- All patients with acute pancreatitis should have an U/S of the gallbladder to exclude gallstones. Acute pancreatitis accompanied by transaminase elevation is characteristic of cholelithiasis.
- All patients with gallstone pancreatitis must have a cholecystectomy prior to discharge.

#### NOTE

Perform ERCP only if there is concurrent ascending cholangitis or no improvement in obstruction.

#### NOTE

Autoimmune pancreatitis typically presents with painless obstructive jaundice or acute pancreatitis (rare). CT scan reveals "sausage-shaped" pancreatic enlargement with indistinct border.

- **Type I** is seen in older men and is associated with pancreatitis, Sjogren syndrome, PSC, bile duct strictures, autoimmune thyroiditis, and interstitial nephritis. Serum IgG4 is increased.
- **Type II** is associated with chronic pancreatitis and IBD and normal IgG4 levels. Most patients respond to corticosteroids.

# CASE 9

## Chief Complaint

"My father is yellow."

## History and Physical Examination

A 45-year-old man presents with a 2-day history of fever, right upper quadrant abdominal pain, and jaundice. The patient's daughter noticed that his skin color changed progressively in the last 2 days. He complains of feeling very tired and has had rigors and diaphoresis. His T is 102.9° F, blood pressure 85/40 mm Hg, and pulse 120/min.

On physical examination the patient has significant tenderness in the right upper quadrant, the sclera are icteric, and the skin is markedly jaundiced. The patient denies any respiratory distress but is difficult to arouse. He has no significant past medical history but did recently have postprandial RUQ pain that self resolved after 30-45 minutes.

## Differential Diagnosis

1. Ascending cholangitis
   - Most likely diagnosis given the findings of jaundice, fever, RUQ abdominal pain, altered mental status and hypotension
2. Cholecystitis
   - An obstruction of the cystic duct does cause RUQ pain, but there would be no AST/ALT changes and a positive Murphy's sign could be seen
3. Choledocholithiasis
   - Predisposing risk factor for the development of cholangitis but given the lack of fever is not inflammatory in nature
4. Primary sclerosing cholangitis
   - Can lead to biliary obstruction but classically occurs in conjunction with inflammatory bowel disease

## Initial Management

**Setting:** emergency room

## Diagnostic/Therapeutic Plan

When dealing with an unstable patient, the initial management plan is the same for all causes: focus on **stabilizing the patient**.

- Insert 2 large-bore IV lines and start fluids (normal saline or crystalloid)
- Saline infusion until systolic BP >90 mm Hg, HR <90, or urine output (if affected) increases
- Obtain CBC, biochemical profile, and PT/PTT
- Consider intubation if patient is markedly obtunded or has unprotected airway
- Insert Foley catheter to monitor urine output

### Test Results

- Hemoglobin 14 mg/dL (normal 13-16 mg/dL)
- WBC 19,100 cells/$mm^3$
- Platelets 80,000/$mm^3$ (normal 140,000-340,000/$mm^3$)
- Sodium 140 mEq/L (normal 135-150 mEq/L), BUN 30 mg/dL (normal 8–18 mg/dL), creatinine 1.4 mg/dL (normal 0.6–1.3 mg/dL)
- Bilirubin 9.5 mg/dL (normal 0.1-1.0 mg/dL), AST 440 U/L, ALT 480 U/L (normal 8-20 U/L), alkaline phosphatase 460 U/L PT/PTT: 17 sec/25 sec (elevated)

### Assessment

Reynolds pentad is a collection of signs and symptoms that indicate ascending cholangitis, a serious infection of the biliary system.

- Jaundice
- Fever
- RUQ abdominal pain
- Altered mental status
- Hypotension (shock)

Ascending cholangitis is caused by an obstruction, most commonly a gallstone; in this patient that is likely as he has a remote history of biliary colic. The patient should be initially resuscitated as he has evidence of hemodynamic instability stemming from his biliary sepsis. Once he has been stabilized, testing and treatment specific to cholangitis can begin.

#### CLINICAL PEARL

*E. coli* is the most common organism implicated in biliary sepsis.

### Further Management Plan/Results

| | |
|---|---|
| • Nothing by mouth | |
| • Piperacillin/tazobactam IV | |
| • Continued IV hydration | |
| • Endoscopic retrograde cholangiopancreatography (ERCP) | • Large radiopaque stone is lodged in the distal common bile duct<br>• Sphincterotomy is performed and stone is removed with a basket retrieval device |

### Discussion

Cholangitis is a rising infection of the biliary tract, with choledocholithiasis as the most common cause of biliary tract obstruction. Less common causes are obstructions due to helminths, occluded biliary stents, and malignancy. The condition most commonly occurs in adults over the age of 60 years and has no predilection to gender.

Patients will present with fever, abdominal (right upper quadrant) pain, and jaundice (the Charcot triad), which is highly suggestive of cholangitis. This triad plus altered mental status and hypotension fulfill the pentad of symptomology that is consistent with cholangitis. Physical examination may reveal fever, icterus, jaundice, and abdominal pain.

The most common aerobic organisms are *Escherichia coli* followed by *Klebsiella* and then *Enterococcus* species. The most commonly reported anaerobic organism is *Bacteroides fragilis.*

Diagnosis of ascending cholangitis is conducted through abdominal U/S that will show a dilated common bile duct with dilated intrahepatic ducts.

Treatment is IV antibiotics and correction of fluid/electrolyte imbalances. Antibiotics can be piperacillin/tazobactam, ampicillin/sulbactam, ertapenem, or ceftriaxone, cefuroxime, cefotaxime, ciprofloxacin, levofloxacin **plus** metronidazole. Patients may present in septic shock and will require intubation, fluid bolus and possible vasopressor therapy. Once vital signs are stable, ERCP is the next best step in management. If patient is too unstable to undergo ERCP, percutaneous transhepatic biliary drainage (PTBD) is an alternative method to decompress the biliary system.

### Follow-up Management and Prevention

Eventual cholecystectomy is needed to treat the underlying nidus of gallstones.

### Final Diagnosis

Cholangitis

# Nephrology 10

## CASE 1

### Chief Complaint

Nausea and malaise

### History and Physical Examination

A 72-year-old woman comes to the emergency department complaining of nausea and generalized malaise for the past day. There is no associated fever, chills, chest or abdominal pain, or other constitutional symptoms. Her past medical history is significant for severe osteoarthritis, which is controlled with ibuprofen. She had a recent flare-up of back pain and had taken "a number of extra pills."

She appears to be in no acute distress. Vital signs are temperature 37° C (98.6° F), blood pressure 100/60 mm Hg, pulse 100/min, and respirations 26/min. Physical examination shows mild jugular venous distension, a heart that is mildly tachycardic but otherwise normal, and left basilar crackles in her lungs. Her abdomen is soft, nontender, and without hepatosplenomegaly. There is 1+ bilateral lower extremity edema.

### Differential Diagnosis

1. Acute kidney injury (AKI)
2. Congestive heart failure
3. Viral gastroenteritis
4. Nephrotic syndrome

### Initial Management

**Setting:** emergency department

### Diagnostic/Therapeutic Plan

- CBC, serum electrolytes, BUN, creatinine
- Urinalysis
- ABGs
- Chest x-ray
- Calcium and uric acid

### Test Results

- CBC normal, sodium 138 mEq/L, potassium 5.8 mEq/L, chloride 106 mEq/L, bicarbonate 12 mEq/L, BUN 78 mg/dL, creatinine 6.3 mg/dL
- Urinalysis: trace proteinuria
- ABGs: pH 7.29, $PCO_2$ 20 mm Hg, $PO_2$ 80 mm Hg
- Chest x-ray: small left pleural effusion
- Calcium and uric acid: normal

**CCS NOTE**

You may not be able to determine a specific diagnosis from the history of present illness. Order the routine admitting labs (CBC, chemistry panel [basic metabolic panel], urinalysis, and chest x-ray) if you don't know what to do.

### Assessment

The clinical presentation of this patient is nonspecific. The history of an older adult person who has taken an excess dose of an NSAID, however, should alert the clinician to the possibility of AKI. This diagnosis becomes quite obvious with measurements of serum electrolytes and BUN.

AKI impairs the excretion of salt and water with alteration of acid-base mechanisms; therefore, it is frequently complicated by fluid overload, hyperkalemia, and metabolic acidosis. The patient should be hospitalized and monitored closely, given the severity of the abnormalities.

AKI is often classified into 2 groups: oliguric (<400 mL/24 hrs) and nonoliguric (>400 mL/24 hrs). The lower the urine output, the worse the prognosis. In cases where hypovolemia contributes to the development of AKI, fluid challenges are often given in an effort to convert a patient from the oliguric to the nonoliguric state. In this patient, however, there are already significant signs of volume overload (jugular venous distension, left basilar crackles, peripheral edema), and adding fluid would not be wise.

It is important to differentiate between prerenal, intrarenal, and postrenal causes. Prerenal azotemia gives a BUN/creatinine ratio of 20:1. This patient's ratio is closer to 10:1, indicating a problem in the kidney itself. There are no crystals in her urine consistent with hyperuricemia or oxalate causing renal failure, and no history of gout. There are no RBCs in the urine. RBCs generally indicate a glomerular disorder. If no urine is produced, an obstructive uropathy must be ruled out by bladder catheterization and renal U/S.

| Further Management Plan | Results |
|---|---|
| U/S of kidneys | Normal |
| Urine stain for eosinophils | Negative |
| Urine sodium | >40 mmol/L |

### Treatment Plan

- Discontinue all NSAIDs, as well as all other possible nephrotoxic agents
- Admit to hospital
- Hemodynamic monitoring
- Close monitoring of electrolytes
- Possible dialysis

### Discussion

NSAIDs can cause renal toxicity (interstitial nephritis, nephrotic syndrome, and prerenal azotemia), although the risk is low. Patients age >60 or with history of renal disease, CHF, ascites, or diuretic use are at higher risk. NSAIDs inhibit prostaglandins, which are vasodilatory in the kidney. Therefore, NSAIDs lead to vasoconstriction.

When assessing AKI, one of the most important decisions is whether hemodialysis is appropriate. Indications for **emergency dialysis** are:

- Refractory hyperkalemia
- Profound metabolic acidosis
- Alteration in mental status
- Refractory fluid overload
- Uremic pericarditis

When BUN remains consistently >100 mg/dL, dialysis is often begun.

Dialysis is used to treat life-threatening complications of renal failure that are not correctable by other means. For example, anemia can be life-threatening, but it is correctable with transfusions or erythropoietin use, and hence does not require dialysis. Pericarditis, however, is not correctable by other means.

Hemodialysis is not without risks, however. The associated volume shifts may predispose patients with underlying cardiac disease to ischemic events. Additionally, the risk of infection is significant.

#### CCS NOTE

If you want to know how the patient is doing and you don't get nurses' notes informing you, click the INTERVAL HISTORY button on the physical exam page.

#### Patient Safety Note

Aspiration precautions should be ordered in uremic patients who complain of nausea and vomiting, and especially in patients with altered mental status, as they are at high risk for aspiration.

There are a few associations that should prompt you to think about specific diagnoses; however, these have to be assessed on a case-by-case basis.

- **Minimal proteinuria with muddy brown casts:** acute tubular necrosis (ATN)
  - Check the fractional excretion of sodium (FENa). Excess sodium is usually lost because of damage in the tubules or glomeruli. Consequently, the calculated FENa would be high (>2%) in ATN, while FENa that is low (<1%) would indicate prerenal causes.
- **Erythrocyte or dysmorphic erythrocyte casts:** glomerulonephritis
  - Investigate the cause by checking dsDNA, ANA, antistreptolysin O antibodies, complement level (C3, C4, CH50), HIV and hepatitis serologies, cryoglobulins, p-ANCA/c-ANCA, and antiglomerular basement membrane antibodies.
- **Eosinophilia, eosinophiluria with or without a rash:** acute interstitial nephritis (AIN)
  - Patient's medication list should be reviewed, as well as history for recent vascular procedure. Another clue for cholesterol emboli is a rash that is described as a "violaceous reticular rash" or "livedo reticularis."

- **Pyuria:** pyelonephritis or AIN, as above
  - Patient's medication list should be reviewed and urine culture checked
- **Nephrotic range proteinuria (urine protein >300 mg/dL):** diabetes and renal vein thrombosis
  - Check patient's blood glucose or HbA1c, and perform renal Doppler study
- **Obstructive uropathy**
  - Check for prostate pathology, kidney stones, retroperitoneal fibrosis, or other malignant obstructing masses; investigations include checking residual bladder volume and taking noncontrast CT or MRI
- **Enlarged kidneys on U/S**
  - Check for obstructive uropathy (as above) or early diabetes, amyloidosis, and HIV nephropathy. Investigations include serum electrophoresis, HIV testing, and blood glucose or HbA1c

**CCS NOTE**

You will not get confirmation of your final diagnosis on the CCS.

### Final Diagnosis

Acute kidney injury, NSAID-induced

# CASE 2

## Chief Complaint

"I feel really weak and confused."

## History and Physical Examination

A 52-year-old woman, who has insulin-dependent diabetes, comes to the clinic because of several months of generalized, progressive weakness. She has not seen you in nearly a year because she has been "scared of what you might tell" her. She comes in now because she is finding it difficult to think clearly. She gets her prescriptions when she needs them from local walk-in clinics. When she was last in the clinic a year ago, she was asymptomatic; lab studies at that time showed hematocrit 34% (normal 38–44%), BUN 42 mg/dL (normal 7–18 mg/dL), creatinine 3.2 mg/dL (normal 0.5–1.3 mg/dL), and potassium 4.9 mEq/L (normal 3.5–5.2 mEq/L).

Her vital signs today are temperature 36.4 C (97.5 F), blood pressure 110/70, pulse 95/min, and respirations 18/min. She has no neck stiffness. Examination of the chest shows mild, bibasilar rales, and cardiovascular examination shows no murmurs or rubs. She has 1–2+ edema of lower extremities bilaterally. Neurologic examination shows no focal defects, but she is somewhat confused. She does not know the exact date or day of the week and cannot do calculations, serial 7s, or remember 3 objects at 5 minutes.

## Initial Management

**Setting:** outpatient workup and treatment

## Differential Diagnosis

1. Hypoglycemia (usually episodic)
2. Hyperglycemia/diabetic ketoacidosis
3. Renal failure
4. Anemia
5. Cerebrovascular accident (unlikely since exam nonfocal)

## Diagnostic/Therapeutic Plan

- Glucose
- BUN, creatinine
- Hematocrit
- Serum bicarbonate
- Potassium
- ABGs

### Test Results

- Glucose: 142 mg/dL (normal 80–120 mg/dL)
- BUN, creatinine: 92 mg/dL, 8.4 mg/dL
- Hematocrit: 29%
- Serum bicarbonate: 15 mEq/L (normal 22–26 mEq/L)
- Potassium: 5.8 mEq/L (normal 3.5–5.2 mEq/L)
- ABGs: metabolic acidosis

### Assessment

This patient has had insulin-dependent diabetes, and she could potentially have any of the end-organ manifestations of the disease. These are all related to damage to the microvasculature.

Manifestations of long-term diabetes are the following:

- Nephropathy
- Stroke
- Myocardial infarction
- Retinopathy (strongly suggests coexisting diabetic nephropathy)
- Neuropathy
- Peripheral vascular disease

This patient had evidence of renal insufficiency in the past, but it was not severe enough to cause symptoms. The renal insufficiency has now progressed and is causing acidosis (decreased bicarbonate), hyperkalemia, mild encephalopathy, and anemia.

The patient's complaints are unlikely to be due to stroke because there is no headache or focal neurologic finding. Meningitis is unlikely in the absence of fever, headache, and neck stiffness. Ketoacidosis is unlikely with a low glucose, but is still possible. Ketoacidosis could also account for the acidosis and the hyperkalemia.

The most immediate concern should always be to address the most life-threatening problem: in this case, the hyperkalemia. The most dangerous effect of hyperkalemia is arrhythmia, and the earliest EKG finding of hyperkalemia is peaked T waves.

| Further Management Plan | Results |
| --- | --- |
| EKG | Normal rate and rhythm; normal T waves; normal QRS |
| Serum acetone | Negative |
| Urinalysis | $3^+$ protein; $1^+$ glucose |
| Renal U/S | Bilaterally large kidneys |

### Treatment Plan

- Correct hyperkalemia
- Continue insulin at present dose
- Refer to nephrologist for institution of dialysis

Treatment of chronic kidney disease is as follows:

- **Hypertension**: an ACEI or ARB in the early stages to prevent further worsening; in late stages when hyperkalemia is evident, caution should be used with ACEI and ARBs. Use calcium blockers and vasodilators.
    - Choose loop diuretic rather than thiazide if GFR< 30 mL/min/1.73 $m^2$
- **Proteinuria (serum protein-creatinine ≥200 mg/mg)**: ACEI or ARB even if patient is normotensive
- **Hemoglobin A1c >7%**: intensive control of DM
- **Anemia:** check iron storage and replete if inadequate; erythropoietin to maintain Hb 10–11 g/dL. **Always check iron studies** before starting erythropoietin.
- **Hyperphosphatemia and hypocalcemia**: phosphate binders (calcium acetate, calcium carbonate, sevelamer) to maintain phosphate levels at 3.5–5.5 mg/dL
- **Hyperlipidemia**: statins with target LDL <100 mg/dL
- **Vitamin D deficiency**: vitamin D analogs

### Discussion

The most important initial management here is to lower the potassium, because that is the most immediate life-threatening problem. Sodium polystyrene sulfonate is a sodium/potassium exchange resin, given orally, which will remove potassium from the body. If the potassium were higher, bicarbonate alone or glucose combined with insulin could be given to lower the potassium more rapidly. With extremely high potassium level and EKG abnormalities, calcium chloride or calcium gluconate is injected intravenously (and given along with the insulin) to protect the heart from arrhythmia.

There are a large number of manifestations of renal failure. These are all due to loss of the excretory, productive, or reabsorptive functions of the kidney. The kidney excretes water, potassium, acid, magnesium, phosphate, uric acid, and nitrogenous waste products. Therefore, kidney failure can result in fluid overload, hyperkalemia, acidosis, hypermagnesemia, hyperphosphatemia, and hyperuricemia. Accumulation of nitrogenous waste products causes encephalopathy, pericarditis, pruritus, and increased infections and bleeding. These last 2 occur because platelets and WBCs don't work well in a uremic environment.

The kidney produces erythropoietin and vitamin D2. Therefore, kidney failure results in anemia and osteodystrophy. Hypocalcemia can occur from insufficient calcium absorption from both the intestine and the kidney.

Although there are many manifestations of chronic renal failure, only a few need emergent dialysis. All are life-threatening and none can be treated well by other means.

- Intractable hyperkalemia (i.e., doesn't respond to sodium polystyrene sulfonate)
- Pericarditis
- Intractable fluid overload

#### CCS NOTE

On the CCS if you order EKG, chest x-ray, urinalysis, and U/S at the same time, they will all be done simultaneously and immediately.

#### CCS NOTE

The consultant will not make specific recommendations. However, asking for a consultation at the appropriate time shows good judgment.

- Acidosis
- Encephalopathy

**Patient Safety Note**

- All patients with ESRD are considered candidates for kidney transplant unless not warranted (chronic infection, neuropsychiatric disease, malignancy, severe cardiovascular disease). Kidney transplant is associated with better quality of life and is less expensive to the health care system than long-term dialysis.
- Advise patients to not use aluminum-containing antacids (aluminum toxicity) or magnesium-containing antacids.

### Final Diagnosis

Chronic renal failure from diabetes

# CASE 3

## Chief Complaint

"I don't want to have diarrhea on my vacation to Thailand."

## History and Physical Examination

A 47-year-old man comes to the office for advice about how to prevent diarrhea on the vacation he is planning to Thailand. He sees you about once a year for minor problems and routine evaluation and is generally quite healthy. His last evaluation the prior year was completely normal. He uses no medications, except occasional vitamins, and smokes 1 pack of cigarettes every 2 days.

Vital signs are temperature 37 C (98.6 F), blood pressure 155/95 mm Hg, and respirations 12/min. He appears not to be in distress. Physical examination shows eye grounds with no hemorrhages or exudates. The remainder of the physical examination is unremarkable.

## Differential Diagnosis

1. Essential hypertension
2. Renal artery stenosis
3. Pheochromocytoma
4. Hyperaldosteronism

## Initial Management

**Setting:** outpatient

## Diagnostic/Therapeutic Plan

- BUN, creatinine
- Urinalysis
- CBC
- Potassium
- EKG

## Test Results

- BUN: 14 mg/dL; creatinine: 0.8 mEq/L (normal)
- Urinalysis: normal
- CBC: normal
- Potassium: normal
- EKG: normal

### CCS NOTE

Office management of non-urgent cases such as this may go on for "months" of simulated time. Do not worry if the case doesn't seem to end. Just keep moving the clock forward and manage the patient.

### Assessment

This patient is in his usual state of good health, except for elevated systolic and diastolic BP. Over 95% of high blood pressure cases are of unknown etiology and are referred to as "essential" hypertension. The most common presentation of essential hypertension is an incidental finding (with no symptoms). When BP is high enough to cause symptoms on presentation, this is often called hypertensive "emergency."

These are poorly defined terms that do not refer to any specific numbers in terms of the pressure. They refer instead to the presence of symptoms—including headache, visual disturbance, dyspnea, chest pain, and mental status changes. Patients with high BP and these symptoms should be treated immediately. A person can have a very high BP and still have no symptoms; this is referred to as hypertensive "urgency."

A single elevation on a single visit is not sufficient to warrant initiation of drug treatment. Up to 1/3 of hypertension is so-called "white-coat" hypertension. This means that the general anxiety of being in the doctor's office can artificially raise BP. When the same patients are given a BP cuff to measure at home, their BP is normal. True hypertension should be defined as an elevation found on several visits over time.

### Further Management Plan/Results

- Diet modification (salt restriction, weight loss), exercise, relaxation methods, and reduction in alcohol intake
- If no response to lifestyle modifications is seen after 6 months, use diuretics first (see Discussion section for choices)

**CCS NOTE**

Do not skip steps such as lifestyle modification just because you don't think they could be effective. Always "advise," "counsel," or "educate" about exercise, weight loss, and diet.

### Discussion

Start with a diuretic. If a diuretic alone does not control the pressure, then add a calcium channel blocker (CCB), ACE inhibitor, or angiotensin-receptor blocker. There are now dozens of medications approved for first-line management of hypertension, but diuretics are still recommended as the first choice—particularly the thiazides, CCBs, and ACE inhibitors.

The goal with BP is <140/90 mm Hg. If BP >160/100, start with 2 medications. If patient has BP >140/90 mm Hg and has diabetes, add 2 medications.

- Diuretics: hydrochlorothiazide
  - Diuretics clearly lower mortality through prevention of stroke and heart disease. They can rarely cause hyperlipidemia, hyperuricemia, hypokalemia, and hyperglycemia. They are not antianginal.
- Beta-blockers: atenolol, metoprolol, propranolol, nadolol, labetalol or carvedilol (a combined nonspecific beta-blocker and central-acting alpha agent)
  - Besides lowering BP, beta-blockers have antianginal effect by decreasing myocardial work. Certain forms are also antiarrhythmic and, for example, can control rate in atrial fibrillation.
  - Disadvantages are occasional depression, memory loss, impotence, and fatigue. In addition, they must be used with caution in diabetics because they mask the symptoms of hypoglycemia and may precipitate bronchospasm in asthmatics. They can cause Raynaud phenomenon and worsen peripheral vascular disease by contributing to constriction of peripheral vasculature (beta-2 stimulation dilates small arteries).

- CCBs: nifedipine, diltiazem, verapamil, amlodipine, felodipine, isradipine, nicardipine
  - Some CCBs are antianginal as well. Verapamil and diltiazem are also useful for tachyarrhythmias. They are used to treat Raynaud syndrome and relieve esophageal spasm.
  - They have relatively few major side effects and there are no lipid effects. They can cause constipation, pedal edema, and reflex tachycardia.
- ACE-inhibitors: captopril, enalapril, lisinopril, fosinopril, ramipril, benazepril, quinapril
  - ACE inhibitors are neither antianginal nor antiarrhythmic. They have few side effects, such as cough, hyperkalemia, angioedema, and rash. They have no significant lipid, CNS, or sexual side effects.
  - ACE inhibitors are all first-choice therapy for those with diabetes, CHF, previous myocardial infarction, and chronic renal failure with proteinuria.
  - Efficacy is an effect of the whole class of medications; it is not based on a specific drug.
- ARBs: losartan, valsartan, irbesartan, candesartan
  - Angiotensin II blockers have the same indications as ACE inhibitors, such as congestive heart failure and diabetes. They are best used if ACE inhibitors cannot be tolerated. Cough is the most common reason why a patient can't tolerate an ACE inhibitor.

Do **not** select beta-blockers as initial monotherapy unless there is a compelling indication present, such as CHF or CAD.

| Drugs | Indications | Contraindications |
|---|---|---|
| Diuretics | Systolic hypertension, heart failure | Gout |
| Beta-blockers | CHF, angina, MI, tachyarrhythmias | Heart block, severe asthma/COPD, pregnancy |
| ACE-Is | CHF, diabetic nephropathy, proteinuria, post-MI | Hyperkalemia, pregnancy, bilateral renal artery stenosis |
| ARBs | ACE-I induced cough, diabetic nephropathy, CHF | Same as ACE-I |
| CCBs | Angina, CAD, cyclosporine induced HTN | Heart block (diltiazem, verapamil) |
| Alpha-blockers | BPH | Orthostatic hypotension |

**Hypertensive urgency** is defined as **systolic BP >180 mm Hg** and/or **diastolic BP >120 mm Hg, with no ongoing end-organ damage**. Management depends on whether or not the patient is on treatment.

- If patient is being treated and is compliant, then adjust medication by either increasing the medication dose or adding a new agent. If patient is noncompliant, restart his home medication and provide counseling.
- If patient is not on treatment and presents with hypertensive urgency, observe for several hours; treatment should include small doses of clonidine or captopril to gradually reduce BP 20–30 mm Hg. Once that is achieved, start a long-acting antihypertensive agent and discharge the patient, with a follow-up appointment in a few days.

**Hypertensive emergency** is defined as **systolic BP >180 mm Hg** and/or **diastolic BP >120 mm Hg, with end-organ damage.** Symptoms may include shortness of breath, chest pain, encephalopathy or stroke, retinopathy, or acute kidney injury.

- Admit the patient and gradually reduce the BP no more than 25% in the first hour; IV medications such beta-blockers (metoprolol), CCB (nicardipine), hydralazine, nitroprusside, and nitroglycerin are preferred.

### CCS NOTE

One of the most anxiety-provoking challenges of the CCS is determining how often to bring a patient back to the office for routine management for a disorder like hypertension. Choose intervals of 2–4 weeks until BP is stable.

Second- and third-line agents are direct vasodilators (hydralazine, minoxidil), central-acting alpha agents (alpha methyldopa, clonidine), and ganglionic blockers (reserpine, guanethidine). These agents are rarely used because of their side effects. The direct vasodilators are typically used in patients with resistant HTN associated with chronic kidney disease.

- Peripheral-acting alpha-blockers: prazosin, terazosin, doxazosin
  - Note these are **not** used routinely for the treatment of hypertension.

An important factor is to rule out the relatively small population that has an underlying cause for their elevation in pressure. Patients presenting at age <25 or >60, or those who have an unusual physical examination finding, such as an abdominal bruit (renal artery stenosis), moonlike facies or striae (Cushing syndrome), hypokalemia (hyperaldosteronism), or signs of acromegaly, should have further investigation for these conditions.

Other indications for which further evaluation may be necessary are:

- Protein in the urine
- Elevation of BUN and creatinine
- Rapidly progressing eye ground abnormalities (hemorrhages, exudates, papilledema)

The EKG abnormalities associated with long-standing hypertension (which are absent in this patient) are most often signs of left ventricular hypertrophy. These are an S-wave in V1 and an R-wave in V5 >35 mm. This is not so much an indication of secondary hypertension as an indication of long-standing disease.

## Final Diagnosis

Essential hypertension

# CASE 4

## Chief Complaint

Headache and high blood pressure

## History and Physical Examination

A 27-year-old woman comes to your office because of a continuous frontal headache for the last several months. You noted her to be hypertensive on examination several months ago, and she has been on nifedipine for the last 8 weeks. Prior to that, she had been healthy her entire life and is on no other medications. The nifedipine dose was raised on her last visit.

Vital signs are temperature 37° C (98.6° F), blood pressure 170/100 mm Hg, and pulse 70/min. Examination of the head, eyes, ears, nose, and throat shows normal eye grounds and no papilledema. The chest is clear bilaterally. She has a regular heart rate and rhythm, with no murmurs or gallops. The abdomen is soft and nontender, with a rhythmic, high-pitched sound in the epigastric area. The extremities are nonedematous.

## Differential Diagnosis

1. Renovascular hypertension (renal artery stenosis)
2. Pheochromocytoma
3. Primary hyperaldosteronism
4. Essential hypertension
5. Coarctation of the aorta

## Initial Management

**Setting:** outpatient

## Diagnostic/Therapeutic Plan

- BUN, creatinine
- Renal U/S
- Potassium

## Test Results

- BUN: 36 mg/dL, creatinine: 1.2 mg/dL
- Renal U/S: bilaterally small kidneys, left smaller than right
- Potassium: 3.4 mEq/L (normal 3.5–5.2 mEq/L)

## Assessment

Over 95% of patients with hypertension have "essential" (or idiopathic) hypertension. Because it is expensive and inefficient to evaluate all patients with new-onset hypertension for causes of secondary hypertension, it is important to develop criteria for determining who to screen.

In general, indications for further evaluation include any of the following:

- Onset of hypertension at age <30 or >55
- Hypertension that remains high despite medication
- Progression from normal to severe hypertension over the course of several months

The list of secondary causes includes those listed in the Differential Diagnosis section above, as well as oral contraceptives, acromegaly, Cushing syndrome, and congenital adrenal enzyme deficiencies. Renal artery stenosis is the most common; in addition, it gives abdominal bruits such as the one in this patient and is common in young women.

| Further Management Plan | Results |
|---|---|
| Magnetic resonance angiography, *or* | Decreased uptake in left kidney |
| Duplex U/S of the renal artery | Renal artery stenosis on left |
| Renal artery arteriography (gold standard) | Stenotic lesion in the distal renal artery on the left |

**CCS NOTE**

There are often multiple pathways to the correct management of individual cases on the CCS. There is more flexibility on the CCS than you might think.

## Treatment Plan

- Balloon angioplasty of stenotic lesion
- Repeat the angioplasty if initial one fails
- Operative repair only if angioplasty is not possible or not effective
- Medical treatment (ACE inhibitors) only if angioplasty and surgery are not possible

## Discussion

The causes of renal artery stenosis can be divided into 2 types:

- Fibromuscular dysplasia of the arterial wall occurs in younger woman, particularly age <30
- Atherosclerotic disease occurs in older men

Although it seldom gives useful specific information, renal sonogram is usually done initially because it is an inexpensive and noninvasive examination. The main finding is of **kidneys different in size**. MRI angiography approaches 95% sensitivity and specificity for stenotic lesions of >50% diameter. The ultimate, and best, test for renal artery stenosis is the arteriogram. This test, however, is not performed, because of its invasiveness, until after the others described above are done.

This patient's hypokalemia is because the high renin-angiotensin state leads to a large amount of aldosterone. The high aldosterone state can cause hypokalemia and alkalosis because aldosterone causes an increased urinary loss of potassium and hydrogen ions in exchange for the reabsorption of sodium.

Treatment is based on reversing the stenotic lesion.

- Balloon angioplasty cures 50% of cases and provides improvement in 30%. If the initial angioplasty fails, it may be repeated.
- If angioplasty repeatedly fails or is not possible, then surgical resection is performed.
- Chronic medical management with ACE inhibitors is used only when these 2 modalities are not effective or possible.
- ACE inhibitors will control the blood pressure, but the kidney will fail in bilateral renal artery stenosis.

### Final Diagnosis

Renal artery stenosis

### CLINICAL PEARL

Consider secondary hypertension in patients with atypical clinical features such as presenting age $<30$ or new onset age $>55$, no family history, hypokalemia, metabolic alkalosis, kidney disease, or persistent hypertension despite the use of multiple medications.

### CLINICAL PEARL

A specific differential diagnosis to keep in mind is primary hyperaldosteronism, which also presents with hypertension and hypokalemia. However, physical examination is usually normal, and patients may present with muscle cramping and muscle pain. Further investigation reveals elevated aldosterone to plasma renin activity ratio.

# CASE 5

## Chief Complaint

"I'm feeling confused. What day is it?"

## History and Physical Examination

A 57-year-old man who is a long-term smoker is brought to the emergency department by his family because of mild confusion that has been developing slowly over the last several days. He was diagnosed with lung cancer by bronchoscopy 2 months ago and is about to undergo chemotherapy. He still has the hemoptysis that led to his original presentation, and his chest x-ray has a left perihilar infiltrate. Besides confusion, he has also been somewhat weaker. There are no other specific complaints. His past medical history is significant for depression and diabetes. He is on an SSRI antidepressant and glyburide.

Vital signs are temperature 37.4° C (99.3° F), blood pressure 120/70 mm Hg, pulse 78/min, and respirations 16/min. There is no neck stiffness. He has a regular heart rate and rhythm, with no murmurs, and his chest is clear to auscultation. Neurologic examination shows that he is awake and alert but disoriented to the exact day. He knows he's in the doctor's office and what the year is. There are no focal deficits, but his muscles are somewhat weak.

## Differential Diagnosis

1. Paraneoplastic syndrome
2. Metastatic cancer to the brain
3. Hyponatremia
4. Hypoxia
5. Meningitis

## Initial Management

**Setting:** emergency department

## Diagnostic/Therapeutic Plan

- Head CT scan with contrast
- Serum electrolytes
- Urine sodium
- Pulse oximetry on room air

## Test Results

- Head CT scan with contrast: normal
- Serum electrolytes: sodium 122 mEq/L (normal 135–145 mEq/L), potassium 4.2 mEq/L (normal 3.5–5.2 mEq/L), chloride 102 mEq/L (normal 98–106 mEq/L), BUN 18 mg/dL (normal 7–20 mg/dL), glucose 90 mg/dL
- Urine sodium: 42 mmol/L
- Pulse oximetry on room air: 96% saturation

### Assessment

Generalized confusion in a patient with a known malignancy should always suggest metastatic disease to the brain. Lung cancer, breast cancer, and melanoma are frequently metastatic to the brain. The absence of focal neurologic findings generally points away from this. However, CT scan or MRI of the head with contrast effectively excludes this as a cause of the symptoms.

There is no neck stiffness indicative of meningitis, and lung cancer is not a specific risk factor for meningitis. Metabolic abnormalities, such as hyponatremia and hypernatremia, can cause confusion, as can hypoglycemia, hypoxia, and drug intoxications. This patient has a focal lung lesion that is unlikely to be large enough to cause lung damage sufficient to lead to hypoxia. Oxygen saturation is normal. Pulse oximetry is acceptable instead of an ABG test when the $CO_2$ does not have to be evaluated. Labs reveal sodium 122 mEq/L (normal 135–145 mEq/L), which is sufficiently low to cause these symptoms.

| Further Management Plan | Results |
|---|---|
| Serum osmolality | 254 mOsm/kg $H_2O$ |
| Urine osmolality | 540 mOsm/kg $H_2O$ |

### Treatment Plan

- Fluid restriction to 1–2 liters per day
- Loop diuretic (furosemide, bumetanide, ethacrynic acid) if there is no improvement with fluid restriction alone and give with normal saline
- Stop the SSRI and sulfonylurea
- Demeclocycline chronically if the underlying cause cannot be corrected

### Discussion

The most common cause of hyponatremia in a patient with a malignancy or any pulmonary abnormality is the syndrome of inappropriate antidiuretic hormone (SIADH). This is a normovolemic form of hyponatremia. A diagnosis of SIADH is confirmed with high urine sodium (>20 mmol/L) and a urine osmolality greater than serum osmolality in the presence of hyponatremia.

In fact, the diagnosis of SIADH is virtually assured if urine osmolarity is >100. In that case anything—except a maximally dilute urine in the presence of hyponatremia—is consistent with SIADH.

The causes of hyponatremia can be divided into 3 categories:

- **Hypervolemic**: occurs in congestive heart failure, nephrotic syndrome, and cirrhosis
- **Hypovolemic**: occurs with Addison disease, GI losses, burns, and diuretic use combined with drinking free water
- **Normovolemic**: SIADH, psychogenic polydipsia, or pseudohyponatremia from hyperglycemia, hypothyroidism

The causes of SIADH can be divided into 4 categories:

- **Pulmonary**: virtually anything—pneumonia, atelectasis, emphysema, embolism, etc.
- **CNS**: virtually anything—tumor, stroke, hematoma, dementia, encephalitis, meningitis, etc.

#### CLINICAL PEARL

Don't forget that severe hyperglycemia causes pseudohyponatremia.

### CLINICAL PEARL

The approach to hyponatremia starts with determining the patient's clinical volume status.

**Hypovolemia (hypotension, dehydration)**

- Spot urine sodium <10 mEq/L
- BUN/creatinine >20:1
- Urine osmolarity >450 mOsm/L
- Renal or GI losses, dehydration, adrenal insufficiency

**Hypervolemia (ascites, edema)**

- Spot urine sodium <10 mEq/L
- BUN/creatinine >20:1
- Urine osmolarity >450 mOsm/L
- Liver cirrhosis, ascites, kidney failure

**Euvolemia: normal volume**

- Spot urine sodium >10 mEq/L
- BUN/creatinine <20:1
- Urine osmolarity; as below
- Urine osmolarity >300 mOsm/L: SIADH, hypothyroidism
- Urine osmolarity: 50–100 mOsm/L: psychogenic polydipsia

### CLINICAL PEARL

Cerebral salt-wasting syndrome causes hypo-osmolar hyponatremia showing similar labs to SIADH. However, this syndrome is associated with hypovolemia and develops within days of a neurological procedure or a subarachnoid hemorrhage.

- **Neoplasm**: only a few are commonly associated with ectopic production, e.g., small-cell (oat-cell) cancer of the lung, thymus, duodenal cancer (although any cancer could be associated)
- **Medications**: any oral hypoglycemic agent can do it, but chlorpropamide is most often associated; cyclophosphamide, clofibrate, and SSRIs (sertraline) are also common causes

Thus, in this patient, oat-cell carcinoma or the involvement of the lung alone can be causing the SIADH. As stated above, the diagnosis of SIADH is confirmed by the finding of a urine osmolarity greater than serum osmolality in the presence of hyponatremia. This is because a healthy person's urine would become maximally dilute (osmolality <100) if they became hyponatremic, in the body's attempt to rid itself of the free water. SIADH is a problem with free water, not a problem with sodium metabolism.

Treatment, therefore, is based on controlling the free water.

- For mild SIADH (sodium level ≥120–125 mEq/L) with few or no symptoms, treatment is fluid restriction.
- For more severe hyponatremia (sodium about 110–120 mEq/L), treatment is normal saline and a diuretic. Saline gives salt, and the diuretic promotes a free water diuresis.
- For profoundly low sodium levels (<110 mEq/L) or severe symptoms, the fastest way to raise sodium is with hypertonic saline.

These numbers are approximations only. The development of symptoms is also highly dependent upon the rate at which sodium declines. In general, whenever there is an altered mental status, you should use hypertonic saline.

Although this patient is symptomatic with disorientation, the symptoms have been present for some time, and the hyponatremia may have developed over several weeks to months. There is no urgency to raise his sodium level over just a few hours. Raising or lowering a patient's sodium too rapidly for therapeutic purposes can also precipitate symptoms.

When you raise the sodium too rapidly, you are at risk for causing central pontine myelinolysis. When you lower it too rapidly, you risk cerebral edema. Mild abnormalities should be corrected at 0.5 mEq/L/hr. With severe symptoms, you can correct it as fast as 1–2 mEq/L/hr.

Because fluid restriction to 1–2 liters can be quite difficult to tolerate on a long-term basis, this patient may need to be maintained on demeclocycline. Demeclocycline is a tetracycline antibiotic that causes a nephrogenic diabetes insipidus and hence makes the kidney insensitive to antidiuretic hormone.

**Patient Safety Note**

Do not correct the serum sodium faster than 0.5 mEq/L/hr (12 mEq over 24 hrs).

### Final Diagnosis

Hyponatremia due to SIADH

# CASE 6

## Chief Complaint

Severe flank pain and blood in the urine

## History and Physical Examination

A 27-year-old woman comes to the emergency department because of severe pain in her left side and dark urine. She denies fever but states that a local internist had seen her several days ago for urinary frequency and burning. She had been treated with 2 double-strength tablets of trimethoprim-sulfamethoxazole at that time, and the dysuria had resolved. The pain she now feels came on very suddenly and is so severe that she cannot walk. There is some nausea, and she vomited twice in the back of her father's car on the drive to the hospital. There is pain in her vaginal area.

Vital signs are temperature 37.2° C (99.0° F), blood pressure 110/70 mm Hg, pulse 95/min, and respirations 14/min. Physical examination of the chest and heart are normal. Her abdomen is soft and nontender with no guarding. Her back is also nontender.

## Differential Diagnosis

1. Nephrolithiasis
2. Pyelonephritis
3. Cystitis

## Initial Management

**Setting:** outpatient or emergency department

## Diagnostic/Therapeutic Plan

- Urinalysis
- Abdominal x-ray
- BUN, creatinine

## Test Results

- Urinalysis: no WBCs, large amount of blood, nitrates negative
- Abdominal x-ray: normal
- BUN, creatinine: normal

## Assessment

A history of very severe flank pain is consistent with an origin in the kidney. Pyelonephritis gives pain in the flank, but there should be clear tenderness, particularly in the costovertebral angle. Pyelonephritis should also give fever and WBCs in the urine, though it can also give RBCs.

### CCS NOTE

Renal colic is a perfect example of when an analgesic such as ketorolac should be ordered with the first screen. It does not matter what order you write in the tests and treatments, as long as they are on the screen at the same time.

Pain as severe as this is profoundly unlikely with cystitis alone, which at most should give some suprapubic tenderness. Pain in the flank without tenderness associated with hematuria is most consistent with stones in the kidney or ureter. It is not possible to tell the difference between these two by history and physical alone.

The major clue to the diagnosis of nephrolithiasis is a characteristic type of profoundly severe pain. Renal colic is said to be the most severe pain a human can experience, even greater in intensity than childbirth. This pain characteristically radiates to the groin, and pain in the vulva or scrotum is classic.

| Further Management Plan | Results |
|---|---|
| CT scan without contrast | 1.4-cm stone visualized in the left renal pelvis |
| Serum calcium and uric acid | Normal |
| 24-hour urine calcium | Normal |
| Urine culture | Normal |

### Treatment Plan

- Hydration to keep urine output 2–3 liters per day
- Analgesia
- Straining the urine
- Shock wave lithotripsy (if available) or percutaneous removal if hydration does not result in passage of the stone. Small stones will pass spontaneously, but they must be small enough to enter the ureter.

**CCS NOTE**

Order all the tests you think are appropriate. The software will tell you which ones need consultations. You won't lose points if the software asks you to order a consult.

### Discussion

Kidney stones are composed of calcium oxalate (70%), calcium phosphate (10%), struvite (10–15%), uric acid (5–10%), and cysteine (1%). Nephrolithiasis affects about 1–5% of the population, with recurrences in 50–80% of those patients.

Alkaline urine predisposes to the formation of calcium-containing stones, whereas acidic urine predisposes to the formation of uric-acid stones. Magnesium-ammonium-phosphate (or struvite) stones are formed in the presence of repeated UTI, particularly with urea-splitting organisms such as *Proteus*.

A patient's history must be explored for causes of increased calcium or oxalate levels, such as abundant milk-product ingestion, vitamin D ingestion, large doses of vitamin C, or a family history of stones. Gout predisposes a person to uric-acid stone formation, but clinical gout is not necessary for the production of these stones. Ten to 30% of patients with hyperparathyroidism present with nephrolithiasis. Serum and urine should be checked for calcium levels in a patient with stones.

The most common initial treatment is **hydration and analgesia**, which allows spontaneous passage of the stones in the majority of patients. The stones must be smaller than 5 mm to have a chance of passing into the ureter. For those patients whose stones do not pass, extracorporeal shock-wave lithotripsy can break up calcium-containing stones that are not excessively large (generally <2 cm). Problems with this technique are its lack of availability, expense, and the entrapment of smaller stone fragments in the ureters later.

Percutaneous removal of stones from the renal pelvis is used when lithotripsy is not an option and the stone does not pass spontaneously. Open procedures are rarely necessary any longer. Ureteral stones can be removed percutaneously or by passing a basket up the ureter via a cystoscope.

Because about 80% of kidney stones contain calcium, about the same amount are visible on an abdominal x-ray. Straining the urine for the stone is also a time-honored method of confirmation. In an emergency room, however, the diagnostic accuracy of the x-ray may be diminished if someone who is not an expert reads the films. Renal sonogram is almost 100% sensitive for stones in the kidney. This sensitivity decreases for stones that are in the ureter: Because the ureters pass posteriorly, they are not well visualized by the anteriorly placed sonogram transducer.

IVP is essentially a historical test and is **a wrong answer choice**. A CT scan is the study of greater sensitivity and specificity. CT scanners are able to perform thin-slice sections through the ureter and can detect even very small stones. When the question asks what the **most accurate diagnostic test** is, answer **CT scan**.

In addition to diagnosing the stone, U/S and CT scan are used to diagnose other anatomic abnormalities such as strictures and obstruction.

### Final Diagnosis

Nephrolithiasis

### CLINICAL PEARL

The best test for nephrolithiasis is CT without contrast.

### CLINICAL PEARL

- To determine the type of stone, straining and checking the urine for stone collection are appropriate.
- Stones $<5$ mm in size tend to pass spontaneously; those $>10$ mm often require invasive intervention.
  - Uric acid stones and hyperuricosuria: allopurinol and decreased animal protein intake
  - Large struvite stones: long-term prophylactic antibiotics and invasive removal
  - If patient is pregnant, choose U/S for the diagnosis of nephrolithiasis (no CT)

# CASE 7

## Chief Complaint

"Why am I swelling up?"

## History and Physical Examination

A 52-year-old woman comes to your office because of generalized edema for the last several weeks. She was recently diagnosed with breast cancer and has had a lumpectomy and axillary lymph node dissection. Her lymph nodes were free of cancer, and she has not had any chemotherapy. Besides the swelling, she has generally been well and offers no other complaints.

Vital signs are temperature 37.2° C (99.0° F), blood pressure 110/70 mm Hg, pulse 95/min, and respirations 14/min. Results of examination of head, eyes, ears, nose, and throat are normal, except for periorbital edema. Her chest is clear to auscultation, and her abdomen is soft, nontender, and without hepatosplenomegaly. Her heart has no murmurs or gallops. Her lower extremities have edema up to the hips, and they are nontender and nonerythematous.

## Differential Diagnosis

1. Nephrotic syndrome
2. Cirrhosis
3. Heart failure
4. Myxedema
5. Other causes of hypoalbuminemia (malabsorption)

## Initial Management

**Setting:** outpatient

## Diagnostic/Therapeutic Plan

- Albumin
- BUN, creatinine
- Urinalysis
- 24-hour urine protein; or protein:creatinine ratio on random sample
- Serum LDL and cholesterol
- Liver function tests

## Test Results

- Albumin: 2.1 g/dL (normal 3.5–5.5 g/dL)
- BUN, creatinine: normal
- Urinalysis: 4+ protein; oval fat bodies seen; few RBC; no casts

- 24-hour urine protein: 5.5 g/24 hours; protein:creatinine ratio on random sample: 5
- Serum LDL and cholesterol: elevated
- Liver function tests: normal

### Assessment

Although the patient has breast cancer, the central problem is generalized edema, or anasarca. Edema forms for one of 2 reasons:

- Plasma protein level is too low to provide enough oncotic pressure to hold fluid in the vessels
- Heart is not pumping well enough, and the hydrostatic forces are increased enough to push the fluid out

This patient gives no cardiac history; there are no murmurs or gallops, and the lungs are clear (arguing against cardiac failure). The low serum albumin with hyperlipidemia and evidence of protein and lipids in the urine are suggestive of nephrotic syndrome. Neither malnutrition, myxedema, nor malabsorption gives proteinuria. Hyperlipidemia is explored when there is already possible evidence for the nephrotic syndrome.

| Further Management Plan | Results |
|---|---|
| Renal biopsy | Light microscopy: thickened glomerular basement membrane with spikes for basement membrane material |
| Electron microscopy | Subepithelial deposits seen |

### Treatment Plan

1. Monitoring of BUN, creatinine, proteinuria, and ACE inhibitors
2. Trial of steroids
3. Cytotoxics (e.g., cyclophosphamide) and steroids

### Discussion

Nephrotic syndrome is a constellation of edema, proteinuria, hypoalbuminemia, hyperlipidemia, and lipiduria. By definition, nephrotic-range proteinuria is >3.5 grams per 24-hour period.

About one-third of adults have nephrotic syndrome on the basis of systemic disease, most commonly diabetes, systemic lupus erythematosus, HIV, or amyloidosis. In this patient, the lack of evidence of any systemic disease besides breast cancer suggests a primary renal cause, such as minimal change disease, mesangial, membranous, focal segmental, or membranoproliferative glomerulonephritis. It is impossible to tell the difference between these on clinical grounds alone. Diagnosis is entirely based on biopsy.

On initial presentation, there is nothing obvious to signal a diagnosis of membranous glomerulonephropathy. However, membranous glomerulonephropathy is a common cause of idiopathic nephrotic syndrome in adults, and this type has an association with malignancies such as breast, lung, and colon cancers. Besides systemic disease, such as lupus erythematosus, diabetes, amyloid, and HIV, virtually any type of glomerulonephritis can develop into nephrotic syndrome. A certain percentage of patients with postinfectious glomerulonephritis, Wegener, Goodpasture, immunoglobulin A nephropathy, polyarteritis nodosa, etc., will eventually develop enough glomerular damage and proteinuria to be diagnosed with nephrotic syndrome.

#### CLINICAL PEARL

Protein:creatinine ratio on random sample is as sensitive and specific as the 24-hour urine protein.

#### CCS NOTE

One of the idiosyncrasies of the CCS is that it allows a patient to simultaneously undergo multiple tests on different parts of the body.

#### CCS NOTE

You do not have to change location to order complex tests. The patient stays in the same location, and the test is done from there.

Membranous nephropathy is more common in whites, and focal segmental glomerulosclerosis is more common in African Americans.

The prognosis of membranous glomerulonephritis is quite variable. One-third will resolve spontaneously; one-third has persistent nephrotic range proteinuria even as BUN and creatinine stay normal; and one-third develops slowly worsening renal function over time. Response to steroids is generally undramatic and disappointing, so this medication is withheld until there is evidence of significant deterioration. Minimal change disease is the most steroid-sensitive glomerular disease.

Current treatment strategies are as follows:

1. **Patients at low risk for progression:** ACE inhibitors or angiotensin receptor blockers (ARBs) to reduce proteinuria, or
2. **Patients at high risk for progression:** Immunosuppressives with or without steroids for those at high risk for progression. Steroids alone are not recommended.

### CLINICAL PEARL

- The most common cause of nephrotic syndrome in adults is FSGS.
- The most common cause of nephrotic range proteinuria (without the 'syndrome') is diabetes.

Immunosuppressive therapy is indicated in patients with the highest likelihood of developing progressive renal failure. These include patients with severe symptoms, those with progressive disease, men age > 50 years with persistent nephrotic syndrome, and patients with thromboembolic complications. Hemodialysis, peritoneal dialysis, and kidney transplantation are indicated in advanced kidney disease from nephrotic syndrome.

## Final Diagnosis

Nephrotic syndrome

### Patient Safety Note

Renal vein thrombosis, DVT, and PE may complicate the disease in patients with nephrotic syndrome, especially those with membranous glomerulonephritis. Special attention should be paid to possible thromboembolism, if renal failure worsens unexpectedly or the patient develops flank/abdominal pain.

# CASE 8

## Chief Complaint

Hematuria

## History and Physical Examination

A 32-year-old man comes for evaluation of painless gross hematuria 2 days after he developed an upper respiratory tract infection. He had a similar episode 3 years ago, but the hematuria resolved after a course of antibiotics. He otherwise feels very well and has no complaints of diarrhea, arthritis, or weight loss. He has not had recent abdominal or pelvic trauma. He has had no previous episodes of pharyngitis. The patient does not drink alcohol, smoke tobacco, or use illicit drugs. His family history is only significant for hypertension and hyperlipidemia. He works as an architect and has had no occupational exposures. He eats a healthy diet but exercises rarely; he has not exercised for the past few weeks.

Vital signs are BP 155/92 mm Hg, pulse 82/min, and respirations 12/min. The patient is afebrile. The head and neck exam are unremarkable except nasal erythema. There are no tonsillar exudates. He has no lymphadenopathy. The heart and lung exam are unremarkable. The abdominal exam is normal with no hepatosplenomegaly. The extremities are normal and without edema. There is no evidence of penile trauma.

## Differential Diagnosis

1. Exercise-induced hematuria
2. Nephritic syndrome: postinfectious glomerulonephritis, rapidly progressive glomerulonephritis, IgA nephropathy
3. Bladder cancer
4. Renal cell cancer
5. Nephrolithiasis
6. UTI with certain bacteria (e.g., Staph)
7. AV malformations
8. Polycystic kidney disease

## Initial Management

**Setting:** outpatient

## Diagnostic/Therapeutic Plan

- Urinalysis
- Creatinine
- Serum albumin
- Urine protein:creatinine (a spot specimen, which is as specific as a 24-hr protein collection)

- Serologies:
  - C3 and C4
  - ANA
  - ANCA
  - anti-GBM antibodies
- HIV
- ESR
- Cholesterol
- Renal U/S and/or CT scan
- Cystoscopy

## Test Results

- Urinalysis: +3 protein and >10 RBCs per high power field, no casts
- Creatinine: 1.2 mg/dL
- Serum albumin: 3.6 mg/dL
- Urine protein:creatinine 1.8 g/dL creatinine
  - CS and C4: normal
  - ANA: negative
  - ANCA: negative
  - anti-GBM: negative
- HIV: negative
- ESR: normal
- Cholesterol: normal
- Renal U/S and/or CT scan: normal size kidneys with no evidence of mass or stone
- Cystoscopy: negative for bladder lesions

## Assessment

First confirm hematuria with dipstick or urinalysis. Next, some experts recommend renal U/S (or CT scan) and cystoscopy to exclude focal process such as bladder and renal cancer. If both of those are negative, then check creatinine, serum albumin, urine protein, and serologies (ANA, ANCA, C3 and C4, ESR, etc.) to exclude or diagnose glomerular disease.

Another approach to hematuria undertakes a twofold urinalysis, simultaneously confirming hematuria and inspecting for protein in the urine. Positive proteinuria indicates the presence of intrinsic renal disease, and it would make sense to check serologies, albumin, etc., before doing a urologic workup with an U/S, cystoscopy, etc. If there is hematuria *without proteinuria*, then proceed to a urologic evaluation.

Several conditions can cause hematuria, most of them not serious.

- Exercise may cause hematuria that goes away in 24 hours, but the negative history in this patient makes this unlikely.
- Nephrolithiasis is a common cause of hematuria but is accompanied by flank pain, absent here.

- UTI (especially Staph) may cause hematuria, but it is accompanied by bladder or flank pain as well as urgency, fever, and pyuria.

When hematuria is the result of a tumor, such as bladder or renal cancer, it is usually painless and gross (unless the tumor causes obstruction). This is why painless hematuria, especially absent evidence of proteinuria, requires urologic evaluation with renal imaging (U/S or CT scan) and cystoscopy (needs referral to urologist).

Glomerular diseases cause hematuria and are associated with proteinuria as well as serologic abnormalities. IgA nephropathy, postinfectious glomerulonephritis, and rapidly progressive glomerulonephritis are some of the more common diseases in this group, but hematuria can also be part of systemic diseases like Goodpasture syndrome, Wegener granulomatosis, or SLE. Confirm glomerular diseases via renal biopsy.

Often, despite extensive workup, no specific cause can be found for hematuria. The following findings are consistent with IgA nephropathy.

| Further Diagnostic Testing | Results |
|---|---|
| Renal biopsy | |
| Light microscopy | • A few glomeruli show complete sclerosis; other glomeruli are mildly enlarged and display mesangial hypercellularity<br>• Tubules and interstitium show regenerative changes including nuclear enlargement<br>• Arterial vessels show medial sclerosis and intimal fibrosis<br>• There is evidence of hyalinosis in arterioles |
| Electron microscopy | Glomerular capillary lumina show widespread attenuation with ischemic-type wrinkling of basement membranes and segmental duplication of basement membranes with cellular interposition and subendothelial immune-type electron dense deposits |
| Immunofluorescence | Diffuse mesangial and segmental glomerular capillary wall staining for IgA ($3^+$) |

## Treatment Plan

- Use ACE-Is or ARBs to optimize BP control and reduce proteinuria; both agents reduce proteinuria and are renoprotective.
- Refer to nephrologist for consideration of corticosteroid treatment with or without immunosuppressive agents (e.g., cyclophosphamide).

## Discussion

IgA nephropathy is the most common glomerulonephritis throughout the world. It occurs when IgA deposits in the kidneys and causes inflammation and scarring of the glomeruli.

### CLINICAL PEARL

Distinguish IgA nephropathy from postinfectious glomerulonephritis as follows:

**IgA nephropathy:**

- Painless hematuria
- Hematuria occurs during the infection
- Proteinuria and hypertension may accompany
- No systemic manifestations
- Normal complement levels
- Diagnose by biopsy

**Postinfectious glomerulonephritis:**

- Painless hematuria
- Hematuria occurs 2 weeks after the pharyngitis
- Proteinuria and hypertension may accompany
- Edema (periorbital)
- Decreased complement levels

Initially IgA nephropathy has no symptoms and can be silent for many years, even decades. IgA nephropathy is more common among Caucasians and Asians. About 25% of adults with IgA nephropathy develop end-stage kidney failure.

The classic presentation of IgA nephropathy is frank hematuria. Hematuria in IgA nephropathy appears during a cold or other infection (pharyngitis here). This presentation is referred to as synpharyngitic hematuria, i.e., the hematuria and infection coincide. (The alternative is postpharyngitic hematuria, typically seen after 2 weeks of poststreptococcal glomerulonephritis.) The gross hematuria resolves after a few days but microscopic hematuria persists. There may also be evidence of proteinuria but it is usually not in the nephritic range. Hypertension and elevated creatinine are also common on presentation, or they may occur later in the disease. If creatinine is high at the time of diagnosis, the patient is more likely to develop kidney failure.

Renal biopsy confirms IgA deposits in the glomeruli. The biopsy can also assess how much kidney damage has already occurred. Remember, other diseases are associated with IgA deposition in the glomeruli (e.g., Henoch-Schonlein purpura), so IgA deposition in the glomeruli is not pathognomonic for IgA nephropathy.

IgA nephropathy cannot be cured. Hence, treatment focuses on slowing the disease and preventing complications. ACE inhibitors and ARBs protect kidney function by controlling BP and reducing proteinuria. Because of this effect, they are the drugs of choice in IgA nephropathy. Drugs such as corticosteroids (prednisone) and immunosuppressive agents (cyclophosphamide, mycophenolate mofetil) may also be helpful.

Patients with IgA nephropathy may develop high cholesterol. Lowering elevated cholesterol may help to slow kidney damage. In research studies, vitamin E and fish oil supplements containing omega 3 fatty acids also slowed kidney damage in some patients.

### Final Diagnosis

IgA nephropathy

# CASE 9

## Chief Complaint

"I feel very tired and my back hurts."

## History and Physical

A 56-year-old woman with a past medical history significant for hypertension comes to your office with complaints of feeling tired and having back pain for the last 3 months. The patient also noticed that her urine appears "frothy" lately, but otherwise denies symptoms of dysuria or signs of blood in her urine. Her medications include metoprolol and a daily multivitamin only.

Vitals signs are: temperature 37° C (98.6° F), blood pressure 127/78 mm Hg, and respirations 22/min. The patient is in no acute distress. Physical examination reveals pallor of the conjunctiva and mucosal membranes. The patient's lower back is tender to palpation, but she does not display any limitations in range of motion. There is no lower extremity edema noted, and no clubbing or cyanosis in the extremities.

## Differential Diagnosis

1. Multiple myeloma
2. Anemia
3. Osteoporosis
4. Renal tubular acidosis

## Initial Management

**Setting:** outpatient

## Diagnostic/Therapeutic Plan

- CBC
- Serum electrolytes
- BUN, creatinine
- Urinalysis
- Plain x-ray film of the lumbosacral region

## Test Results

- CBC: WBC count 7,400/$mm^3$, hemoglobin 9.6 mg/dL, platelets 221,000/$mm^3$
- Serum electrolytes: sodium 135 mEq/L, potassium 3.1 mEq/L, chloride 109 mEq/L, bicarbonate 16 mEq/L, glucose 98 mg/dL
- BUN: 28 mg/dL, creatinine: 2.1 mg/dL
- Urinalysis: 2+ protein, 1+ glucose, pH 5.6, protein:creatinine ratio 4.2
- Lumbosacral x-ray: lytic lesions present

### Assessment

The patient presents with fatigue, back pain, and frothy urine. She was found to have anemia, elevated BUN and creatinine, hypokalemia, low bicarbonate, and significant proteinuria along with a normal anion gap, metabolic acidosis, and alkalotic urine pH. She also has glucosuria with normal blood glucose.

Although the clinical picture clearly points to a diagnosis of multiple myeloma, the underlying findings (low bicarbonate, alkalotic urine pH, and hypokalemia) point to a renal tubular acidosis (likely, type 2) secondary to multiple myeloma in view of her clinical presentation and lab results.

| Further Management Plan | Results |
|---|---|
| ABGs | pH 7.31, $PCO_2$ 30 mm Hg, bicarbonate 18 |
| Serum protein electrophoresis (SPEP) | IgG monoclonal spike |
| Urine protein electrophoresis (UPEP) | Positive for Bence-Jones proteins |

### Treatment Plan

This patient should be worked up further for multiple myeloma. The next step would be peripheral smear, bone marrow biopsy, and skeletal survey for further evaluation of her bone pain.

RTA (type 2 in this case) is usually treated with bicarbonate and thiazide diuretics because thiazide diuretics will cause volume depletion, thus enhancing bicarbonate reabsorption.

### Discussion

**Renal tubular acidosis type 2 (proximal RTA)** is caused by an inability to reabsorb bicarbonate at the level of the proximal tubules. The body excretes bicarbonate in the urine until the supply is so depleted that the distal tubule can absorb the rest.

Initially the urine pH is basic, and then it becomes acidic (pH <5.4). Patients with type 2 RTA usually present with hypokalemia and serum bicarbonate 18–20. The major cause of proximal RTA in adults is proximal tubular damage due to increased excretion of light chain immunoglobulins; this is seen in patients with multiple myeloma. This final defect impairs all sodium-coupled transport processes and can produce Fanconi syndrome, as in this case. Such patients can present with hypophosphatemia, renal glucosuria with normal glucose level, and hypouricemia.

**Renal tubular acidosis type 1 (distal RTA)** is caused by the body's inability to excrete acid or hydrogen ions at the distal tubule. The results are alkaline urine and inability to lower the urine pH (kidney stones will develop in alkaline urine), hypokalemia, and hyperchloremic metabolic acidosis. The failure of the H+/K+-ATPase leads to urinary potassium loss, which explains the hypokalemic hyperchloremic metabolic acidosis.

**Renal tubular acidosis type 4** is a normal anion gap metabolic acidosis with hyperkalemia, resulting from a hypoaldosterone-like state that highlights the major role of aldosterone in urinary potassium excretion.

**Normal anion gap metabolic acidosis:** RTA and diarrhea (loss of bicarbonate) are the most common causes of RTAs. Other causes include ileostomy fluid loss and carbonic anhydrase inhibitors (acetazolamide). The challenge is to differentiate between diarrhea and RTAs. Urine pH alone is not enough to distinguish between them: urine pH in GI loss is low, but it is also low in proximal RTA.

In the case of diarrhea, the kidney still has the ability to excrete acid. In distal RTA, the problem is inability to excrete acid. In proximal RTA, the problem is inability to reabsorb bicarbonate.

To differentiate between diarrhea and RTA, calculate the urinary anion gap.

UAG = **urine sodium** + **urinary potassium** − **urinary chloride**

UAG is positive in RTA, suggesting the inability to excrete acid in the urine. If UAG is negative, ability to excrete acid is intact, suggesting diarrhea as a cause of the acidosis.

### CLINICAL PEARL

In cases with a normal anion gap metabolic acidosis, UAG can help distinguish the cause for the acidosis.

- RTA has positive UAG
- Diarrhea has negative UAG
- **RTA + ↑ potassium = type 4 RTA** (most common type)

### Different Types of RTA

| Type | Findings | Treatment |
|---|---|---|
| **Type 1: Distal RTA** | Normal anion gap metabolic acidosis, **hypokalemia**, urine pH >5.5, low serum bicarbonate, positive urine anion gap, nephrolithiasis, associated with autoimmune disorders (SLE, Sjögren) | Bicarbonate |
| **Type 2: Proximal RTA** | Normal anion gap metabolic acidosis, with positive urine anion gap, **hypokalemia**, urine pH <5.5, low bicarbonate with a higher range than in type 1 (16–18), Fanconi syndrome with loss of glucose, amino acids, phosphate, uric acid, and tubular proteinuria | High dose of bicarbonate, thiazide diuretics |
| **Type 4: Hyperkalemic RTA** | Normal anion gap metabolic acidosis, **hyperkalemia**, positive UAG and urine pH <5.5. Seen in DM, UTI | Fludrocortisone |

# CASE 10

## Chief Complaint

Altered mental status

## History and Physical Examination

A 66-year-old man with history of alcohol abuse is brought to the emergency department because of confusion and unresponsiveness. Family members state that he was in his usual state of health the day before. On physical examination the patient is confused.

Vital signs are temperature 37 C (98.6 F), blood pressure 110/68 mm Hg, heart rate 117/min, respirations 26/min, and $O_2$ saturation at 98% on room air. Physical examination of the heart reveals tachycardic, normal S1/S2, no S3, no murmurs or rubs. Chest examination is clear bilaterally, with no wheezing or rales. Neurologic exam is non-focal.

## Differential Diagnosis

1. Remember the differential diagnosis of altered mental status (confusion) in a patient with nonfocal neurologic exam (mnemonic "DIM"):
   - **D**rugs (drugs of abuse as well as side effects of prescription drugs especially in geriatric patients)
   - **I**nfections
   - **M**etabolic (hypernatremia, hyponatremia, hyperglycemia, hypoglycemia, renal failure, etc.)
2. In this patient, specifically consider ethanol toxicity; methanol toxicity; ethylene glycol toxicity; other drug ingestion; infectious process (aspiration pneumonia, lung abscess)

**CLINICAL PEARL**

In a patient with alcohol abuse, remember to consider "other" toxic alcohols that are of medical and toxicological importance as they cause various syndromes; the principal ones are ethylene glycol and methanol.

## Initial Management

**Setting:** emergency department

## Diagnostic/Therapeutic Plan

- Initial antidote
- ABG
- CBC
- Basic metabolic panel
- Chest x-ray
- EKG
- Urinalysis
- Blood alcohol
- Plasma osmolarity

### Test Results

- Initial antidote: dextrose, thiamine, naloxone
- ABG: pH 7.3, $PCO_2$ 20 mm Hg, $PO_2$ 99 mm Hg
- CBC: normal
- Basic metabolic panel: glucose 105 mg/dL, sodium 142 mEq/L (normal 135–145 mEq/L), potassium 3.6 mEq/L (normal 3.5–5.2 mEq/L), chloride 105 mEq/L (normal 99–106 mEq/L), bicarbonate 7 mEq/L (normal 18–22 mEq/L), BUN 10 mg/dL, creatinine 2.2 mg/dL
- Chest x-ray: normal
- EKG: tachycardia
- Urinalysis: >50 RBCs per high-power field, trace bacteria, unidentifiable crystals; urine toxicology screen: negative
- Blood alcohol: <10 mg/dL
- Plasma osmolarity: 316 mOsm/kg $H_2O$

### Assessment

This patient presents with an anion gap metabolic acidosis—note the bicarbonate of 7. The next step is to **calculate the anion gap** as follows:

Anion gap = **serum sodium** – (**serum chloride** + **serum bicarbonates**)

$$142 - (105 + 7) = 30$$

The patient has a high anion gap metabolic acidosis (anion gap = 30). The next step is to look at the expected respiratory compensation using Winter's formula:

Expected $PCO_2$ = **1.5 × [bicarbonate] + 8 ±2 mm Hg**

This patient's predicted $PCO_2$ is 18 ±2 mm Hg, while the measured $PCO_2$ is 20 mm Hg. Therefore, only the high anion gap acidosis accounts for the acid base abnormality.

#### CCS NOTE

You may not be able to determine a specific diagnosis from the history and physical. Initial management of any altered mental status includes administration of dextrose, thiamine, naloxone. Order routine admitting labs (CBC, chemistries, urinalysis) and chest x-ray simultaneously.

### Further Management Plan

When considering alcohol toxicity, serum osmolar gap must be calculated. The serum osmolar gap is the difference between measured and calculated plasma osmolarity. The **calculated** plasma osmolarity is as follows:

$$2 \times [\text{serum sodium}] + [\text{blood urea nitrogen}] \div 2.8 + [\text{plasma glucose}] \div 18$$

Normal osmolar gap is <10 mOsm/kg $H_2O$. If the gap is >10, consider alcohol poisoning as the source of the unmeasured osmoles. Ethanol is the most common cause of alcohol poisoning, but in this case ethanol levels were low. The osmolar gap is roughly 23.

#### CLINICAL PEARL

Activated charcoal and nasogastric lavage have no role in toxic alcohol poisoning. Typically the alcohols will be absorbed too quickly for either of these modalities to have any efficacy.

### Treatment and Management Plan

Many patients with ethylene glycol ingestion are extremely obtunded and are at high risk of aspiration; endotracheal intubation may need to be considered. Immediately obtain intravenous access and laboratory specimens.

- Ethylene glycol level
- Aggressive IV fluids to enhance renal clearance and to limit deposition of oxalates in renal tubules
- Monitored setting for symptomatic patients
- EKG for detecting arrhythmias resulting from hypocalcemia
- Low serum calcium may induce a prolonged QT interval
- Foley catheterization for patients with altered mental status to monitor urinary output and allow serial examination of urine for crystals or fluorescence

If the serum osmolal gap is elevated, begin empiric antidotal therapy with fomepizole (**more common**) or ethyl alcohol. (Ethyl alcohol is usually given as IV but may be given orally when emergency hospital care is not immediately available).

- Fomepizole is commonly used in EDs. It causes no alteration in mental status, hypoglycemia, or respiratory depression. Additionally, it only needs to be administered every 12 hrs. The main disadvantage is its extremely high cost.
- Oral or parenteral ethanol (less common) is used as a temporizing measure while awaiting test results.

Hemodialysis is used to treat severe metabolic acidosis or to prevent renal insufficiency. Early in the intoxication, the toxin is present as the parent compound, ethylene glycol. As time passes, toxic metabolites accumulate and metabolic acidosis develops. Eventually, oxalate is deposited in the kidney and elsewhere, leading to possible renal insufficiency. Once any of these manifestations occur, antidotal therapy alone (used to block alcohol dehydrogenase with ethanol or fomepizole) is insufficient to treat the poisoning.

Consequently, alcohol dehydrogenase–blocking therapy must be accompanied by dialysis in these cases to remove the metabolites. Traditional dialysis indications include acute renal failure and ethylene glycol level >50.

| Further Results | Treatment |
|---|---|
| Serum ethylene glycol | Level of 112 mg/dL (15.6 mmol/L) reported from outside laboratory approximately 7 hours after the blood sample taken |
| Nephrology consult initiated | Acute hemodialysis |

### Discussion

Alcohol poisoning causes high anion gap metabolic acidosis, typically with anion gap above 25. Ethylene glycol is an automotive radiator fluid added to prevent overheating or freezing, depending on the season. Ethylene glycol is extremely toxic and ingestion can be fatal if untreated. Fluorescein dye is often added to radiator fluid to help mechanics identify the source of a radiator leak. The fluorescein in the fluid fluoresces when viewed under ultraviolet light.

### Basic Science Correlate

The toxic alcohols (ethanol, ethylene glycol, and methanol) are parent compounds that exert most of their toxicity by conversion to metabolites. Although the parent compound, ethylene glycol, may cause some alteration of mental status, it is relatively nontoxic. It is the metabolites that cause the distinctive toxicity associated with this compound. Ethanol is metabolized by the enzyme alcohol dehydrogenase (ADH) pathway, which is located in the liver and gastric mucosa, and by the cytochrome P-450 mixed function oxidase (MFO) system in the liver.

As with ethyl alcohol and methanol, ethylene glycol is metabolized by the enzyme alcohol dehydrogenase. In this step it forms glycolaldehyde.

- Through interaction with aldehyde dehydrogenase, ethylene glycol is metabolized to glycolic acid (GA).
- A profound acidosis often ensues with this intoxication, attributable to the glycolic acid in circulation.
- This glycolate is then transformed into glyoxylic acid. At this point, the molecule may be transformed into the highly toxic oxalate.
- With the formation of oxalate crystals in the urine, calcium oxalate crystals form and accumulate in blood and other tissues.
- The precipitation of calcium oxalate in the renal cortex results in decreased glomerular filtration and renal insufficiency.
- Calcium is consumed in circulation, and hypocalcemia may occur.
- The rate-limiting step of ethylene glycol metabolism is the alcohol dehydrogenase–catalyzed step.

Common ethyl alcohol (ethanol) binds much more easily to alcohol dehydrogenase than either ethylene glycol or methanol. Because ethanol is the preferred substrate for alcohol dehydrogenase, the presence of ethanol may essentially block metabolism of ethylene glycol. In addition, this enzyme is blocked by the administration of fomepizole (4-methylpyrazole [4-MP]).

When the diagnosis of alcohol poisoning is suspected, obtain the following:

- Serum ethylene glycol level
- Osmolar gap and anion gap
- Baseline creatinine and BUN level
- Urine examination for evidence of fluorescence (Fluorescein is excreted in the urine faster than ethylene glycol, but fluorescence can be eliminated before the patient even arrives in the ED. Thus the presence of fluorescence of urine under a Wood's lamp is not a sensitive test, but it is highly specific.)
- Both a serum calcium level and EKG, since hypocalcemia may occur as calcium combines with oxalate in the form of calcium oxalate crystals

Ethylene glycol produces CNS depression similar to that of ethanol. Symptoms of ethylene glycol toxicity include confusion, ataxia, hallucinations, slurred speech, and coma. Symptoms are most severe 6–12 hrs after ingestion, when the acidic metabolites of ethylene glycol are at their maximal concentration. If the patient presents early or has consumed small amounts of ethylene glycol, presentation may be similar to ethanol intoxication. However, an ethanol odor will be absent, and serum or respiratory ethanol levels will be too low to account for the degree of CNS depression. **Absence of a strong odor of alcohol** in a patient who appears intoxicated should raise the suspicion of ethylene glycol ingestion.

### Patient Safety Note

Begin aspiration precautions in every comatose patient.

Following a period of CNS depression, metabolic acidosis and cardiopulmonary symptoms become prominent. Renal involvement becomes apparent within 24 to 72 hours after ingestion. (Ethylene glycol needs time to be metabolized into oxalate before urinary crystals can form.) Calcium oxalate formation depletes serum calcium levels and deposits in intestinal mucosa, liver, brain, heart, lung, and kidney. Calcium oxalate crystals are usually present in the urine, but not always.

Summary of the different types of alcohol poisoning:

| Isopropyl Alcohol | Methanol | Ethylene Glycol | Ethanol |
|---|---|---|---|
| Somnolence or coma with normal acid-base status | Pancreatitis and retinal toxicity<br>Severe anion gap metabolic acidosis with acute visual changes or severe abdominal pain | Acute kidney failure and calcium oxalate nephrolithiasis<br>Severe anion gap metabolic acidosis and acute kidney failure | Anion gap metabolic acidosis with osmolar gap >10 mOsm/kg $H_2O$ |
| Treat with IV fluid and gastric lavage; if severe, hemodialysis | Treat with fomepizole and hemodialysis | Treat with fomepizole and hemodialysis | Treat with IV normal saline and dextrose |

## Final Diagnosis

Ethylene glycol toxicity

# Rheumatology 11

## CASE 1

### Chief Complaint

Joint pain and stiffness for 1 year

### History and Physical Examination

A 32-year-old woman presents to your office with complaints of joint pain and swelling, along with significant weakness, fatigue, and malaise that have been present for the last year. She has been using multiple over-the-counter medications that have not helped her symptoms including acetaminophen and naproxen. She states she has significant difficulty grabbing objects in the morning due to stiffness in the joints of her hands, and she has symptoms causing pain and disability in her knees as well. Her symptoms improve as the day progresses, and in the afternoon her joint stiffness improves and she tends to feel better. The patient denies any history of insect bites, rashes, low back pain, or diarrhea.

On examination the woman is pale and thin, with BMI 21. Her temperature is 37.0° C (98.6° F), pulse is regular at 98/min, and blood pressure 115/75 mm Hg. The hands reveal mild swelling and tenderness of the proximal interphalangeal and metacarpophalangeal joints, bilaterally. The distal interphalangeal joints are unremarkable. The knees are slightly swollen and tender to touch. Incidentally you find some rounded nodules on the extensor surface of the elbows, which are non-tender and rubbery in consistency, measuring 2 cm in diameter.

### Differential Diagnosis

1. Rheumatoid arthritis (RA)
   - Presents with bilateral joint pain, involving 3 joint areas simultaneously (including one of the hand joints) and the presence of inflammatory symptoms
2. Systemic lupus erythematosus (SLE)
   - Can present with bilateral joint pain indistinguishable from RA, but this patient does not meet criteria for a diagnosis of SLE
3. Lyme disease
   - Can present with symptoms similar to RA, so it should be included in the differential diagnosis of this patient; initial lesion in Lyme is characteristic skin rash, erythema chronicum migrans

4. Viral infection
    - Can present with symmetrical joint pain, but is usually of shorter duration than what is seen in this patient
5. Osteoarthritis
    - Usually presents with hand joint involvement, but spares the metacarpophalangeal joints and mainly affects the distal and proximal interphalangeal joints
    - Not associated with inflammatory symptoms as seen in this patient
    - Does not present with symmetrical polyarthritis

### Initial Management

**Setting:** outpatient

### Diagnostic/Therapeutic Plan

- Assess the number of symptoms for diagnostic criteria of RA (diagnosis is based upon clinical criteria met)
- ESR/CRP
- CBC
- Comprehensive metabolic panel
- X-ray of the hands

### Test Results

- Patient's criteria for RA:
    - Morning stiffness >1 hr
    - Three joint areas affected simultaneously
    - Proximal interphalangeal joint, metacarpophalangeal joint, or wrist affected
    - Joints affected bilaterally
    - Probable rheumatoid nodules
- ESR elevated at 88 mm/h
- CBC: WBC 7,385/mm$^3$, RBC 5.3 $\times$ 10$^6$, platelet count 155/mm$^3$, hemoglobin 9.6 g/dL, MCV 78 µm$^3$, RDW 16.5
- CMP: albumin 3.2 g/dL

### Assessment

This patient is experiencing bilateral joint pain with stiffness in the morning lasting until the afternoon, as well as fatigue, malaise, and other systemic evidence of inflammation. She has no findings or history of a rash, which is usually present with SLE and initially with Lyme disease. She also has no history of diarrhea, which would be likely in a patient with IBD.

The sparing of this patient's DIP joints and lack of back pain/symptoms make this clinical picture characteristic of RA. The other significant findings here include the appearance of suspected rheumatoid nodules on the extensor surfaces, as well as the presence of at least 3 simultaneous joint areas affected, which is typical for RA.

In patients with RA, it is important to follow disease activity with radiography of the hands as well as inflammatory markers such as ESR or CRP to determine if there is progression of the disease and if the current treatment regimen is effective.

Because this patient is complaining of fatigue, it is important to determine her hemoglobin level to see if she has anemia of chronic disease, which is commonly seen in patients with chronic inflammatory conditions.

### Basic Science Correlate

TNF-α, interleukin-1 (IL-1), and interleukin-6 (IL-6) mediate most of the pathogenic features of RA. Most of the biological treatment agents used today will inhibit these cytokines. TNF and IL-1 are 2 cytokines that are released by cells involved in the inflammatory process.

- TNF causes fatigue and weight loss
- IL-1 causes fever and inflammation, as well as vasodilation (vasodilation stimulates histamine release, which can lead to edema formation in the inflammatory process)
- IL-6 stimulates the production of hepcidin, which is the primary mechanism for the cause of anemia of chronic disease in RA patients
- IL-6 also stimulates the activation of osteoclasts, which will lead to the bony erosions seen in many patients

## Further Management Plan

- Anti-inflammatory agent, usually an NSAID with a corticosteroid, until a disease-modifying agent starts to take effect
    - Gold standard for treatment of RA is methotrexate
- If methotrexate has been started, follow CBC and LFTs; if transaminitis develops, **discontinue methotrexate immediately**
- Periodic symptoms assessment, ESR/CRP levels, and radiographs of the hands to assess response to treatment; frequency of follow-up appointments depends on severity of disease

## Discussion

RA is a chronic inflammatory disease affecting small and large joints, as well as the surrounding soft tissue including cartilage. It is usually bilateral and most often spares the distal interphalangeal joints and lumbar spine. The joints are usually swollen, soft, and tender to touch. Patients have excessive bony erosions and cartilage damage mediated by tumor necrosis factor (a therapeutic target for this disease).

When progressive joint deformity of the hands occurs, alignment of the joints can be compromised with a characteristic ulnar deviation of the digits and radial deviation of the wrists.

To diagnose RA, one needs **4 of the diagnostic criteria** listed below.

- Morning stiffness (>1 hr) for 6 wks
- Swelling of wrists, MCPs, PIPs for 6 wks
- Swelling of 3 joints for 6 wks

- Symmetric joint swelling for 6 wks
- Rheumatoid factor positivity or anti-cyclic citrullinated peptide
- Elevated CRP or ESR

Risk factors for RA include inherited alleles such as HLA-DR1, DR4, and DR14, as well as TNF promoter gene polymorphism and transcription factor stimulation. Smoking is strongly associated with RA and the risk reduces after smoking cessation. Environmental factors and hormonal factors are also implicated in the risk for developing RA.

Usually RA is associated with rheumatoid factor and anti-cyclic citrullinated peptide, but these antibodies by themselves do not indicate disease, and if absent do not rule out the disease. Usually patients with RA will have elevated ESR/CRP and possible anemia of chronic disease. A plain radiograph of the affected joints usually reveals periarticular osteopenia, joint space narrowing, and bony erosions. Bony erosions may not be present initially in the disease, but baseline radiographs of the hands and feet should always be obtained to follow disease progression. MRI can detect bone erosion earlier than plain radiography.

Extra-articular manifestations include:

- Damage to the ligaments and tendons: radial deviation of the wrist with ulnar deviation of the digits, Boutonnière deformity, and swan-neck deformity
- Rheumatoid nodules: due to focal vasculitis, usually in areas of mechanical stress (olecranon, occiput, Achilles tendon). Methotrexate therapy may cause flare-ups in this process.
- Felty syndrome: RA, splenomegaly, and granulocytopenia
- Caplan syndrome: RA with pneumoconiosis

## Follow-up Management and Prevention

- Assess the response to treatment with the patient's signs and symptoms, ESR/CRP, and x-ray of the hands
- If poor response to methotrexate, consider adding another biological agent, eg, TNF-alpha inhibitor such as adalimumab, etanercept, infliximab. (Be sure to get a PPD before starting patients on a biological agent.)
- If patient responds poorly to TNF-alpha inhibitor, consider replacing it with another biological agent such as abatacept (can cause lymphoma, lung cancer, and COPD exacerbation) or rituximab (anti-CD20 agent), used in combination with methotrexate.
- Care should be taken for patients needing intubation due to the significant damage that RA can cause to the cervical spine (atlanto-axial subluxation). Do a neck x-ray before intubation to determine if significant cervical spine disease exists, to avoid significant morbidity in the patient.

## Final Diagnosis

Rheumatoid arthritis

# CASE 2

## Chief Complaint

Pain and swelling in the left ankle for 1 day

## History and Physical Examination

A 50-year-old man comes to the clinic with swelling of the left ankle joint. He recently started a new exercise regimen after joining a gym. The swelling and pain of the ankle joint developed overnight. He denies any trauma. Six months ago he had similar attacks, for which he took over-the-counter painkillers. He never sought medical help, and the symptoms resolved spontaneously after a week or so. He denies any other significant past medical history and has not had recent sexual contact or trauma to the area.

Vital signs are T 37.3 C (99.1 F), BP 120/85 mm Hg, and pulse 88/min. The left ankle is swollen, warm, tender, and erythematous. A small effusion is present, and movement of the ankle is very painful. The other joints are normal. No skin rash is noted.

## Differential Diagnosis

1. Gout
2. Pseudogout
3. Septic arthritis
4. Osteoarthritis

## Initial Management

**Setting:** outpatient

## Diagnostic/Therapeutic Plan

- Joint aspiration
- X-ray of left ankle

## Test Results

- Arthrocentesis of the left ankle: WBC 37,000/mm$^3$, negative Gram stain, needle-shaped crystals
- X-ray: soft tissue swelling with minimal effusion in the left ankle but no dislocation or fracture

## Assessment

Joint aspiration is the single most important test in a patient with acute monoarthritis. X-ray of the ankle is helpful to rule out a fracture, dislocation, or bony abnormality; x-ray may also show chondrocalcinosis in patients with pseudogout, which could help in the diagnosis of the condition.

**CLINICAL PEARL**

- **Acute monoarthropathy:** septic arthritis, crystal-induced arthropathy, trauma
- **Chronic monoarticular arthritis:** osteoarthritis until proven otherwise

Acute monoarthropathy is due to septic arthritis or crystal-induced arthropathy, such as gout or pseudogout, but can be due to trauma as well. In this case, a similar history of arthropathy that resolved in the past makes the most likely cause a crystal-associated arthritis such as gout or pseudogout. Gouty attacks can be precipitated by excessive activity, weight loss, and increase in consumption of food with high purine content.

Septic arthritis and gonococcal arthritis are other possible diagnoses that may be associated with fever and leukocytosis, but gonococcal arthritis tends to present more frequently as a migratory polyarthritis. The only way to differentiate between these conditions is to do an arthrocentesis of the affected joint.

- Septic arthritis is diagnosed by WBC count $\geq$50,000/mm$^3$ in the synovial fluid and can be associated with other joint diseases such as crystal-induced arthritis. Culture of the synovial fluid for *Staphylococcus* is positive in >90% of cases, while gonococcus is usually negative.
- Gonococcal arthritis is the most common cause of septic arthritis. Staphylococcal septic arthritis is more commonly seen in older patients and in those with pre-existing rheumatic disease.

Osteoarthritis may present as a chronic monoarthropathy, but not acutely like in this patient, and does not include the signs of inflammation present in this case.

### Basic Science Correlate

Hyperuricemia leads to precipitation of urate crystals in the joints and causes an inflammatory process by:

- Phagocytosis of crystals by macrophages releases inflammatory cytokines such as IL-1 among others, which recruit other inflammatory cells. This recruitment causes further damage to the joint specifically by activation of proteases.
- Activation of complement and the kinin system, with recruitment of neutrophils which will ingest the urate crystals and produce inflammatory cytokines such as LTB4, prostaglandins and free radicals. Eventually the neutrophils will lyse, which then releases lysosomal enzymes into the tissue exacerbating the tissue damage.

## Further Management Plan/Results

1. NSAIDs (indomethacin) or colchicine, continued until the pain is no longer present
2. If NSAIDs are contraindicated, glucocorticoids orally or via intra-articular injection
3. Once acute attack resolves, consider urate lowering therapy with allopurinol (first-line) or febuxostat in patients with a history of $\geq$2 episodes per year or to patients with tophaceous gout.

With acute gout, do not give allopurinol because it can increase the severity of the attack.

## Discussion

The crystal-induced arthropathies (monosodium urate, calcium pyrophosphate, calcium oxalate, and calcium hydroxyapatite) are due to microcrystal deposition in the joints. Despite differences in crystal morphology, they have identical clinical presentations and can only be distinguished by synovial fluid analysis.

Gout primarily affects middle-aged men and presents most commonly with acute monoarthritis. (Women represent only 5–15% of all patients with gout; premenopausal women make up 17% of all women with gout). As gout becomes chronic, multiple joints may be involved, and deposition of urate crystals may occur in connective tissue (tophi) and the kidneys.

The metatarsophalangeal joint of the first toe is most commonly affected in patients with gout (podagra), but other joints like the knee, ankle, PIP, or DIP joints may also be initially involved. The first episode commonly occurs at night with severe joint pain that wakes the patient from sleep. The joint rapidly becomes warm, red, and tender (similar to cellulitis). Without treatment, the joint pain usually goes away spontaneously within 3–14 days.

Certain events that precipitate gout sometimes precede the attack: excessive alcohol ingestion, trauma, surgery, infection, steroid withdrawal, certain drugs (diuretics [hydrochlorothiazide and furosemide], anti-tuberculosis medications [pyrazinamide and ethambutol]), and serious medical illnesses.

Serum uric acid level is of no value in the diagnosis of acute urate arthropathy. Serum uric acid during an acute attack at times may be normal or even low, while many people with an elevated serum uric acid level may never develop gout. This is why the diagnosis is made by the analysis of synovial fluid and presence of needle-shaped negatively birefringent crystals under polarized light microscopy.

In treating acute gouty arthritis, the goal is to decrease inflammation and thus prevent erosions and joint destruction. An NSAID (e.g., indomethacin), colchicine or corticosteroid is the treatment of choice.

Lowering the serum uric acid should not be done during an acute attack since it can worsen the attack. Indomethacin is preferred because it has fewer side effects when compared to colchicine (causes GI disturbance). However, if colchicine is used, it should be given within the first 24 hours of the acute attack. If the patient has a contraindication to or cannot tolerate NSAIDs or colchicine, glucocorticoids can be given orally, intramuscularly, or as an intra-articular injection.

For chronic hypouricemic therapy, the goal is to decrease uric acid levels to <6 mg/dL, and this treatment is usually required for life. It is initiated in patients who have had recurrent gouty attacks that cannot be corrected by a low-purine diet, limitation of alcohol, avoiding diuretics, etc. Patients started on urate-lowering therapy should be given prophylactic anti-inflammatory medication for the first 6 months due to the increased risk of acute gouty attack that occurs in these patients initially. Unlike in acute gout, the uric acid level may be helpful in following the effect of hypouricemic treatment. Treatment options include:

- Allopurinol or febuxostat is used for "overproducers" by inhibiting xanthine oxidase and blocking production of uric acid. It can also be used for patients with renal failure and/or kidney stones.
- Pegloticase is a potent recombinant uricase (given IV) which metabolizes uric acid to a much more soluble substance (allantoin), which does not precipitate, and it is indicated for treatment-refractory cases.
- Probenecid (rarely used) can be used for "undersecretors" (>80% of adults), those that have high uric acid levels in the blood and low uric acid levels the in urine. Probenecid is contraindicated in patients with renal insufficiency and nephrolithiasis.

### CLINICAL PEARL

If the patient develops acute gouty arthritis while on allopurinol (prevention), do not discontinue allopurinol. Simply add NSAIDs (preferably) or colchicine to the regimen and continue until the flare-up resolves.

Overall, allopurinol is the most commonly used drug to prevent gouty arthritis. Allopurinol can be used in "undersecretors" as well as "overproducers." It is given once a day and can be used in patients with renal insufficiency.

Patients with gout and coexisting renal insufficiency should not use NSAIDs or colchicine. These patients are better treated with corticosteroids.

### Final Diagnosis

Gout

## CASE 3

### Chief Complaint

Joint pain for several months

### History and Physical Examination

A 28-year-old woman comes to the office complaining of intermittent joint pain for several months, plus discrete swelling of the joints only recently. She points to her wrists and metacarpophalangeal and proximal interphalangeal joints. She has also suffered from intermittent fevers, morning stiffness for longer than 1 hour, and weight loss of 15 lb. Several months ago after being at the beach, she noted a rash on her face, which took 1 month to resolve. She denies a history of diarrhea. There is no history of known insect bites. Her prior medical history is significant for 2 spontaneous abortions. She is afebrile.

Her BP is 145/90 mm Hg, pulse 70/min, and respirations 14/min. Examination of the head, eyes, ears, nose, and throat is normal. There is no cervical lymphadenopathy noted. There is good air entry in both lungs. The heart has a regular rate and rhythm, with no murmurs or rubs appreciated. There is no splenomegaly, but her liver is mildly enlarged. There are no rashes. Neurologic examination is nonfocal.

### Differential Diagnosis

1. Systemic lupus erythematosus (SLE)
2. Rheumatoid arthritis (RA)
3. Hepatitis or other viral polyarthropathies
4. Lyme disease

### Initial Management Plan

**Setting:** outpatient

### Diagnostic/Therapeutic Plan

- Antinuclear antibodies (ANA)
- CBC
- Chest x-ray
- BUN/creatinine
- Urinalysis
- Rheumatoid factor
- ESR or C-reactive protein
- LFTs
- Viral titers and Lyme titers

### Test Results

- ANA: positive 1:640
- WBCs: 3,000/mm$^3$; hemoglobin 11 mg/dL; platelets 120,000/mm$^3$
- Chest x-ray: no effusions or infiltrates
- Creatinine: 2.1 mg/dL
- Urinalysis: mild proteinuria
- Rheumatoid factor: negative
- ESR: moderate elevations
- LFTs: WNL
- Viral titers and Lyme titers: both negative

### Assessment

This patient has a nonspecific history of joint pain and rash, but laboratory results show renal insufficiency with proteinuria, leukopenia, anemia, and mild thrombocytopenia. This picture is most consistent with systemic lupus, although another collagen vascular disease such as RA is possible.

A positive ANA is a sensitive test for lupus; $<3\%$ of patients with systemic lupus are ANA-negative if the HEP-2 substrate is used. However, it is relatively nonspecific, particularly at a low titer. A positive ANA may be seen in other autoimmune diseases and in up to 10% of the normal population.

Generally with RA, the physical findings for joint disease are more prominent. Hepatitis can present with arthropathy, but in this case the titers were negative, and in fact there are multiple other organs involved.

### Further Management Plan

- 24-hour urine protein measurement
- Double-stranded DNA antibodies (specific for SLE)
- Anti-Smith antibodies (specific for SLE)
- Anti-Ro/SSA and anti-La/SSB (associated with neonatal lupus)
- Complement levels (C3, C4, or CH50)

### Results

- Urine protein: 4 gm/24 hours
- Double-stranded DNA antibodies: positive
- Anti-Smith antibodies: positive
- Anti-Ro/SSA positive and anti-La/SSB: negative
- Complement levels: decreased

### Basic Science Correlate

The complement system is activated by an antigen/antibody complex in the classical pathway, and directly by pathogens leading to C3 attachment to antigens in the alternative pathway. In SLE, there is autoimmune-mediated complement activation by both the classical and alternative pathways, so it will lead to low levels of C3, C4 and CH50.

## Treatment Plan

- Prednisone (immediately) at 1 mg/kg/day
- Kidney biopsy to diagnose the type of lupus nephritis (prednisone will not affect the kidney biopsy for about 6 wks)
- Possible immunosuppressant such as azathioprine, mycophenolate mofetil, methotrexate, or cyclophosphamide (to be reserved only for lupus nephritis due to its severe toxicity)
- Possible hydroxychloroquine (most patients will benefit from the antimalarial since it will prevent lupus flares and decrease organ damage, thrombosis and bone loss even for those on immunosuppressive therapy)

## Discussion

SLE is a systemic disease in which tissues and multiple organs are damaged by pathogenic autoantibodies and immune complexes.

- Unknown etiology
- Women 90% of cases
- Abnormal immune response probably depends upon interaction between susceptible host and environmental factors
- Ultraviolet-B light is the only environmental factor known to cause flares

To diagnose SLE, one needs **4 of the 11 diagnostic criteria** listed below:

1. Malar rash
2. Discoid rash
3. Photosensitivity
4. Oral ulcers
5. Arthritis (identical to RA except that it is nonerosive)
6. Serositis (pleuritis or pericarditis)
7. Renal involvement
8. Neurologic disorder (seizures or psychosis)
9. Hematologic disorder (hemolytic anemia)
10. Immunologic disorder (anti-dsDNA, anti-Smith) or antiphospholipid antibody
11. Positive ANA

**NOTE**

How do you know if a patient with known SLE has an exacerbation of the disease? Order complement levels and ESR (and dsDNA if positive). A flare-up will reveal decreased complement levels and elevated ESR and dsDNA antibodies.

Both the malar rash and photosensitivity rash (diffuse, maculopapular) flare with exposure to ultraviolet-B light (thus, patients are considered photosensitive) and resolve with no scarring of the skin. Discoid lupus is a circular rash with a raised rim that occurs over the scalp and face; it can be disfiguring because of central atrophy and scarring. Only 5% of patients with discoid lupus will go on to develop SLE.

The dsDNA and anti-Smith antibodies are specific for lupus. These occur only with lupus, so if found, think lupus only. Complement levels (C3, C4, or the more sensitive CH50) are depressed in patients with active lupus. Remember, when dsDNA antibody levels are elevated, this is very specific for the diagnosis of lupus; they also increase the likelihood of lupus nephritis. Also, a change of personality and psychosis may be manifestations of central nervous system lupus.

An associated syndrome often seen with systemic lupus is the antiphospholipid syndrome. This is a syndrome of recurrent arterial and venous thrombosis, spontaneous abortions, thrombocytopenia, and a false-positive Venereal Disease Research Laboratory test. It is also associated with an elevated PTT. Libman-Sacks endocarditis is a noninfectious endocarditis rarely seen in lupus patients.

All patients with renal involvement must undergo renal biopsy; prompt use of steroids is indicated since it will not change the outcome of the biopsy for at least 6 wks.

**Drug-induced lupus** is a limited form of lupus that occurs with exposure to certain drugs. Procainamide, hydralazine, isoniazid, and methyldopa are the most common. There is no major organ involvement (kidney or CNS involvement is typically absent); it presents only with a rash and antihistone antibodies and resolves after the offending agent is removed. There is also no hypocomplementemia with this condition.

With respect to **pregnancy** and **SLE,** fertility rates are normal in patients with SLE, though spontaneous abortions and stillbirths are more common. One reason for the spontaneous abortions may be the antiphospholipid antibodies causing placental infarcts. This is treated with low molecular weight heparin.

- It is unclear if lupus worsens with pregnancy.
- If there is a lupus flare during pregnancy, steroids may be used safely to suppress the disease.
- All pregnant patients with lupus need to be screened for anti-Ro/SSA and anti-La/SSB antibodies. These cross the placenta and are passively transferred to the fetus, causing neonatal lupus and, rarely, permanent heart block.

### Final Diagnosis

Systemic lupus erythematosus

# CASE 4

## Chief Complaint

"My skin feels funny."

## History and Physical Examination

A 34-year-old woman comes to the office complaining of swollen hands for the past few months. She has had some itchiness and tightness of the skin of the hands for 6–9 months. She also complains of discoloration of the hands and some difficulty swallowing solids and liquids. Her past medical history is significant for gastroesophageal reflux disease, for which she takes omeprazole. She has no other symptoms.

Her temperature is 37.0° C (98.6° F), BP is 110/90 mm Hg, and pulse is 82/min. On physical examination the skin over her fingers is shiny and has a slight cyanotic appearance distal to the PIP joints. Lung exam reveals good air entry without rales. Heart exam reveals a loud S2 but otherwise normal. The remainder of the physical exam is within normal limits.

## Initial Management

**Setting:** outpatient

## Diagnostic/Therapeutic Plan

- CBC
- Comprehensive metabolic panel
- Urinalysis

## Test Results

- Hematocrit 28% (normal: 36–42%)
- BUN 34 mg/dL and creatinine 1.9 mg/dL; electrolytes and LFTs normal
- Urinalysis: 2+ proteinuria

## Assessment

Systemic sclerosis (SSc), previously called scleroderma, is divided into limited and diffuse forms.

- **Limited cutaneous systemic sclerosis** (formerly called **CREST syndrome**) affects the skin distal to the elbows and knees, as well as the face.
  - Associated with high risk for development of pulmonary hypertension
  - Progression to interstitial lung disease is less common
- **Diffuse cutaneous systemic sclerosis** is a progressive form of SSc that usually affects the skin proximal to the elbows and knees.
  - Characterized by diffuse organ involvement, commonly affecting the lungs leading to interstitial lung disease, and the kidneys causing SSc renal crisis
  - Diffuse pulmonary fibrosis, cardiac involvement, and renal disease are common

### CLINICAL PEARL

**Raynaud Associations**

**Secondary**

- 90% of patients with scleroderma
- Other collagen vascular diseases: SLE, polymyositis, RA
- Arterial occlusive disease (atherosclerosis of the extremities)
- Drugs ($\beta$-adrenergic blockers, ergot derivatives)

**Primary, or Idiopathic**

- Usually women age 20–40 and otherwise normal

To differentiate primary from secondary, look for systemic manifestations in secondary disease (renal failure, arthritis, anemia, fever).

CREST syndrome (calcinosis, Raynaud's phenomenon, esophageal dysmotility, sclerodactyly, telangiectasia) is a limited form of SSc, with a better prognosis and more indolent course.

A diagnosis of SSc should be considered in a patient who has Raynaud's phenomenon and symptoms of skin thickening. Laboratory findings which are nonspecific, but can be found in SSc patients, are anemia of chronic disease, elevated ESR, and elevated creatinine kinase or aldolase (signifies muscle involvement). In limited cutaneous systemic sclerosis, **anti-centromere antibodies** are seen. In diffuse cutaneous systemic sclerosis, **antibodies to topoisomerase I (Scl-70)** are seen.

### Basic Science Correlate

CD4 lymphocytes respond to an unknown offending antigen and release cytokines in different organs activating inflammatory cells and fibroblasts. TH2 cells have been isolated from the skin of patients with scleroderma and were found to produce TGF-$\beta$ and IL-13, which stimulate collagen production and extracellular matrix proteins, which ultimately will lead to fibrosis.

## Further Management Plan

- Antinuclear antibody test; specifically, Scl-70 (antibody to topoisomerase 1) and anti-centromere antibodies

## Results

- Positive anti-centromere antibodies

## Treatment Plan

1. Calcium channel blockers (nifedipine) and avoid cold exposure
2. ACE inhibitor for kidney involvement and hypertension
3. Methotrexate

## Discussion

SSc is a rare connective-tissue disease characterized by widespread vessel obliterative disease and fibrosis of the skin and multiple internal organs that include heart, lung, kidney, and GI tract. Women > men.

The etiology is unknown. Vascular endothelial-cell injury, mediated by different mechanisms, appears to be the process in systemic sclerosis. There is vascular endothelial damage, fibroblast proliferation, vascular hyperreactivity, and renin-angiotensin axis damage.

Management of SSc is targeted at the organ-specific condition affecting the patient. Almost all patients (95%) have skin involvement, as well as Raynaud's phenomenon, which should be treated with avoidance of cold exposure, CCBs and phosphodiesterase-5 inhibitors such as sildenafil. Patients at risk for gangrene of any of their fingers should receive aggressive inpatient treatment with prostacyclin analogs, which has shown some promise as a treatment modality.

Patients also have telangiectasias, subcutaneous calcifications, and skin chancres and ulcers. Esophageal motility dysfunction and reflux are common features of the disease, and PPIs are indicated to avoid intestinal metaplasia of the lower esophagus and risk of adenocarcinoma in the esophagus. Small bowel involvement leads to intestinal hypomotility.

Pulmonary alveolitis should be treated with cyclophosphamide to reduce progression to interstitial lung disease.

Renal failure and malignant hypertension were once the leading causes of death in patients with SSc, but now they may be treated with ACE inhibitors. The major causes of morbidity and mortality today are pulmonary hypertension, interstitial lung disease, and cardiac disease.

Pulmonary hypertension can be treated with phosphodiesterase-5 inhibitors such as sildenafil, as well as with prostacyclin analogs such as iloprost, epoprostenol, or treprostinil. Nonselective and selective endothelin receptor antagonists such as bosentan and ambrisentan have also been shown to delay progression of pulmonary hypertension in these patients.

There is no current treatment for systemic sclerosis. Raynaud's phenomenon is treated with CCBs (nifedipine). Methotrexate and other immunosuppressants are helpful for some symptoms.

## Final Diagnosis

Systemic sclerosis, limited cutaneous form

# CASE 5

## Chief Complaint

"I feel pain in my left knee and in my hands."

## History and Physical Examination

A 60-year-old man comes to the office complaining of increasing left knee pain. He states that he chronically has had knee pain that he attributes to an "old football injury." It is sensitive to changes in weather and it becomes bothersome after overuse. Over the last 6 months he has started to experience similar pain in both of his hands. He has noticed swelling in the right-second and left-third distal interphalangeal joints. He complains of morning stiffness lasting approximately 20 minutes. He otherwise feels and appears well.

There is swelling of the distal interphalangeal joints with no effusion or erythema. On the left knee, there is crepitation but no effusion, warmth, or erythema. The remainder of the physical examination is normal.

## Differential Diagnosis

1. Osteoarthritis
2. Seronegative arthropathies (e.g., ankylosing spondylitis)
3. Crystal-induced arthropathy and septic arthritis
4. Rheumatoid arthritis (RA)
    - Unlikely since it presents as polyarticular symmetric arthritis

## Initial Management

**Setting:** outpatient

## Diagnostic/Therapeutic Plan

- CBC
- Erythrocyte sedimentation rate
- Plain films of the knee and hands
- Rheumatoid factor and antinuclear antibodies (ANA)

## Test Results

- CBC: normal
- ESR: normal
- Loss of joint space and presence of osteophytes and eburnation of the subchondral bones
- Rheumatoid factor and ANA: negative

## Assessment

Osteoarthritis should be the first consideration in **chronic, asymmetric, oligoarticular arthritis** or **monoarticular** arthritis. Because osteoarthritis is not an inflammatory disease, significant morning stiffness is not evident. Also, since osteoarthritis is a disease that affects articular cartilage without visceral involvement, there are **no constitutional symptoms**, such as malaise, fatigue, weakness, and the **lab tests are normal**, including the ESR and CRP.

The seronegative arthropathies (e.g., ankylosing spondylitis) commonly present with asymmetric joint involvement. In these diseases, there is always lower back involvement and morning stiffness usually lasting >30 minutes because there is a significant inflammatory component.

Crystal-induced arthropathy and septic arthritis present with monoarthritis. They are rarely misdiagnosed as osteoarthritis because of the intense inflammatory reaction of the joints and short duration of symptom manifestation before the patient seeks medical help.

In RA, there is always symmetric involvement, as well as evidence of significant joint inflammation and morning stiffness >1 hr. There is never distal interphalangeal joint involvement.

### Basic Science Correlate

The pathogenic mechanism of osteoarthritis can be divided into 3 stages:

1. Chondrocyte injury
2. Chondrocyte proliferation intended to remodel the cartilaginous matrix causes changes in the synovium and subchondral bone
3. Repetitive injury leads to cartilage dropout and extensive subchondral bone changes

## Further Management Plan

- Non-pharmacologic therapy, e.g., patient education regarding joint protection and an assistive device such as cane or walker; dietary recommendation for weight loss; hydrotherapy; and rehabilitation therapy
- If not adequate, trial of acetaminophen on PRN basis
- If not adequate, trial of NSAIDs on PRN basis (trial of opiates also possible if no improvement with acetaminophen and NSAIDs)
- If not adequate, joint replacement
- Hyaluronic acid injection into knee joint may provide relief of osteoarthritis for up to 3–6 mos

### Discussion

Osteoarthritis is the most common joint disease in humans. The major target tissue is articular cartilage, and there is failure of cartilage along with secondary remodeling and hypertrophy of the bone. Osteoarthritis, unlike RA, is **not an inflammatory disease**.

Knee osteoarthritis is the leading cause of chronic disability in the older adult in the Western world. Major risk factors include the following:

- Age
- Female sex
- Genetic factors
- Major joint trauma (potentially modifiable)
- Repetitive stress (potentially modifiable)
- Obesity (potentially modifiable)

Osteoarthritis can be categorized as idiopathic or secondary. Secondary osteoarthritis is pathologically indistinguishable from the idiopathic type.

- **Idiopathic osteoarthritis** is the most common form, where no predisposing factor is evident.
- **Secondary osteoarthritis** is attributable to an underlying cause, e.g., other arthropathies (gout), endocrine disease (DM, acromegaly), deposition disease (hemochromatosis), or mechanical factors (valgus/varus deformity, unequal lower extremity length).
  - Any disease that causes stress or trauma to a joint may eventually cause secondary osteoarthritis.

**CLINICAL PEARL**

In osteoarthritis, the severity of radiographic findings is not related to severity of symptoms. Treat the symptoms, not the findings!

The most common joint to be affected is the knee, while the second most common is the thumb base. The major joints involved are the weight-bearing joints (hip and knee) and the small joints of the fingers (proximal interphalangeal and distal interphalangeal).

- Osteoarthritis **spares the metacarpophalangeal joints**. The joints are affected in an oligoarticular/asymmetric or monoarticular pattern.
- Joint involvement is very slow, progressive, and irreversible.
- Because the cartilage "fails" and there is increased pressure on articular bone, **joint pain increases with exercise** and is **relieved by rest**.
- **Morning stiffness** is always **<20–30 min**.
- Crepitations may be noted with movement of the joint.
- There are no systemic manifestations with osteoarthritis.
- Laboratory tests are always normal, especially indices of inflammation.
  - Thus, ESR and C-reactive protein levels are always normal. If ESR is elevated, then another process is complicating osteoarthritis (e.g., septic joint) or it is not osteoarthritis at all.

X-ray findings include **osteophytes, eburnation and loss of joint space**. Osteophytes (spurs) are the reparative efforts by the bone; when these occur in the proximal interphalangeal joints, they are called **Bouchard's nodes**. Similar changes occurring in the distal phalangeal joints are called **Heberden's nodes.**

Diagnosis is made clinically and with x-ray findings. Treatment is aimed at reducing pain and maintaining mobility. Non-pharmacologic measures involve reduction of joint loading by correction of **poor posture and weight loss, and physical therapy and exercise** programs to maintain range of motion, strengthen periarticular muscles, and improve physical fitness. Drug therapy is palliative because no agent has been shown to change the natural course of the disease.

- The first drug to use for pain in osteoarthritis is **acetaminophen**.
- If no response, add an **NSAID**.
  - Use caution with dosing for older adult patients because they are at the highest risk for side effects associated with NSAIDs, especially GI problems (ulcers, hemorrhage).
- COX-2 inhibitors may be used in patients who are high risk for GI complications.
- In patients with **refractory disease, judicious treatment with opioid analgesics** is an option to maintain joint function and relieve pain.

Another modality that has been shown to be of great benefit with osteoarthritis is capsaicin cream, which depletes the local sensory nerve endings of substance P. Consider **orthopedic surgery and joint arthroplasty** for cases where aggressive medical treatment has been unsatisfactory and if the quality of the patient's life has been decreased.

Chondroitin and glucosamine therapy for osteoarthritis have not shown significant benefits in randomized controlled trials.

### Final Diagnosis

Osteoarthritis

# CASE 6

## Chief Complaint

"Could my back pain be due to osteoporosis?"

## History and Physical Examination

A 72-year-old woman comes to your office worried about osteoporosis. She asks if there is anything she can do to diagnose and prevent it. She is also concerned that her back pain, which she has had on and off for 2 years, is due to osteoporosis. Her mother had osteoporosis when she was in her early seventies. She does not smoke or take any medications, and she reports no weight loss. Her back pain usually gets better with rest, and she has not noticed symptoms consistent with sciatica.

Her vital signs are stable. Physical examination is within normal limits, except for mild lower back pain on palpation.

### CLINICAL PEARL

- **T score** compares bone density to a young population; it is abnormal if >2.5 SD below mean, ie, there is significant risk for osteoporotic fracture.
- **Z score** compares bone density to an age-matched population; it is helpful when considering secondary osteoporosis, eg, from steroids, warfarin.

## Differential Diagnosis

1. Osteoporosis
2. Osteoarthritis
3. Musculoligamentous back pain
4. Cancer with metastases

## Initial Management

**Setting:** outpatient

## Diagnostic/Therapeutic Plan

- Plain x-ray of the back (although not sensitive, the x-ray may give us information on osteoporosis, osteoarthritis, or metastatic disease involving the spine)

## Test Results

- X-ray: probable compression fracture of L5 and significant osteopenia

## Assessment

Musculoligamentous back pain is considered the most common form of back pain and usually resolves within 3 wks with appropriate treatment. Cancer with metastases should be considered in a patient with prior history of cancer or with symptoms consistent with cancer, e.g., weight loss, loss of appetite, smoking history, and anemia.

After sudden bending, lifting, or jumping movements in older patients with osteoporosis, vertebral collapse is common in the lower dorsal or upper lumbar regions. Pain usually subsides after several days, and patients can be ambulatory in 4–6 wks. Collapse that is not associated with pain can cause dorsal kyphosis and exaggerated cervical lordosis. In the absence of fracture, a 30% decrease in bone mass may not be evident on standard x-rays. More sensitive studies, such as dual-energy x-ray absorptiometry (DEXA) scan, may determine whether the patient is at risk for fracture.

**Osteoporosis** is diagnosed as a **T-score <–2.5** and **osteopenia** a **T-score <–1.1**. Remember, it is a negative value so "less than" here is equal to a more negative number.

### Further Management Plan/Results

| | |
|---|---|
| • DEXA scan | Density T-score –2.7 |
| • CBC | Normal |
| • Electrolytes (Cushing's) | Normal |
| • Phosphorus (hyperparathyroidism) | Normal |
| • Creatinine (chronic renal failure) | Normal |
| • Alkaline phosphatase | Normal |
| • TSH | Normal |

### Treatment Plan

1. Oral calcium 1.5 grams per day and vitamin D supplementation
2. Alendronate

### CLINICAL PEARL

Diagnostic studies should focus on excluding secondary causes of osteoporosis. In males, obtaining a morning testosterone level (before 10 AM) is also recommended.

### Discussion

Osteoporosis is defined as a reduction of bone density below a level required for mechanical support. Remodeling of bone is continuous. Density decreases whenever the rate of resorption exceeds formation. Vertebrae, wrists, hips, humeri, and tibiae are the bones most commonly prone to fractures.

- Type I osteoporosis
  - Disproportionate loss of trabecular bone
  - Associated with fractures of the vertebrae and distal forearms
  - Usually occurs in middle-aged and postmenopausal women
- Type II osteoporosis
  - Associated with fractures of the femoral neck, proximal humerus, proximal tibia, and pelvis
  - Usually occurs in men and women age >75

The gold standard is the dual-energy x-ray absorptiometry (DEXA) scan. A diagnosis of osteoporosis is made for anyone with **bone density >2.5 standard deviations below the mean**. Further evaluation may include parathyroid hormone, urinary calcium, and plasma 1,25-dihydroxy and 25-hydroxy vitamin D levels

Management is directed at preventing bone loss and reducing the risk of fracture. This could be achieved by the following:

- Smoking cessation
- Muscle-strengthening exercises
- Reduction of caffeine intake
- Correction of existing metabolic abnormalities

Pharmacologic treatments seek to minimize osteoclast-mediated resorption of bone. Estrogens have fallen out of favor, with studies demonstrating a possible association with breast cancer, and should not be used for the treatment of osteoporosis.

Treatments that have been shown to prevent or improve osteoporosis and decrease the risk of fractures are bisphosphonates (alendronate).

- Alendronate, a short-acting bisphosphonate, is the most commonly used drug in the United States for the treatment and prevention of osteoporosis.
  - Given daily or weekly for osteoporosis and osteopenia
  - Esophagitis (most common side effect) can be prevented by taking alendronate while standing up and following with a tall glass of water.
- Patients receiving treatment with bisphosphonates should also take 1,000–1,500 mg/d of calcium (1,200 mg/d is usual recommendation) with or without 800 IU/d of vitamin D in order to build bone mass.

Treatment with calcium alone will not improve or reverse existing osteoporosis.

- Raloxifene is for patients who cannot tolerate bisphosphonates or women with osteoporosis and an increased risk of invasive breast cancer. It is a tissue-selective estrogen receptor modulator.
- Teriparatide (recombinant human PTH) is currently the only available anabolic agent for osteoporosis approved in the United States.
- Denosumab is a monoclonal antibody directed against the receptor activator of nuclear factor κB (RANK) ligand causing a decrease in osteoclastic activity.

### Basic Science Correlate

There is constant balance between bone resorption and bone deposition, which maintains normal bone health. The interaction of RANK with RANKL stimulates bone resorption.

- Osteoprotegerin (OPG) is a decoy receptor for RANK, competing for RANKL, which will inhibit bone resorption, favoring bone formation.
- The mechanism behind control of bone remodeling involves the interaction between the RANK-RANKL-OPG signaling pathway, which regulates osteoclast activation, and differentiation.
- Estrogen, testosterone, glucocorticoids, and PTH are hormones that regulate the RANKL:OPG ratio, and this will lead to alteration and balance in bone resorption.
- This balance is also controlled in part by vitamin D, inflammatory cytokines (i.e. IL-1), and growth factors.
- Osteoblasts control bone resorption by overexpression of either RANKL or OPG in different circumstances.

### CLINICAL PEARL

- HRT should not be used routinely for the prevention of osteoporotic fractures; recent trials show an increased risk for breast cancer and CV disease in those taking it.
- Bisphosphonates (alendronate) are the most common agent used to treat osteoporosis.

### Final Diagnosis

Osteoporosis

# CASE 7

## Chief Complaint

Proximal muscle weakness

## History and Physical Examination

A 42-year-old woman presents with proximal muscle weakness for 5 weeks. She reports an inability to comb her hair, climb stairs, get up from a chair, and get in and out of the bath. She is able to button her shirt and write without difficulty. She also reports no ocular symptoms. Generally she feels very tired; tasks that were normally easy are now exhausting. Her symptoms do not improve or worsen with repetitive activity. She also has noted a 10-lb weight loss. She takes no medications, and her family history is significant only for psoriasis in a maternal uncle.

She is afebrile; BP is 112/64 mm Hg, pulse 86/min and regular, and respirations 16/min. There is a violaceous discoloration of the upper eyelids associated with some periorbital edema. She has pinkish plaques with scales on the extensor surface of some joints, including the elbows, MCP and PIP joints, and knees. Heart and lung exams are unremarkable. Abdominal exam is normal, and the liver and spleen are within normal limits. The joints show no evidence of erythema or swelling. Neurologic exam reveals normal reflexes and sensation, but significant weakness affecting the quadriceps muscles and deltoid muscle groups with 3/5 strength bilaterally.

## Differential Diagnosis

1. Dermatomyositis
2. Polymyositis
3. Inclusion body myositis
4. Corticosteroid induced myositis
5. Myasthenia gravis
6. Lambert-Eaton syndrome
7. Polymyalgia rheumatica (an inflammatory disorder that causes muscle pain and stiffness [not weakness]; associated with temporal arteritis)

## Initial Management

**Setting:** outpatient

## Diagnostic/Therapeutic Plan

- CPK
- TSH
- ESR
- CBC

### Test Results

- CPK: 3,000 units/L
- TSH: normal
- ESR: 70 mm/hr (elevated)
- CBC: normal

### Assessment

When evaluating patients with proximal muscle weakness and elevated muscle enzymes (>1,000 IU/L), consider inflammatory myopathies as the cause.

- Dermatomyositis presents with the typical heliotrope rash.
- Polymyositis presents with isolated muscle weakness and no evidence of dermatologic manifestations.
- Inclusion body myositis characteristically affects older males and affects both the proximal and distal muscles (distal muscle weakness not present in this patient).
- Typically, dermatomyositis and polymyositis spare the ocular muscles.
- Steroid-induced myositis presents with normal CPK and ESR in patients using steroids.
- Myasthenia gravis characteristically involves the ocular muscles. The weakness associated with myasthenia typically worsens with activity; the patient typically reports that the symptoms are worse at the end of the day and improve with rest.
- Lambert–Eaton syndrome, seen as part of the paraneoplastic syndromes associated with small-cell cancer, has proximal muscle weakness that improves with repetitive activity and improves at the end of the day.

#### Basic Science Correlate

- In dermatomyositis, there is perimysial inflammatory infiltrate.
- In polymyositis, there is endomysial inflammatory infiltrate.
- In inclusion body myositis, there are inclusions of amyloid in the muscle fibers and diffuse inflammatory infiltrate in the muscle cells.

### Further Management Plan/Results

| | |
|---|---|
| • Muscle biopsy | Diffuse inflammation around muscle fascicles and perivascular walls; the inflammatory infiltrate is predominantly lymphocytic |
| • EMG | Increased spontaneous activity, repetitive discharges and positive sharp waves |
| • ANA | Positive in 1:360 |
| • Anti-Jo-1 | Positive |

## Treatment Plan

1. High-dose corticosteroids until CPK normalizes, then gradually taper
2. Monitor clinical improvement of weakness and CPK levels
3. In refractory cases, consider methotrexate and azathioprine
4. Hydroxychloroquine is effective for the rash of dermatomyositis as well as topical corticosteroids or tacrolimus
5. Physical therapy

## Discussion

Polymyositis and dermatomyositis are inflammatory myopathies. They present with progressive proximal weakness (involvement of large muscle groups) but spare fine motor movement initially (writing, etc.). **Inclusion-body myositis presents with both proximal and distal muscle weakness.** No ocular involvement is evident (ocular involvement is so rare that if eye muscles are involved, other causes should be considered).

The first test should be to check muscle enzymes: CPK and aldolase, which are increased (typically in the thousands). Antinuclear antibodies are positive in 80% of cases but are non-specific; anti-Jo-1 antibodies are specific for the inflammatory myopathies but occur only in a small percentage of patients. The confirmatory test is the muscle biopsy, which shows the typical lymphocytic infiltrate involving the muscles. The EMG is also helpful in that it shows characteristic positive sharp waves and repetitive discharges and can show which muscles are affected and should be biopsied to confirm the diagnosis.

Treatment is high-dose steroids (oral) following CPK to monitor the response. If no response, consider methotrexate or azathioprine.

Remember that dermatomyositis, especially, is associated with cancer (typically adenocarcinoma—ovarian cancer being the most common in women, but also breast cancer and colon cancer). **Screening for occult malignancy is mandatory in adults who are diagnosed with inflammatory myopathies.** Assessment for cancer should include urinalysis, chest radiography, colonoscopy, PSA in men, and Pap smear and CA-125 in women. Additional testing usually includes pelvic ultrasonography or CT to exclude ovarian cancer. CT of the chest, abdomen, and pelvis is often performed in patients at high risk for cancer.

## Final Diagnosis

Dermatomyositis

# CASE 8

## Chief Complaint

Headaches, fever, and proximal muscle stiffness

## History and Physical Examination

A 70-year-old man presents with excessive fatigue, fever, muscle aches, headaches, and shoulder–hip pain. He had been in good health until 6 weeks ago, when he began experiencing mild headaches, described as 'throbbing,' mostly on the right side of the head. They were relieved by acetaminophen and ibuprofen. He also has had some joint and shoulder stiffness with considerable morning pain, which prevents him from brushing his teeth or combing his hair. Additionally, his legs feel heavy in the mornings and he needs help getting out of bed. The symptoms improve as the day goes on. He has no abdominal pain, early satiety, diarrhea, visual difficulties, jaw claudication, arthritis, or joint swelling.

His temperature is 37.9° C (100.2° F), BP 126/72, pulse 102/min, and respirations 14/min. Skin has no rashes. There is no lymphadenopathy. Joints have no synovitis or erythema. Heart and lung exams are normal. Abdominal exam is normal, including normal liver and spleen. The pulses are intact in the lower extremities and there is no edema. Neurologic exam is non-focal.

## Differential Diagnosis

1. Temporal arteritis with polymyalgia rheumatica
2. Tension headache
3. Migraine headache

## Initial Management

**Setting:** outpatient

## Diagnostic/Therapeutic Plan

- Erythrocyte sedimentation rate (ESR)
- Hb
- WBC
- Platelets
- MCV
- Comprehensive panel

## Test Results

- ESR: 102 mm/h
- Hb: 11.5 g/dL
- WBCs: 9,500 /mm$^3$ (normal differential)

- Platelets: 325,000 /$mm^3$
- MCV: 78 $\mu m^3$
- Comprehensive panel: normal

## Assessment

Consider temporal arteritis (TA) in all patients presenting with new-onset headache who are age ≥50. In this patient it is the likely diagnosis, since he has proximal muscle pain and stiffness (polymyalgia rheumatica is seen in ~30% patients with TA) as well as elevated ESR (always >60).

Migraine and tension headaches are very common but should be considered a less-likely diagnosis in older patients with new-onset headache. Also, neither migraine nor tension headache is associated with the systemic symptoms that this patient is experiencing (weight loss, fever, proximal pain, etc.).

### Basic Science Correlate

In temporal arteritis there is segmental granulomatous inflammation of the media of large vessels causing narrowing of the lumen and possible thrombosis of the affected section of the vessel leading to distal ischemia and necrosis.

## Further Management Plan/Results

| | |
|---|---|
| • **Start prednisone (60 mg daily)** | |
| • Get surgical consult for temporal artery biopsy | A 2 cm specimen of right temporal artery shows evidence of inflammation, fibrosis, lymphocytic infiltration, and giant cell infiltration. |

Remember, always **start prednisone before the biopsy!**

## Treatment Plan

1. Continue prednisone until patient improves clinically and the ESR is normal

## Discussion

Temporal arteritis (TA), also known as giant cell arteritis, is a vasculitis affecting the large arteries that supply the head, eyes, and optic nerves. New-onset headache in any patient age >50 prompts consideration of this diagnosis; if left untreated, TA may result in permanent vision loss.

The most common symptoms of giant cell arteritis are headache and pain, which usually occur in one or both temples. Other common symptoms include scalp tenderness (pain when combing hair), jaw claudication (jaw pain when chewing), decreased or blurry vision, tongue numbness, or rarely, sudden loss of vision. Sometimes the patient may have proximal muscle pain and stiffness (neck, arms, hips) due to polymyalgia rheumatica, a coexisting condition with TA.

ESR is the first test to do when TA is suspected. Since ESR is always increased in TA, all patients will have an elevated ESR (100% sensitive). Diagnosis is always confirmed by biopsy of the temporal arteries in which the characteristic giant cells are demonstrated.

- When TA is suspected and ESR is elevated, start corticosteroids immediately, even before the temporal artery biopsy is performed.
- Follow the ESR for response to treatment.
- Taper off the corticosteroids when the ESR normalizes.

Patients should be followed for possibility of aortic aneurysm in the future.

## Final Diagnosis

Temporal arteritis with associated polymyalgia rheumatica

# CASE 9

## Chief Complaint

Lower back stiffness and pain

## History and Physical Examination

A 25-year-old man comes to the office with complaints of joint pain of 5 years duration. After periods of inactivity it has now worsened. He has started to exercise every morning to improve the back pain and stiffness. The back pain is non-radiating and there are no neurologic complaints. He recently developed painful swelling in the left ankle, which causes considerable morning stiffness lasting a few hours.

He is afebrile. His blood pressure is 110/74 mm Hg, pulse 82/min and regular, and respirations 14/min. The chest is clear to auscultation. The heart has normal S1 and S2, with no gallop, lift, or murmurs. Abdominal exam is unremarkable. The left ankle is swollen and painful to motion. There is a reduced range of motion of the lumbar spine.

## Differential Diagnosis

1. Ankylosing spondylitis
2. Psoriatic arthritis
3. Reactive arthritis
4. Inflammatory bowel disease
5. Osteoarthritis

## Initial Management

**Setting:** outpatient

## Diagnostic/Therapeutic Plan

- X-ray of lumbar spine and sacroiliac joints
- ESR
- Rheumatoid factor

## Test Results

- X-ray: bamboo spine and bilateral sacroiliitis
- ESR 70 mm/h
- Rheumatoid factor negative

## Assessment

Back pain with inflammatory features, along with asymmetric joint involvement, make seronegative arthropathy the likely diagnosis. Ankylosing spondylitis is the likely diagnosis given the fact that this condition is inflammatory in nature, and affects the lower back, with bilateral sacroiliitis. This patient has none of the clinical characteristics of other seronegative spondyloarthropathies, such as inflammatory diarrhea with IBD, small joints of hands with psoriatic arthritis, or conjunctivitis/urethritis/diarrheal illness with reactive arthritis.

Osteoarthritis sometimes presents as an asymmetric arthropathy, but evidence of inflammation makes this diagnosis unlikely.

### Basic Science Correlate

Ninety percent of patients with ankylosing spondylitis have HLA-B27 positivity. The human gene encoding for major histocompatibility antigens (MHC) and human lymphocyte antigen (HLA) is coded in a small section of chromosome 6.

- MHC Class 1, which presents antigens to CD8 lymphocytes, is composed of 3 main sections: A, B, and C, named HLA-A, HLA-B, HLA-C.
- The section that codes for MHC class II, which present antigens to CD4 lymphocytes, has one main group D or HLA-D.
  - HLA-D is further divided into 3 subsections: P, Q, and R.
  - Thus, we have HLA-DQ, HLA-DR, and HLA-DP.
- Each individual has a unique set of HLA genes that makes it challenging to match individuals for organ transplantation.

## Further Management Plan

- NSAIDs
- Methotrexate, sulfasalazine, cyclosporine, antimalarials, penicillamine. azathioprine, retinoic acid derivatives, anti-TNF-alpha agents

## Discussion

The seronegative spondyloarthropathies are a group of related multisystem disorders that affect the spine, peripheral joints, and periarticular structures. They may also show extra-articular manifestations. They include ankylosing spondylitis, reactive/Reiter arthritis, psoriatic arthritis, and arthritis associated with inflammatory bowel disease.

Absence of antinuclear antibodies and the rheumatoid factor are the hallmark of these diseases; hence the name seronegative. They involve the lower back and sacroiliac joints and present with lower back pain and stiffness; hence the name spondyloarthropathies. They commonly have extra-articular manifestations and can also affect the aortic valve, the lung parenchyma (often apices), the eye (anterior inflammation), and the skin.

The presence of HLA-B27 is seen in most patients who have seronegative arthropathy. However, HLA-B27 is not used to confirm the diagnosis.

Ankylosing spondylitis is an inflammatory disorder of unknown etiology that primarily affects the axial skeleton.

- Usually starts age 20–30 and is very rare age >40
- Men > women by 3–4 times (one of the few collagen vascular diseases that affect men more than women)
- Ninety percent of cases are HLA-B27 positive

- Usually presents with chronic lower back pain in a young man
  - The giveaway is morning stiffness lasting >1 hr and improves with exercise
  - Cervical spine is rarely, if ever, affected, and happens only late in the disease

Extra-articular manifestations are common in ankylosing spondylitis:

- Anterior uveitis
- Aortic insufficiency that may sometimes lead to CHF
- Third-degree heart block

On examination there will be evidence of decreased spine mobility (positive Schober's test, which measures spine flexion, and sometimes obliteration of the lumbar lordosis). Because of this, spine fractures are sometimes seen in patients with ankylosing spondylitis after minimal trauma.

X-rays show evidence of sacroiliitis (the earliest finding) and eventual fusing of the sacroiliac joints. Chronic spine inflammation will eventually cause "bamboo spine and squaring" of the vertebral bodies.

A diagnosis of ankylosing spondylitis is based on clinical and x-ray criteria. HLA-B27 is not used for diagnostic purposes. Treatment is NSAIDs, physical therapy, exercise, and disease-modifying agents such as methotrexate and infliximab.

Reactive arthritis is a seronegative arthropathy that occurs as a complication from an infection somewhere in the body. There are mainly 2 types of infection causing 2 different syndromes.

- **Reiter's syndrome**: follows an incident of non-gonococcal urethritis (*Chlamydia, Ureaplasma*), causing a syndrome of conjunctivitis and arthritis
  - Patients may also have distinct mucocutaneous manifestations, such as keratoderma blennorrhagica, circinate balanitis, and oral/genital ulcers.
- The other type occurs after an infectious diarrhea caused by *Campylobacter, Shigella,* or *Salmonella* (think of the organisms that cause enteroinvasive diarrheas); *Campylobacter* is most common.

Reactive arthritis, like ankylosing spondylitis, is a clinical diagnosis. X-ray findings will be consistent with a seronegative spondyloarthropathy.

Treatment for reactive arthritis is the same as for ankylosing spondylitis. There are studies which support an accelerated recovery of Reiter's syndrome due to a chlamydial infection after prolonged treatment with tetracycline (~3 weeks' duration). There are also studies that indicate that prompt antibiotic use in urethritis will decrease the chance of Reiter's syndrome.

A severe form of Reiter's syndrome and reactive arthritis has been described in HIV patients. The skin manifestations are particularly aggressive in these patients and improve with antiretroviral medications.

### Final Diagnosis

Ankylosing spondylitis

#### CLINICAL PEARL

Spine fractures occur:

- With minimal stress in older people who have osteoporosis
- With long-standing inflammatory diseases of the spine in young people

# CASE 10

## Chief Complaint

Fever, body aches and pain, and weight loss for 6 weeks

## History and Physical Examination

A 33-year-old male who uses IV drugs presents with complaints of fever and chills with associated muscle aches and joint pain. He has been losing weight and is concerned. He takes no medication and was in good health until about 6 weeks ago when he started to develop his current symptoms.

On examination his temperature is 37.9 C (100.2 F), blood pressure 175/95 mm Hg, pulse 95/min, and respirations 20/min. Lungs are clear to auscultation and the heart has a regular rate and rhythm with no murmurs. Examination of the abdomen reveals mild abdominal discomfort with no organomegaly. The skin shows a mottled, reticulated vascular pattern, and there is a lace-like purplish discoloration of the skin with the presence of ulcerations and nodules.

## Differential Diagnosis

1. Polyarteritis nodosa (PAN)
2. HIV
3. Dermatomyositis
4. Chronic viral hepatitis

## Initial Management

**Setting:** outpatient

## Diagnostic/Therapeutic Plan

- CBC with differential
- Urinalysis and creatinine
- ESR
- HIV test
- CPK
- Viral hepatitis titers

## Test Results

- Hematocrit 31%, WBCs 13,000/mm$^3$, platelets 160/mm$^3$
- Urinalysis: no casts, creatinine 1.9 mg/dL
- ESR 75 mm/h
- HIV negative
- CPK 233 U/L
- HAV-IgM and IgG–negative, HCV antibodies–negative, HBsAg-positive, HBsAb-negative, HBeAg-positive, HBcAg IgG–positive

### Assessment

This patient appears to have chronic active hepatitis B, likely due to his history of IV drug use. Patients with PAN usually present with the following symptoms:

- Fever
- Weight loss
- Myalgias and arthralgias with presence of cutaneous nodules and livedo reticularis
- Ulceration of the nodules
- Renovascular hypertension (when renal artery is affected)

The ESR is elevated here, indicating an inflammatory condition. The HIV test is negative, and, given that the symptoms started 6 weeks ago, it is unlikely that this patient has HIV. The elevation of CPK is only mild, and usually CPK is very elevated in patients with dermatomyositis (typically >1,000 IU/l). Viral titers are negative for hepatitis A and C.

### Further Management Plan/Results

| | |
|---|---|
| • Mesenteric and renal angiography | Mesenteric angiography reveals aneurysms of the mesenteric and renal arteries |
| • Biopsy of cutaneous lesion | Segmental transmural fibrinoid necrosis of arteries in different stages |
| • Prednisone 1mg/kg/day | |
| • Antiviral therapy for hepatitis B (entecavir) | |
| • If no response to steroids, try cyclophosphamide | |

### Discussion

PAN usually presents with fever, arthralgias/myalgias, and weight loss associated with skin manifestations including cutaneous nodules—which tend to ulcerate—and livedo reticularis.

- Associated with chronic hepatitis B infection in about 50% of cases
- Affects mainly medium-sized muscular arteries (less frequently, small-size vessels)
- Can affect any organ but **spares the lung**
- Biopsy findings show segmental transmural necrotizing inflammation forming aneurysms with fibrinoid necrosis

Symptoms depend on the organ involved.

- In the kidneys, PAN can cause renovascular hypertension by affecting the medium-size renal artery. This can lead to kidney atrophy. Patients with PAN typically do not have glomerulonephritis.
- In the GI system, PAN can cause abdominal pain and melena.
- Skin manifestations include cutaneous and livedo reticularis.
- In the nervous system, PAN can present with peripheral neuropathies, including tingling, numbness, and/or pain in the hands, arms, feet, and legs, and **mononeuritis multiplex** (e.g., foot drop).

Diagnosis is suspected when angiography of mesenteric and renal arteries shows evidence of aneurysms. A diagnosis of PAN is confirmed with biopsy of the affected skin lesions or involved organs showing transmural necrotizing fibrinoid arteritis.

Treatment consists of corticosteroids or cyclophosphamide for refractory cases. If the patient is HBsAg-positive (50% of the cases), antiviral treatment for hepatitis B is mandatory. Drugs for hepatitis B include entecavir, adefovir, tenofovir, telbivudine, and lamivudine.

#### Basic Science Correlate

Antivirals such as the ones used for herpes virus, hepatitis B and C, and HIV can be nucleotide or nucleoside analogs. These drugs function as purine or pyrimidine bases in the synthesis of DNA. Once these drugs are phosphorylated, they act as a nucleotide and are incorporated into the growing DNA of the virus causing faulty DNA to form.

### Follow-up Management and Prevention

This patient should be counseled to avoid sharing needles and should be referred to a detox center for drug abuse. Additionally, he should be educated on the risk of IV drug use causing hepatitis C and HIV disease.

- Follow patient with serial LFTs, as well as hepatitis B viral load and hepatitis B titers to assess response to antivirals for his condition
- Check patient for markers of inflammation such as ESR or CRP

Vaccination for hepatitis A is necessary in this patient, as well as hepatitis B vaccination to any household contact of the patient that is not immune to hepatitis B.

### Final Diagnosis

Polyarteritis nodosa with chronic hepatitis B infection

# Dermatology 12

## INFLAMMATORY CONDITIONS

### Erythema Nodosum

**Pathogenesis.** Erythema nodosum is a localized inflammatory condition of the skin or panniculitis. It is secondary to recent infections or inflammatory conditions. It is also associated with pregnancy. The most common causes of erythema nodosum are recent streptococcal infections, coccidioidomycosis, histoplasmosis, sarcoidosis, inflammatory bowel disease, syphilis, or hepatitis. Enteric infections such as *Yersinia* also cause the disorder.

**Clinical Presentation.** Erythema nodosum consists of *multiple painful, red, raised nodules* on the *anterior* surface of the *lower extremities*. They are extremely tender to palpation. They do not ulcerate, and they generally last about *6 weeks*.

## FUNGAL INFECTIONS

### Tinea Pedis, Cruris, Corporis, Versicolor, Capitis, and Onychomycosis

**Clinical Presentation and Diagnosis.**

Superficial fungal infections of the skin, hair, and nails are primarily diagnosed by their visual appearance and confirmed by a potassium hydroxide (KOH) test of the skin.

- The leading edge of the lesion on the skin/nails is scraped with a scalpel to remove some of the epithelial cells or some of the nail and hair.
- KOH has the ability to dissolve the epithelial cells and collagen of the nail, but not the ability to melt away the fungus.
- Hence, a KOH preparation gives an immediate diagnostic answer by revealing fungal hyphae. This is particularly characteristic in tinea versicolor, where the *Malassezia furfur* (*Pityrosporum orbiculare*) organism appears in a "spaghetti and meatballs" pattern.

**Treatment.** For onychomycosis (nail infection) or hair infection (tinea capitis), the medications with the greatest efficacy are oral terbinafine or itraconazole. These medications are used for 6 weeks for fingernails and 12 weeks for toenails. Terbinafine is potentially hepatotoxic, and it is important to periodically check liver function tests. Griseofulvin must be used for 6 to 12 months in the treatment of fingernails and has much less antifungal efficacy than terbinafine. Griseofulvin is no longer recommended in the treatment of onychomycosis of the toenails. In the treatment of tinea capitis, griseofulvin is recommended for 6 to 8 weeks.

**CCS NOTE**

For oral antifungal treatment, the drugs of choice for **tinea capitis** and **onychomycosis** are terbinafine and itraconazole.

*All other fungal infections* of the skin that don't involve the hair or nails may be treated with a topical medication: ketoconazole, clotrimazole, econazole, terbinafine, miconazole, sertaconazole, sulconazole, tolnaftate, or naftifine.

### Clinical Correlate

**Tinea versicolor** presents with altered pigmentation, i.e., lesions of different colors from light brown to pink (hence the name *versicolor*). The lesions often do not undergo color changes when exposed to sun, and therefore present with pale areas in the middle of a normal tan. The organism may also be contagious. A KOH preparation and fungal culture are used in the same manner as for the other dermatophytes.

Treatment for tinea versicolor is oral therapy with itraconazole or fluconazole—not because of antifungal resistance but because the condition typically involves large amounts of body surface area and thus is difficult to cover with an ordinary topical cream/lotion.

**Vitiligo,** on the other hand, is a complete absence of pigmentation. Treatment is topical selenium sulfide every 2–3 weeks to reduce the difference in color between the affected and normal areas.

# VIRAL INFECTIONS

## Herpes Simplex

**Pathogenesis.** Herpes simplex infections of the genitals are characterized by multiple, painful vesicles.

**Clinical Presentation.** The vesicles are usually obvious by examination, and antibiotic therapy should be initiated immediately without waiting for results of the tests.

**Diagnosis.** This is done with active lesions only. In the event that the diagnosis is not clear or the lesions have become confluent into an ulcer, the best initial test is a Tzanck smear. Tzanck smears detect *multinucleated giant cells* and are similar in technique to a Pap smear.

The most accurate diagnostic test is a viral culture, which will grow in 24 to 48 hours. Serology is *not* a useful test for diagnosing herpes infections.

**Treatment.** Immediate therapy is with oral acyclovir, famciclovir, or valacyclovir.

## Herpes Zoster/Varicella

Episodes of dermatomal herpes zoster, also known as shingles, occur more frequently in the older adult and in those with defects of the lymphocytic portion of the immune system (i.e., leukemia, lymphoma, HIV, or those on steroids).

**Clinical Presentation.** The vesicles are 2 to 3 mm in size at all stages of development and are on an erythematous base.

**Diagnosis.** Although the Tzanck prep and viral culture are the best initial and most accurate diagnostic tests, they are generally not necessary because little else will produce a band of vesicles in a dermatomal distribution besides herpes zoster.

**Treatment.** Patients with shingles benefit from oral antiviral therapy, as evidenced by accelerated healing of lesions and resolution of zoster-associated pain with acyclovir, valacyclovir, or famciclovir. Acyclovir is typically administered at a dosage of 800 mg, 5x/day for 10 days. Compared with acyclovir, both famciclovir and valacyclovir offer the advantage of less frequent administration with equal (if not better) efficacy. Also, for the skin lesions, aluminum acetate soaks can be comforting.

In severely immunocompromised hosts (transplant recipients) and in patients with disseminated herpes zoster, treatment at the outset should be with IV acyclovir rather than oral. In these cases, IV acyclovir will reduce the risk of visceral complications, but has no effect on healing of the skin lesions or pain.

The management of postherpetic neuralgia can be particularly difficult. Analgesics such as non-narcotics and narcotics and drugs such as gabapentin, amitriptyline, lidocaine patch, and pregabalin are typically used. In one study, glucocorticoid therapy started early in the course of the disease significantly accelerated return to usual activities and termination of analgesia. Glucocorticoids should not be used in immunocompromised patients and without concomitant antiviral therapy (risk of dissemination).

Prevention of herpes zoster with the vaccine is recommended in individuals age >60. The incidence of shingles in those given the vaccine has been shown to reduce by 50%, and the incidence of post-herpetic neuralgia by 66%.

### CLINICAL PEARL

In Ramsay Hunt syndrome, zoster affects the geniculate ganglion of the sensory branch of the facial nerve. Vesicles and pain appear on the external auditory canal, and patients lose their sense of taste in the anterior 2/3 of the tongue. At the same time, they develop ipsilateral facial palsy.

**Facial palsy + pain = zoster**

**Facial palsy — pain** (especially bilateral), consider **Lyme disease** and other processes.

# BACTERIAL INFECTIONS

## Lyme Disease

**Pathogenesis.** Lyme disease is caused by an infection of the *Borrelia burgdorferi* spirochete, transmitted by the deer tick (*Ixodes scapularis*).

**Clinical Presentation.** More than 85% of patients who have Lyme disease develop a rash. By definition, the rash must be erythematous with central clearing and be at least 5 cm in diameter. It usually occurs 7 to 10 days after the tick bite.

**Diagnosis.** This rash is so characteristic of Lyme that it is more important than serologic testing in terms of confirming a diagnosis.

**Treatment.** If the rash is described, then go straight to therapy with oral doxycycline, amoxicillin, or cefuroxime. Without treatment, the rash will resolve in the vast majority of cases in a few days to a few weeks. The problem is that without therapy, two-thirds of these patients will develop joint disease. A smaller number will develop neurologic or cardiac disorders.

In patients with Lyme and neurologic/cardiac conduction abnormalities (atrioventricular block, PR interval increase), administer IV ceftriaxone for 14–28 days. With cardiac conduction abnormalities, cardiac monitoring is necessary at least for part of the course, but a permanent pacemaker is usually not recommended.

## SEXUALLY TRANSMITTED DISEASES

### Syphilis

**Pathogenesis.** Both primary and secondary syphilis mainly present with cutaneous disorders. The causative organism is *Treponema pallidum*.

**Clinical Presentation.** The chancre of primary syphilis is an ulceration with heaped-up, indurated edges that is painless the majority of the time. Secondary syphilis presents with a generalized copper-colored, maculopapular rash that is particularly intense on the palms and soles of the feet. The other manifestations of secondary syphilis are predominantly dermatologic as well, such as the mucous patch, alopecia areata, and condylomata lata.

**Diagnosis.** The best initial test of primary syphilis is a darkfield examination because there is a false-negative rate of 25% for both the VDRL and RPR. In other words, these serologic tests need several weeks to become positive, and they are only 75% sensitive in primary syphilis. For secondary syphilis, the VDRL and RPR tests have nearly 100% sensitivity.

**Treatment.** Both primary and secondary syphilis are treated with a single, intramuscular dose of penicillin. In those patients allergic to penicillin, doxycycline orally for 2 weeks is the alternative therapy.

## MALIGNANT LESIONS

### Melanoma

**Pathogenesis.** Superficial spreading melanoma is the most common type of malignancy, accounting for ~70% of cases.

**Clinical Presentation.** Malignant lesions grow in size, have irregular borders, are uneven in shape, and have inconsistent coloring. Lentigo maligna melanoma arises on sun-exposed body parts in the older adult. Acral-lentiginous melanoma arises on the palms, soles of feet, and nail beds.

**Diagnosis.** Biopsy diagnosis is best performed with a full-thickness sample because tumor thickness is by far the most important prognostic factor.

**Treatment.** Excision

### Squamous Cell Carcinoma

**Pathogenesis.** Develops on sun-exposed skin surfaces in older adult patients

**Clinical Presentation.** It is particularly common on the lip, where the carcinogenic potential of tobacco is multiplicative. Ulceration of the lesion is common.

**Diagnosis** is with a biopsy, and the **treatment** is surgical removal. Radiotherapy can be used for lesions that cannot be treated surgically.

### Basal Cell Carcinoma

**Pathogenesis.** Far more common than squamous cell carcinoma (80% of all skin cancer cases)

**Clinical Presentation.** Basal cell carcinoma has a shiny or "pearly" appearance.

**Diagnosis** is confirmed by shave or punch biopsy.

**Treatment** is with surgical removal. Mohs microsurgery has the greatest cure rate. In this technique, instant frozen sections are done to determine when enough tissue has been removed to give a clean margin; 5-FU can be used in treatment of superficial lesions.

## SCALING DISORDERS/PAPULOSQUAMOUS DERMATITIS

### Psoriasis

**Clinical Presentation.** Silvery scales develop on the extensor surfaces. It can be local or enormously extensive. Nail pitting is a common accompaniment.

**Treatment.** Salicylic acid is used to remove heaped-up collections of scaly material so that the other therapies can make contact. If the disease is relatively localized, topical steroids are used. Severe disease also needs coal tar or anthralin derivatives. To avoid the long-term use of steroids, which can cause skin atrophy, and to avoid coal tars, which are messy to use, we can substitute topical vitamin D and vitamin A derivatives. The vitamin-D derivative most frequently used is calcipotriene. Tazarotene is a topical vitamin A derivative.

### Eczema

**Clinical Presentation.** Eczema is a disease of unknown etiology that is characterized by itchy, erythematous, vesicular, at times weeping and crusting patches. The term *eczema* is also commonly used to describe atopic dermatitis and atopic eczema.

Eczema is broadly applied to a range of persistent skin conditions. These include dryness and recurring skin rashes that are characterized by redness, itching/dryness, crusting, flaking, blistering, cracking, or bleeding. Areas of temporary skin discoloration may appear and are sometimes due to healed lesions. Scratching a healing area may result in scarring and may enlarge the rash.

Specific types:

- **Atopic dermatitis** is an allergic disease believed to have a hereditary component; it often runs in families whose members also have asthma. It is particularly noticeable on the head/scalp, neck, inside of elbows, back of knees, and buttocks.
- **Contact dermatitis** (2 types):
    - Allergic: resulting from a delayed reaction to an allergen, such as poison ivy, poison oak, nickel
    - Irritant: resulting from direct reaction for example to a detergent

**Treatment.** There is no known cure for eczema. Treatment aims to control symptoms by reducing inflammation and relieving itching, typically with moisturizers and corticosteroid creams. If these are not effective, creams based on calcineurin inhibitors (tacrolimus) may be used.

# Radiology 13

## APPEARANCES OF COMMON DISORDERS ON CHEST X-RAY

### COPD/Emphysema

The most common appearance of COPD on a chest x-ray is related to hyperinflation of the lung. This leads to a darkening of the lung fields because more air is present. This trapped air also flattens the diaphragm and gives the impression of an elongated or tubular-shaped heart because it has been stretched down. There is an increased anterior/posterior diameter, or "barrel chest." Further, bullae are large, air-filled cavities that can give thin, white lines on a chest x-ray as the walls of the cavities press up against each other.

### Pneumonia

Lobar pneumonia causes a whitening of each individual lobe of the lung because of the greater density of the lung. The "silhouette" sign is present, which is when the border between the affected lobe and the surrounding denser structure is obscured. (The density of the lung increases because of alveolar infiltration to the point where it takes on the density of the nearby heart or diaphragm; hence, one can no longer tell where the lung ends and the denser structure nearby begins. Lower lobe pneumonia gives a silhouette over each half of the diaphragm. Right middle-lobe pneumonia obscures the right heart border and will not pass the minor or horizontal fissure seen on a PA chest x-ray. Upper-lobe infiltration will not pass the major fissure, and this is more easily seen on a lateral x-ray. You cannot determine a specific microbiologic etiology from the x-ray alone.

Disease of the lung outside the airspace but in the interstitial membrane gives a fine, lacy appearance visible in most, if not all, of the lobes. Examples of disorders that give interstitial infiltrates are *Pneumocystis* pneumonia, *Mycoplasma*, viruses, chlamydia, and sometimes *Legionella*. Noninfectious etiologies of an interstitial infiltrate are pulmonary fibrosis secondary to silicosis, asbestosis, mercury poisoning, berylliosis, byssinosis (from cotton), or simply idiopathic pulmonary fibrosis. As the long-standing disorders become worse and more chronic, a greater degree of fibrosis occurs. This leads to greater thickening of the membrane. The terms that are used for this more chronic, thicker appearance are *reticular-nodular* and, later, *honeycombing*.

**CCS NOTE**

Interstitial syndromes of the lung include:

- **S**arcoidosis
- **H**istiocytosis X
- **I**PF (Interstitial Pulmonary Fibrosis)
- **T**umor
- **F**ailure
- **A**sbestosis
- **C**ollagen Disorders
- **E**nvironmental
- **D**ust
- **D**rugs

### Congestive Heart Failure

The majority of pulmonary vascular flow is normally at the base of the lungs because of gravity. When there is fluid overload, the blood vessels toward the apices become fuller. This is known as pulmonary vascular congestion, or cephalization of flow. The term *cephalization* is used because more flow is moving toward the head. The other findings associated with congestive heart failure are cardiomegaly, effusions, and Kerley B lines.

Kerley B lines are the least important. They are small, horizontal lines at the bases that represent fluid in the interlobular septa. Each lung has several lobes. When fluid builds up outside the lobes, this is known as a pleural effusion. When fluid builds up within each lobe, in between the lobules, this is known as a Kerley B line. This type of subtle radiologic finding is less important in the evaluation of congestive heart failure since the advent of the widespread use of echocardiography.

## Position of Lines and Tubes

Chest x-rays are routinely used to determine the appropriate position of central venous lines and both endotracheal and chest tubes. The proper position of the tip of an endotracheal tube is 1 to 2 cm above the carina. It is important to keep some space above the carina so that when the head moves forward, the tube does not push into the carina, which is extremely uncomfortable and will provoke coughing. The tip of central venous lines is at the junction of the superior vena cava and the right atrium, at the point where the right mainstem bronchus is seen. The tip of the line should not be fully inside the atrium because this can irritate the heart and may provoke an arrhythmia.

## Air Under the Diaphragm

When there is perforation of an abdominal hollow organ, such as the duodenum, air is released and is visible under the diaphragm. The proper film to detect this is a chest x-ray taken in the upright position. This will allow the air to collect under the diaphragm, which should be easily visible. Abdominal x-rays do not always visualize the top of the diaphragm because of differences in body size. Chest x-rays always visualize the top of the diaphragm.

# Ophthalmology 14

## RETINAL DISEASES

### Diabetic Retinopathy

The etiology of diabetic retinopathy is based on damage to the endothelial lining of the small blood vessels of the eye. This is identical in pathogenesis to the damage that diabetes causes to all blood vessels in the body, as in the heart, kidney, brain, and peripheral nervous system. The endothelial lining of the retinal vessels becomes damaged, leading to progressive occlusion on a microscopic level. The occlusion leads to obstruction and increased pressure.

- **Nonproliferative (or background) retinopathy** is the earliest form of this adverse effect of the retina. It is characterized by dilation of veins, microaneurysms, retinal edema, and retinal hemorrhages. Hemorrhages into the retina are not as damaging as intravitreal hemorrhages because they do not obstruct sight.
- **Proliferative retinopathy** is a more advanced form of the disease and is markedly more serious, e.g., it progresses more rapidly to blindness.
  - As the microvascular damage to the vessels worsens, the vessels secrete increased amounts of an angiogenesis factor. The vessels are not providing sufficient nutrition to the retina, i.e., they are exerting increased effort to have more of them produced in an effort to deliver more nutrition and oxygen to the retina. Unfortunately, this "neovascularization," or new blood vessel formation, leads to the optic nerve getting covered with abnormal new vessel formation.
  - In addition, hemorrhages protrude into the vitreous chamber. Vitreal hemorrhages are much more serious than microaneurysms or intraretinal hemorrhages because they are much more sight-threatening.
  - The goal of treatment with diabetic retinopathy is (a) to prevent the patient from ever progressing to the proliferative phase and (b) to slow down the disease's progress with laser photocoagulation, should it occurs.

### Retinal Detachment

Retinal detachment is usually spontaneous, but it may result from trauma. The term *rhegmatogenous*, which is used to describe the detachment, is from the Greek word for "tear." The most common predisposing factors are myopia and surgical extraction of cataracts. Traction on the retina can also occur from proliferative retinopathy from diabetes, retinal vein occlusion, and age-related macular degeneration.

The most common presentation is blurry vision in one eye without pain or redness. The patient may complain of seeing "floaters," as well as flashes at the periphery of vision. Sometimes it is described as a "curtain coming down," as the retina falls off the sclera behind it. Diagnosis is made by ophthalmologic examination.

Treatment includes various methods of trying to reattach the retina.

- The patient leans the head back to promote the chance that the retina will fall back into place.
- The retina is mechanically reattached to the sclera surgically, by laser photocoagulation, cryotherapy, or the injection of expansile gas into the vitreal cavity (the gas presses the retina back into place).
- A "buckle" (or belt) is placed around the sclera to push the sclera forward so that it can come into contact with the retina.
- As a last resort, the vitreous is removed and the retina is surgically attached to the sclera. Most cases (80%) of uncomplicated rhegmatogenous retinal detachments can be cured with one operation, with 15% needing a second one.

### Central Retinal Artery Occlusion

The etiology of the disorder can be from carotid artery embolic disease, temporal arteritis, cardiac thrombi or myxoma, or any of the usual causes of thrombophilia, such as factor V Leiden mutation.

There is a sudden, painless, unilateral loss of vision. There is no redness of the eye. Ophthalmoscopy reveals a pale retina, with overall diminished perfusion and a "cherry-red" spot at the fovea. There is also "box-car" segmentation of the blood in the veins.

Diagnosis is made with carotid artery imaging, echocardiography, and evaluation for thrombophilia.

### Central Retinal Vein Occlusion

Patients have a clinical presentation similar to those with retinal artery occlusion. There is the sudden loss of vision without pain, redness, or abnormality in pupillary dilation. Ocular examination by funduscopy reveals disk swelling, venous dilation, tortuosity, and retinal hemorrhages.

Retinal hemorrhages are the main way to distinguish venous versus arterial obstruction.

### Closed-Angle Glaucoma

Closed-angle glaucoma is often an ophthalmologic emergency precipitated by the use of medication that has anticholinergic properties.

Patients present with an eye that is red, painful, hard to palpation, and associated with a fixed midpoint pupil. The cornea has a hazy cloudiness, and there is marked diminishment of visual acuity.

Acute angle-closure glaucoma is an ophthalmologic emergency. IV acetazolamide, urea, and osmotic diuretics (mannitol, glycerol) are used acutely. Pilocarpine is used to open the canal of Schlemm, and beta-blockers are used to decrease humor production. If ineffective, consider laser trabeculoplasty.

# KERATITIS

## Herpes Simplex Keratitis

Herpes simplex keratitis is characterized by severe pain in the eye and a sensation that something is caught under the eyelid. Diagnosis is based on finding a characteristic dendritic pattern over the cornea on fluorescein staining of the eye with examination under a blue light.

Treatment is oral acyclovir, famciclovir, or valacyclovir plus topical trifluridine 1% solution or idoxuridine.

Never use oral or topical steroids in an attempt to relieve inflammation

# Neurology 15

## CASE 1

### Chief Complaint

"My back hurts."

### History and Physical Examination

A 55-year-old woman with chronic back pain and history of breast cancer comes to the office because of worsening back pain. The pain has recently become worse after doing some heavy lifting during a spring cleaning of the house, and it has begun to radiate around her body like a tight belt. The pain has continued to increase, and she has gone from using increasing amounts of ibuprofen over the last week to an oxycodone and acetaminophen combination.

Physical examination shows spinal tenderness over the lower thoracic spine and poor effort on motor examination due to pain. Tone in lower extremities is increased. There is a sensory level at T10 to pain and temperature. Deep tendon reflexes are increased, and plantar responses are extensor bilaterally.

### Differential Diagnosis

1. Metastatic cancer
   - Prostate, breast, and lung cancer (**most common**)
   - Lung cancer (**most common inter-medullary cancer**)
   - Renal cell carcinoma, non-Hodgkin's lymphoma, multiple myeloma
2. Intra-medullary primary tumor: ependymomas, astrocytomas, oligodendrogliomas
3. Transverse myelitis
4. Epidural abscess
5. Epidural hematoma
6. Herniated disc
7. Spondylosis
8. Intradural extramedullary tumor: meningioma, schwannoma, neurofibroma
9. Extradural primary tumor: sarcoma, chondrosarcoma, chondroma

## Initial Management

**Setting:** outpatient

## Diagnostic/Therapeutic Plan

- Chest x-ray
- Spinal x-ray

## Test Results

- Chest x-ray: large tumor on right lower lobe
- Spinal x-ray: destruction of vertebral body at T10

## Assessment

Spinal cord compression is a neurologic emergency. The time course is crucial in making the diagnosis and in successful treatment. Acute paraplegia without trauma is the result of a vascular accident involving a bleed compressing the spinal cord. Surgical intervention might be necessary.

In this patient, a history of low back pain should not be dismissed if the pain is changing in character, increasing in intensity, and accompanied by neurologic deficits. A history of cancer must be taken seriously.

- A crescendo pattern to the pain is characteristic, along with an increase in the strength and dosage of analgesia.
- In 95% of cases, the initial symptom of epidural cord compression is unifocal back pain.
- Pain commonly precedes other neurologic symptoms by several weeks. Pain is initially local, progressively increasing over time and developing a radicular quality.
- Myelopathy is characteristic of cord compression with spastic paraparesis, increased deep tendon reflexes, and extensor plantar responses.
- Bladder/bowel dysfunction is generally a late finding.

MRI is the study of choice to look for epidural disease due to metastases. Gadolinium is not needed but is helpful for identifying other metastatic lesions (even asymptomatic). Once the tumor is found, restaging of the disease may be necessary, especially if this is the first evidence of recurrence.

Alarm symptoms include:

- Age >50
- Prior cancer history
- Pain: unremitting back pain; constant pain at night; pain worse with recumbency; pain >1 month
- Neurologic symptoms
- Sexual function deficits
- Unexplained weight loss
- No improvement in condition following conservative therapy

### CCS NOTE

Consider spinal cord compression when there are complaints of back pain in a patient who has a history of cancer or fever. The next appropriate test in this case is MRI, even in the absence of neurologic deficits on physical examination.

### CLINICAL PEARL

An epidural abscess might explain this patient's symptoms, but there would generally be point tenderness over the spine and fever or other signs of infection. Although rare now, TB used to commonly involve the spine (Pott's disease). Injection drug abuse is an important predisposing factor to epidural abscess; consider it in IV drug abusers presenting with back pain.

### Further Management Plan/Results

| | |
|---|---|
| • CT scan of chest, abdomen, and pelvis | Liver and lung metastases |
| • MRI | Multilevel replacement of bone by tumor with epidural disease causing cord compression at T10 |

### Treatment Plan

- Steroids
- Radiation therapy to spine
- Chemotherapy in selected forms of cancer, such as lymphoma

### Discussion

Acute treatment involves the use of high-dose steroids. Long-term treatment depends on the stage of disease. If the lesion is unifocal and the tumor is radiation-sensitive, then urgently initiate radiation.

- If the single lesion does not respond to radiation, consider surgery. Indications for decompressive surgery for metastatic epidural spinal cord compression include situations where a tissue diagnosis is necessary, where there is spinal instability, or where the tumor is known to be highly resistant.
- If the lesion is caught early, i.e., before the presence of neurologic deficits, chemotherapy might be used to shrink the tumor.

Use caution when performing a myelogram below the level of a "block" created by a condition such as a tumor. Decreasing the pressure below the block by removing CSF might cause the tumor to shift downward, worsening the neurologic deficit.

### Final Diagnosis

Spinal cord compression; epidural spinal cord compression

#### CLINICAL PEARL

With a prior history of breast cancer, metastatic disease would be the expected pathology, but occasionally one can see a primary spinal cancer develop. A meningioma also might be considered in a middle-aged woman.

# CASE 2

## Chief Complaint

"I can't walk."

## History and Physical Examination

A 42-year-old man who has developed ascending weakness in the lower extremities and paresthesias after a recent episode of gastroenteritis comes to the emergency department. His weakness has increased over the last week to the point that he can't walk.

Physical examination shows flaccid paralysis of lower extremities and loss of ankle jerks. The weakness is symmetric, and there is a mild sensory disturbance. Cranial nerve examination is normal.

## Differential Diagnosis

1. Acute inflammatory polyneuropathy (Guillain-Barré syndrome)
2. Poliomyelitis
3. Transverse myelitis
4. Botulism
5. Tick paralysis
6. Tetrodotoxin
7. Charcot-Marie-Tooth disease

## Initial Management

**Setting:** emergency department (early in the disease, may be an office visit)

## Diagnostic/Therapeutic Plan

- Lumbar puncture

### CLINICAL PEARL

- Consider Guillain-Barré as the primary diagnosis in a patient who has evolving paralysis with areflexia and no other systemic manifestations.

## Test Results

- Lumbar puncture: elevated protein; no WBCs

## Assessment

Although a number of illnesses are listed in the differential, this patient's history is characteristic of Guillain-Barré syndrome. The ascending weakness, which has occurred over the course of a week or so with accompanying paresthesias, is the classic combination. Symptoms typically appear after a viral illness.

Poliomyelitis occurs in the setting of an epidemic and has accompanying meningeal symptoms, fever, and asymmetric areflexic paralysis without sensory loss but with WBC in the CSF. Acute myelopathy has sphincteric paralysis and a marked sensorimotor paralysis below a given spinal level. Transverse myelitis gives a clear motor and sensory level, with hyperreflexia below that level, and the patient presents with loss of anal sphincter tone.

Botulism leads to early loss of pupillary reflexes and is dominated by cranial nerve abnormalities. The paralysis in botulism is descending, not ascending.

Tick paralysis is hard to distinguish from Guillain-Barré unless one finds the tick. Tetrodotoxin found in the puffer fish can cause tachypnea and iridoplegia, as well as motor paralysis.

Charcot-Marie-Tooth disease usually has a very slow onset, and rarely gets very severe. Patients may present with a foot drop/weakness or sensory loss in a stocking distribution.

## Further Management Plan/Results

| | |
|---|---|
| • Mean inspiratory pressures | −30 cm $H_2O$ |
| • EMG/nerve conduction velocity | Delayed F-wave responses |
| • Vital capacity | 30 mL/kg (decreased) |

## Treatment Plan

- Plasmapheresis
- IV high-dose immunoglobulin therapy
- Respiratory support as needed

## Discussion

There are about 3,500 cases of Guillain-Barré syndrome in North America each year. Recent infection with *Cytomegalovirus*, Epstein-Barr virus, or *Campylobacter jejuni* are common, but the specific etiology is often not documented. The usual findings are:

- Areflexic paralysis of the lower extremities
- Mild sensory disturbance
- Acellular rise of CSF protein without WBCs

Careful monitoring of vital signs is critical because respiratory failure, cardiac arrhythmia, and autonomic instability can occur. Vital capacity should be followed carefully, because when it drops, intubation will be needed.

Acute intermittent porphyria can be associated with a demyelinating motor neuropathy that can mimic Guillain-Barré. Attacks can be precipitated by medication (sulfa drugs, phenobarbital, alcohol, phenytoin). Abdominal pain is often associated, and the urine will turn dark.

Treatment is plasmapheresis or IV immunoglobulins, initiated within 2 wks of onset. (There is no benefit to combining these treatments.) Physical therapy also plays an important role early in the disease.

About 25% of patients will need ventilatory support at some point, thus all patients require hospitalization for monitoring. Glucocorticoids have not been shown to be effective.

The prognosis is good; 85% of patients gain complete recovery within weeks to months.

## Final Diagnosis

Guillain-Barré syndrome

# CASE 3

## Chief Complaint

"My memory is failing me."

## History and Physical Examination

A 64-year-old man with no significant medical history comes to the office because of a gradual onset of forgetfulness. He initially noted that he forgot where he had placed things and then found that he couldn't remember certain words. His wife is worried about his hearing because he keeps asking her the same questions again and again. Most recently, he seems to get lost on the way to the bathroom and has difficulty dressing himself. His wife states that he is not quite himself.

His vital signs are normal. There is a decreased ability in the naming of objects and in calculations. None of the objects were remembered at 5 minutes. When asked to name as many objects that one can buy in a grocery store, the patient was only able to name 15 objects in 1 minute. There are no focal neurologic deficits.

## Differential Diagnosis

1. Alzheimer's disease
2. Normal pressure hydrocephalus
3. Chronic subdural hematoma
4. Vitamin B12 deficiency
5. Hypothyroidism
6. Tertiary syphilis
7. Pseudodementia of depression
8. Pick disease (frontotemporal dementia)
9. Multiinfarct dementia
10. Prion disease
11. Dementia with Lewy bodies

## Initial Management

**Setting:** outpatient

## Diagnostic/Therapeutic Plan

- CT or MRI

## Test Results

- CT: mild atrophy; periventricular leukomalacia

## Assessment

An extensive number of diseases can cause dementia, though Alzheimer's disease is the most common. This diagnosis is essentially made when a patient both (a) is older adult and (b) has had dementia that has developed over a prolonged period of several months to many years, ranging from mild forgetfulness to a vegetative state.

Normal pressure hydrocephalus presents with a triad of dementia, gait ataxia, and urinary incontinence. It often occurs after head trauma, meningitis, or an SAH. The ataxia and urinary incontinence often precede the dementia.

Vitamin B12 deficiency produces a peripheral neuropathy and defects of position and vibratory sense on examination, as well as hypersegmented polymorphonuclear leukocytes on CBC. B12 deficiency can occur with anemia, with neurologic disease, or with both. Although chronic subdural hematoma and multiple previous infarctions could present like this, CT scan should easily detect those.

Hypothyroidism can cause dementia and psychiatric changes, vestibular changes, and auditory changes.

Pick disease is also known as "lobar atrophy" because the brain lesions tend to be localized to a specific lobe, rather than generalized as seen with Alzheimer's. In addition, Pick is characterized by defects in judgment, hygiene, social appropriateness, and language dysfunction first, with memory loss occurring later.

Prion disease is Creutzfeldt-Jakob disease, and there is usually a rapid deterioration over several months with myoclonic jerks found on physical exam.

If our patient were younger (age 30–50s), you would need to consider other etiologies:

- HIV/AIDS (**most common cause of dementia in younger patients**)
- Huntington disease (characteristic chorea-athetoid movements and personality changes [progressing to psychosis] accompany dementia); look for atrophy of the caudate nuclei on CT/MRI ["boxcar" ventricles])

Consider **prion disease** in rapid progressive dementia associated with myoclonus and motor rigidity.

## Further Management Plan/Results

| | |
|---|---|
| • CBC, B12 level, thyroid function tests, VDRL tests | Normal |
| • Drug screen | Negative |

## Treatment Plan

- Social support and prevention of injury and illness
- Donepezil, rivastigmine, or galantamine (cholinesterase inhibitor). Memantine is added to cholinesterase inhibitors in moderate to severe dementia.

## Discussion

The diagnosis of Alzheimer's can be confirmed only by findings on biopsy of the brain or at autopsy. The characteristic lesions are neurofibrillary tangle and cerebrovascular amyloidosis.

### CLINICAL PEARL

With dementia syndromes:

- **Exclude possible reversible causes:** B12 deficiency; hypothyroidism; CNS syphilis; normal pressure hydrocephalus
- **Look for depressive signs:** weight loss, insomnia, recent sentinel event (death of family member)

None of this is directly treatable. New medications (acetylcholinesterase inhibitors) can transiently improve symptoms by increasing acetylcholine concentrations in the brain.

The only eventual treatment is the avoidance of injury at home by instituting social supports and avoiding the toxicities of medication often used for other illnesses in the older adult, e.g., antihypertensives and psychotropics.

## Final Diagnosis

Alzheimer's disease

### CLINICAL PEARL

Other common causes of dementia include:

- **Normal pressure hydrocephalus**
  - Clinical triad of gait abnormalities, incontinence, and dementia
  - Clinical findings should be supported by CT/MRI, revealing hydrocephalus and LP (shows normal pressure)
  - Improvement in gait speed, stride length, reaction time, and tests of verbal memory and visual attention after removal of 30-50 mL of CSF (called Fisher test)
  - Responds to CSF shunting if caught early
- **Chronic subdural hematoma**
  - Consequence of remote trauma, sometimes mild
  - Ruling this out is a very good reason to get imaging study of the brain in any demented patient, even if no clear history of trauma
  - A tear in the bridging veins of the dura can lead to a slow accumulation of blood, which leads to deformation of the brain and gradual loss of cognition (reversible with surgery)
- **Pseudodementia (depression)**
  - Common in the older adult
  - "Low moods" may not manifest as depressive symptoms in the older adult; instead, may be physical signs such as poor memory, fatigue, insomnia, and weakness
  - Most demented patients make an effort in the mental status exam and try to mask their failures, whereas depressed patients tend to give up quickly (i.e., "What year is this?" "I don't know.")

# CASE 4

## Chief Complaint

"My husband isn't talking right and doesn't have control of his right hand."

## History and Physical Examination

A 72-year-old man is brought to your office by his wife. She reports observing multiple episodes of speaking difficulties and language comprehension, as well as multiple episodes of dropping objects held in his right hand. The problems have been developing slowly over a year. The patient is a former actor who appeared in a number of Western movies prior to giving up acting for a career as a politician. He and his wife have noted his gradually increasing forgetfulness over the last year. He has recently been doing a lot of horseback riding. He denies headaches.

Vital signs are T 36.8 C (98.2 F), blood pressure 130/87 mm Hg, pulse 70/min, and respirations 12/min. Physical examination shows that the pupils are normal and chest is clear. The abdomen is benign. Neurologic examination reveals that the patient is alert but disoriented to year: He thinks it's 1957 and that Eisenhower is president. Some right-hand and leg weakness are present. Calculations and judgment are intact, but short-term memory is poor.

## Differential Diagnosis

1. Alzheimer's disease
2. Transient ischemic attack
3. Subdural hematoma
4. Epidural hematoma
5. Cerebrovascular accident (stroke)
6. Brain cancer
7. Neurosyphilis

## Initial Management

**Setting:** emergency department or outpatient

## Diagnostic/Therapeutic Plan

- CT scan

## Test Results

- Concave fluid collection in a crescent along left side of the brain; some compression of left lateral ventricle; no midline shift; there is a smaller collection on right

### CLINICAL PEARL

A chronic subdural hematoma may cause a "change in personality" and fluctuating "confusion." A history of trauma may or may not be elicited (30% of patients recall no head injury), particularly the older adult with bleeding diathesis. The injury in this population may be trivial or forgotten because it was remote.

Look for mild hemiparesis on the exam (pronator drift).

### Assessment

This patient has a chronic subdural hematoma that has slowly increased in size over the last 2 mos. Symptoms arise as blood accumulates.

Alzheimer's is unlikely here because of the focal neurologic deficit, as is cerebrovascular accident (stroke) which is more sudden in onset and less likely to cause a gradual decline in memory.

It would be hard to reconcile a single brain tumor with deficits of both motor and cortical (memory) function. Also, there should be more headaches and nausea with a tumor. Chronic subdural hematomas accumulate slowly and are therefore less likely to cause headaches, nausea, vomiting, and acute alterations in mental status.

### Further Management Plan

- Surgical drainage to relieve pressure on the brain
- Neurology consult

### Discussion

As people age, it is normal for the brain to decrease in size. As the brain shrinks, the bridging veins between the brain and the draining structures become stretched. The added tension on these veins makes them more sensitive to traumatic rupture. Hence, in the older adult, even small amounts of head trauma may predispose to leakage and subdural hematomas.

As the blood accumulates, pressure on the surrounding structures can result in dementia in the older adult. Associated focal neurologic deficits develop, depending on the size and location of the collection. In this case, the left-sided collection can compress the speech areas on the left, making it difficult for the patient to speak.

If the collection of blood were larger, we might expect to find evidence of herniation, such as unequal pupils, respiratory compromise, and lethargy. Because this collection has developed over a year and these findings are absent, there is no need for acute treatment such as hyper-ventilation and mannitol.

Steroids are of little use in any case of intracranial bleeding.

### Final Diagnosis

Subdural hematoma

## CASE 5

### Chief Complaint

"I have the worst headache of my life."

### History and Physical Examination

A 39-year-old woman with no significant past medical history comes to the emergency department because of an excruciating headache. She states that it started suddenly in the occipital area while she was in the bathroom defecating. She has never experienced anything like it before, describing it as the "worst headache of her life." She has concomitant nausea and vomiting, but denies fever, chills, neck stiffness, weakness and paresthesia.

On physical examination the patient is in acute distress due to pain. Her temperature is 36.7° C (98.0° F), blood pressure 151/89 mm Hg, pulse 101/min, and respirations 14/min. Her $O_2$ saturation is 100% on room air. Examination of the head is normocephalic with no signs of trauma; the neck is supple and negative for JVD or bruits. Pupils are equal and reactive to light. Cardiac examination reveals a slight tachycardia with normal S1/S2 and normal rate and rhythm with no murmurs. Auscultation of the lungs is clear bilaterally, and abdominal exam is benign. On neurologic examination the patient is alert and oriented; cranial nerves II–XII are intact, and there are no motor or sensory deficits.

### Differential Diagnosis

1. Subarachnoid hemorrhage (SAH)
2. Pituitary apoplexy
3. Acute complicated sinusitis
4. Migraine headache
5. Ischemic stroke

### Initial Management

**Setting:** emergency department

### Diagnostic/Therapeutic Plan

- Non-contrast CT scan of the head

### Test Results

- An extensive SAH filling the basilar cisterns; findings consistent with ruptured intracranial aneurysm

**CLINICAL PEARL**

If the CT scan is negative (<10% of SAH), further investigate with an LP to exclude SAH.

### Assessment

Subarachnoid hemorrhage presents commonly as a sudden, severe headache, often described as the worst headache of the patient's life. Nausea, vomiting, meningismus, or loss of consciousness may or may not be associated with the headache. The sudden-onset headache should certainly raise concern for subarachnoid hemorrhage regardless of severity, associated symptoms, or patient's previous history of prior headaches.

Non-contrast CT with or without lumbar puncture will effectively rule in (or out) the diagnosis of SAH; however, if one is still doubtful, CT angiography can be considered. A thunderclap headache is a neurologic emergency that necessitates urgent imaging of the cerebral vasculature with either magnetic resonance or CT angiography.

This patient should undergo CT angiography of the head and neck. She has experienced a thunderclap headache. Most of the other causes of thunderclap headache include:

- Unruptured cerebral aneurysm
- Carotid or vertebral artery dissection
- Cerebral venous sinus thrombosis
- Reversible cerebral vasoconstriction syndrome

All of these causes can be excluded by noninvasive angiography. CT angiography can detect un-ruptured aneurysms as small as 3 mm in diameter and thus is adequate to exclude this diagnosis. Magnetic resonance angiography (MRA) would also be appropriate in this setting.

Both CT angiography and MRA can be performed with a venous phase to exclude cerebral venous sinus thrombosis.

**Patient Safety Note**

First-degree relatives of patients with subarachnoid hemorrhage have a high risk for aneurysm. Screening should be considered on an individual basis.

### Further Management Plan

The patient should be admitted to the ICU once the diagnosis of SAH is established. Neurosurgery consult should be ordered as ruptured aneurysms should be treated with surgical clipping and coiling within 48–72 hours.

**CLINICAL PEARL**

Genetic syndromes associated with aneurysm include dominant polycystic kidney disease and Ehlers-Danlos syndrome.

There are 3 major complications of SAH:

- Re-bleeding
- Delayed brain ischemia from vasospasm
- Hydrocephalus

Nimodipine, a dihydropyridine calcium channel blocker, should be prescribed for 21 days to prevent post-SAH vasospasm and ischemia. Re-bleed and hydrocephalus are treated with ventricular drainage. Monitor the patient very closely with neurologic checks; any change in mental status should prompt repeat imaging to rule out the above-mentioned complications.

## Discussion

The most common cause of spontaneous subarachnoid hemorrhage is a ruptured saccular aneurysm in the Circle of Willis. Less commonly, it is due to cocaine, arterial dissection, coagulopathy, and rupture of an AVM.

Sentinel hemorrhage occurs in 40% of cases and usually presents with severe headache for the past few wks. Non-contrast CT establishes the diagnosis in >90% of cases. The clot is demonstrated in the subarachnoid space if the scan is performed within 24 hours of the bleed. The head CT should be performed with thin cuts through the base of the brain to detect smaller bleeds. Lumbar puncture is the next step if there is a high clinical suspicion and CT brain is negative.

Lumbar puncture will demonstrate a high opening pressure and elevated RBCs that do not diminish from CSF tube 1 to tube 4. If the lumbar puncture is negative, CT angiography or MRA should be the next step.

Once the diagnosis of subarachnoid hemorrhage has been made, the etiology of the hemorrhage must be determined with vascular imaging. Repeat angiography is necessary if the initial study is negative. Up to 24% of all subarachnoid hemorrhage patients with negative initial angiography will have an aneurysm found on repeat angiography.

## Final Diagnosis

Subarachnoid hemorrhage

### CLINICAL PEARL

Patients with subarachnoid hemorrhage are admitted to the ICU.

- Place on bed rest, DVT prevention with pneumatic compression devices; avoid all antithrombotic medications; put on telemetry and manage electrolytes closely. Hypoxemia, hyperglycemia, metabolic acidosis and cardiac instability are associated with a worse outcome.
- If there is acute hydrocephalus with elevated ICP, perform a ventriculostomy.
- Re-bleed is associated with high mortality.
- Significant vasospasm is associated with delayed cerebral ischemia and poor neurologic outcome.
- Hyponatremia is a common complication and thought to be secondary to SIADH.

# CASE 6

## Chief Complaint

"The room is spinning around me."

## History and Physical Examination

A 58-year-old man was outside gardening when his wife called out to him. As he looked over his shoulder to respond, he experienced a sudden onset of dizziness. He presents to your office 4 days later with the same symptoms of dizziness and concomitant nausea, stating that the symptoms recur each time he turns his head to look back. When asked what he means by "dizziness," he states that it feels like the room is spinning around him. There are no other aggravating factors, but his symptoms are usually alleviated after a few minutes when he lies down and stays still. He reports no sensory deficits, visual changes, ringing in the ears, ear pain or discharge. His hearing is intact. He has a past medical history significant for hypertension, which is well-controlled on amlodipine. He denies any prior surgeries and has no significant past family history.

On physical exam the patient is afebrile, with blood pressure 124/76 mm Hg, pulse 72/min, respirations 14/min, and $O_2$ saturation 100% on room air. Cardiac examination reveals normal S1/S2 with no S3 and no murmurs or rubs. Auscultation of the chest is clear bilaterally with no wheezing or rales present. The abdomen is soft, non-tender, and non-distended with no organomegaly. The extremities show no edema, clubbing, or cyanosis. On neurologic examination the patient is alert and oriented x3, and cranial nerve exam is unremarkable. There are no motor or sensory deficits, and deep tendon reflexes are intact.

## Differential Diagnosis

1. Benign positional vertigo
2. Meniere's disease
3. Vestibular neuritis
4. Vertebrobasilar TIA

## Initial Management

**Setting:** outpatient

## Diagnostic/Therapeutic Plan

- Dix-Hallpike test

## Test Results

- Patient's symptoms recur and the presence of a peripheral nystagmus is noted

### Assessment

Vertigo in a patient usually represents a vestibular dysfunction. It usually presents as a transient feeling of spinning, dizziness, or a sense of swaying or tilting. Vertigo can be caused by disorders of the peripheral vestibular system, or by CNS lesions in the brainstem, or cerebellar pathology.

| Peripheral Causes | Central Causes |
|---|---|
| • Benign positional vertigo: induced by change of position, attacks are brief (10–30 seconds), and recur frequently during the day<br><br>Diagnosis: Dix-Hallpike test | • Cerebellar hemorrhage: more common in older patients with risk factors, presents with gait impairment, limb dysmetria, dysphagia may occur, and no auditory symptoms are present<br><br>Diagnosis: CT, MRI |
| • Meniere's disease: recurrent tinnitus, severe vertigo with progressive sensorineural hearing loss<br><br>Diagnosis: Audiometry shows unilateral sensorineural hearing loss | • Vertebrobasilar insufficiency: multiple brainstem findings including facial weakness, dysarthria, diplopia and central vertigo<br><br>Diagnosis: MRI |
| • Vestibular neuritis (labyrinthitis): acute and severe, symptoms of unsteadiness with GI symptoms including nausea and vomiting, and symptoms may last for hours<br><br>Diagnosis: Head thrust test | • MS: characteristic remitting and relapsing neurological symptoms<br><br>Diagnosis: MRI |

The Dix-Hallpike maneuver helps to differentiate the different types of vertigo based on the patient's symptoms of nystagmus.

- In the central causes of vertigo, the nystagmus develops immediately, does not stop rapidly, and does not decrease with repeated testing; it is non-fatigable.
  - Vertical nystagmus is the most common type.
- In the peripheral causes of vertigo, the nystagmus begins within a period up to 40 seconds, stops within 30 seconds, and tends to decrease with repeated testing; it is fatigable.
  - Horizontal or rotary nystagmus is the most common type.

#### Patient Safety Note

- Treatments for vertigo should emphasize safety and reduction of risk factors.
- Consider fall precautions and assessment of safety at home, reduction of polypharmacy, physical therapy evaluation, and assessment of gait.
- Provide assistive devices if necessary.
- Evaluate patients for hearing and vision impairment.

## Discussion

The patient has benign paroxysmal positional vertigo. This is suggested by the exacerbation of symptoms with head movement, the duration and recurrence of the vertigo, and the reproduction of symptoms and peripheral nystagmus with a Dix-Hallpike maneuver. The absence of hearing loss, tinnitus, and neurologic findings is also consistent with the diagnosis.

The Epley maneuver to reposition otolith debris (canalith repositioning) within the patient's affected semicircular canal is effective for eliminating symptoms and has minimal adverse effects. Audiometry is indicated in all patients with ear fullness, tinnitus and hearing loss.

Meniere's disease is associated with a fluctuating, low frequency hearing loss. It is usually treated with meclizine, salt restriction, and diuretics. If symptoms are refractory to treatment, then surgery is the next step in treatment. If asymmetric hearing loss is detected, this suggests retrocochlear pathology such as meningioma or acoustic neuroma, and MRI of the auditory canal would be next step in management.

Neuroimaging should usually be reserved for patients with cerebellar or focal neurologic symptoms or vertical nystagmus.

## Final Diagnosis

Benign positional vertigo

# CASE 7

## Chief Complaint

Loss of consciousness

## History and Physical Examination

A 28-year-old man arrives at your office after an earlier incident at work. His coworkers on a construction site noticed that his arm started to "jump" and his face began to twitch. He then lost consciousness and his muscles contracted repeatedly. The patient has no memory of the event but does recount a previous episode of his hand jumping out of control. He denies intravenous drug use but has used cocaine and marijuana on a regular basis. He denies head trauma. He does not have sex with men, but he has paid for sex with women.

Physical examination shows a right visual-field defect, right facial droop, right pronator drift, increased tone, and hyperreflexia on the right, with an upgoing toe on the right side.

## Differential Diagnosis

1. Seizure with Todd paralysis
2. Stroke with seizure
3. Arteriovenous malformation with seizure
4. Brain tumor with seizure
5. Metabolic cause of seizure
6. Cocaine overdose or alcohol/benzodiazepines withdrawal

## Initial Management

**Setting:** emergency department

## Diagnostic/Therapeutic Plan

- Electrolytes, serum glucose, arterial blood gases, CBC, urinalysis, toxicology screen
- CT scan with and without contrast

## Test Results

- Negative
- CT scan: ring-enhancing lesion

## Assessment

The patient has had a focal seizure with secondary generalization. Many partial seizures are due to a focal brain lesion. Age is an important factor in determining the etiology of a seizure. In the pediatric population, a host of diseases can lead to a seizure and most involve inborn errors of metabolism. In the very old, vascular events are the most common causes. In younger and middle-aged adults, mass lesions are more common, and brain tumors are a major concern.

**CLINICAL PEARL**

- New-onset focal seizures in the adult patient (with or without generalization) are due to CNS focal processes until proven otherwise (past trauma and scar, space-occupying lesion, as in this case).
- Imaging, usually MRI with contrast, is necessary.

Anterograde and retrograde amnesia can occur with seizures that generalize.

- The progression of seizure activity occurring from limb to face to limb on one side is referred to as a "Jacksonian march."
- A hemiparesis that resolves within hours of a seizure is called a "Todd paralysis."

Cocaine use can lead to seizure activity from a stroke, so do a toxicology screen. This patient has had sex with prostitutes, which puts him at increased risk for HIV and AIDS and would mean that toxoplasmosis and primary CNS lymphoma would need to be considered.

Metabolic causes of seizures need to be considered, so workup includes assessing electrolytes including sodium, calcium, and magnesium. Check glucose, LFTs, and BUN. If there are other meningeal signs/symptoms, do an LP. Arterial-venous malformations can also occur in this age group and can cause seizures due either to an increase in size or to a small bleed. In this case, a ring-enhancing lesion was found; the differential diagnosis includes abscess, tumor, lymphoma, or toxoplasmosis.

### Further Management Plan/Results

- HIV serology
- IV lorazepam 5 mg if seizure persists; phenytoin load of 18 mg/kg and standing dose of 300 mg/day
- If HIV-negative, biopsy of lesion
- If HIV-positive, empiric therapy for toxoplasmosis, pyrimethamine and sulfadiazine plus folinic acid; if no improvement, then biopsy of lesion
- Rule out secondary causes of seizure and treat accordingly

### Discussion

Start medications only if the patient is considered at risk for recurrence. Medications are usually started after second seizure. In this situation, phenytoin should be started. Because the patient is not actively seizing, the patient can be loaded orally with 500 mg, given twice, and then a single dose of 300 mg orally each day.

For long-term treatment, if phenytoin as a single agent does not control the seizures, add a second agent such as levetiracetam, lamotrigine, or valproic acid. Lamotrigine is associated with serious cutaneous hypersensitivity (Steven-Johnson syndrome).

With pregnancy, there is no clear indication for any one anticonvulsant. Maintain a pregnant woman on monotherapy and at the lowest dose of medication possible. Uncontrolled seizures can cause placental disruption. The risk of uncontrolled seizure outweighs the risk of teratogenicity. Because most of the anticonvulsants cause depletion of folate, it is important to provide continuous folic acid supplementation and monitor serum levels regularly.

In seizure patients with ring-enhancing lesion on CT, it is equally important to determine the patient's immune status to help narrow the diagnosis. Workup must be done for HIV status in order to guide the management of the patient. For a ring-enhancing lesion, one must differentiate between 2 causes: infectious cause and malignancy.

If the patient is HIV-positive, initiate antitoxoplasmosis therapy as soon as possible with CT scan follow-up in 2 wks to monitor treatment response. If the lesion fails to respond, biopsy might be needed. Biopsy might also be needed if the tumor workup is negative. Because risk factors for AIDS were mentioned specifically in the history, keep a very low threshold of suspicion for AIDS-related pathology.

### Basic Science Correlate

**Phenytoin toxicity** acts like a class Ia antiarrhythmic by blocking voltage-sensitive sodium channels. Phenytoin administration can be associated with acute or chronic toxicity, depending on the time and route of administration.

- Acute toxicity mostly presents after IV administration, with signs and symptoms of cardiac toxicity (hypotension, bradycardia, myocardial depression, arrhythmias).
- Susceptible patients could develop hypersensitivity reaction after 2–4 wks of treatment; patients usually present with fever, rash, lymphadenopathy, and in some instances hemolytic anemia or interstitial nephritis.
- Chronic use has been associated with hirsutism and a characteristic gingival hyperplasia.

## EMERGENCY TREATMENT FOR STATUS EPILEPTICUS

Status epilepticus is defined as a continuous, unremitting seizure lasting >5 min, or recurrent seizures in a patient unable to regain consciousness between seizures for >5 min.

**Step 1** for any acutely seizing patient is to secure the airway, breathing, and circulation. Once adequate airway and breathing is ensured and the patient is hemodynamically stable, Step 2 is to simultaneously evaluate and treat any precipitating cause of seizure.

- The best initial therapy in a patient actively seizing is IV bolus of a benzodiazepine such as lorazepam or diazepam.
- If the seizures persist, administer phenytoin or fosphenytoin (the latter has fewer side effects and faster IV administration).
- If the patient continues to seize, add phenobarbital.
- Finally, for severely refractory seizures, use a neuromuscular-blocking agent such as vecuronium or pancuronium to prepare the patient for endotracheal intubation and general anesthesia with midazolam or propofol.

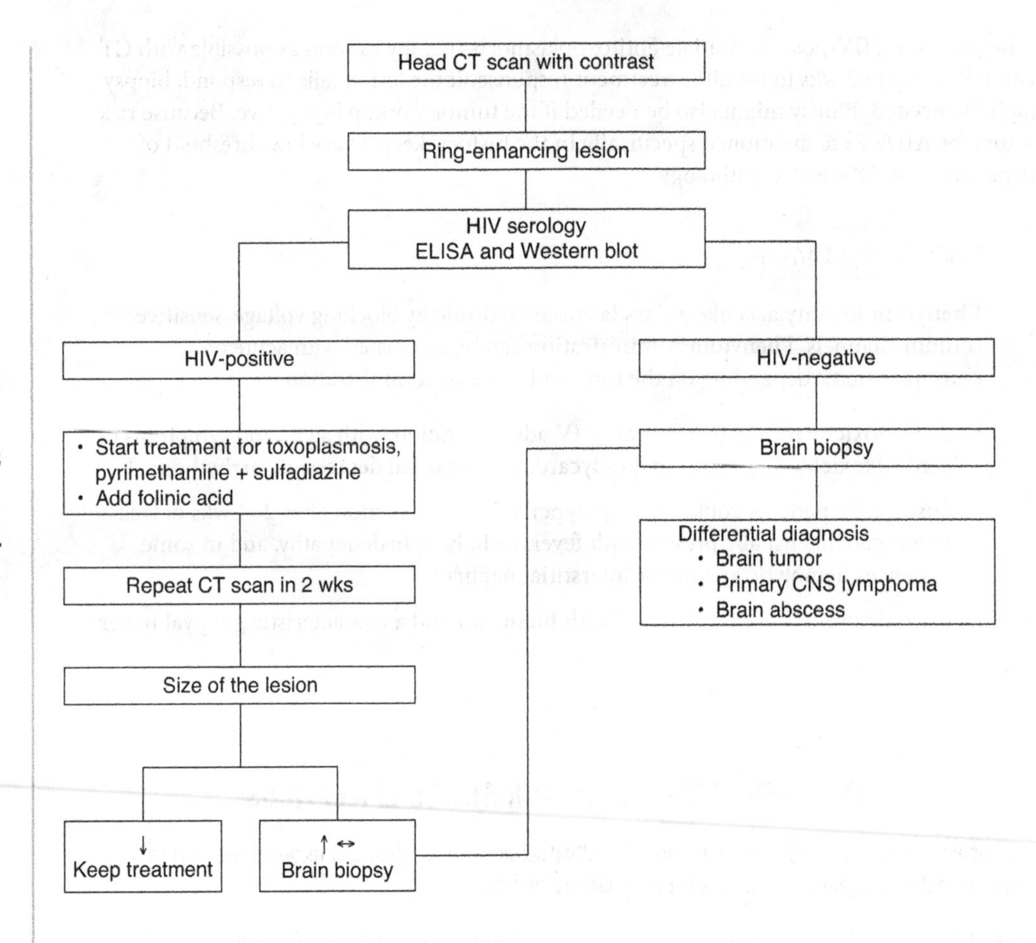


**Algorithm for the Management of Ring-Enhancing Lesions**

### CLINICAL PEARL

Consider any metabolic causes of seizure.

- Screen for the initial work-up.
- In every work-up for new onset of seizure, include a complete metabolic profile (to exclude hyponatremia, etc.), as well as a drug/toxicology screen.
- Opiates and amphetamines in particular will lower the seizure threshold.

### Final Diagnosis

Seizure disorder

# CASE 8

## Chief Complaint

"My hand is weak and I can't talk right."

## History and Physical Examination

A 54-year-old man with a history of high blood pressure, non-insulin-dependent diabetes mellitus, and hypercholesterolemia is brought to the emergency room because of hand weakness and "garbled speech." His wife reports that these symptoms came on suddenly 24 hours ago. He does not like doctors much but recently had come under the care of a medical doctor for control of his blood pressure and diabetes. Two weeks earlier, he had a loss of vision in the left eye, which resolved after a few hours.

Physical examination shows his speech to be fluent but with frequent errors. For example, he uses the word "thumb" for "tongue" and is unable to repeat the phrase "Today is a nice day." There is a right visual field defect and a widened palpebral fissure, with flattening of the nasolabial fold on the right. Right pronator drift and weakness is noted in the right upper and lower extremities, with increased tone. Reflexes are brisk on the right, and he has a Babinski sign on the right. Pupils are equal and reactive to light.

## Differential Diagnosis

1. Hemorrhagic stroke
2. Ischemic stroke
3. Hyperviscosity syndrome
4. Bland infarction in middle cerebral artery distribution from thrombotic or embolic source
5. Amyloid angiopathy, producing lobar bleed
6. Brain tumor

### CLINICAL PEARL

Look for these other classic stroke syndromes:

**Pure Motor Hemiplegia**

- Face, arm and leg are equally involved
- Due to internal capsule lesion (lacunar stroke involving penetrating vessels in patients with hypertension)

**Pure Sensory Loss**

- Usually due to a thalamic lesion

## Initial Management

**Setting:** emergency department

## Diagnostic/Therapeutic Plan

- CT of the head without contrast

## Test Results

- Negative

### Assessment

With no evidence of a bleed at the time of presentation to the emergency room on head CT, the most likely etiology is a bland infarct that is too early to see on the initial CT of the brain. Because of the sudden onset of symptoms, this is most likely an embolic phenomenon. Motor function is on the right-hand side of the body and is controlled by the left cortex, and because speech is also controlled most often by the left brain, we know the defect is on the left in the temporoparietal lobe—even if we can't see it on the CT scan.

Always try to localize the affected area in the brain on the basis of the physical findings. Then use the CT scan to confirm your suspicion. Don't just get the scan to 'take a look.' The transient ocular defect is amaurosis fugax, which often precedes a stroke. That is because the ophthalmic artery is the first branch of the carotid, and small emboli often affect this area first (although this is more often seen in carotid stenosis).

The head CT is most often normal in the first 24–48 hours. It takes 3–5 days for 90% of cerebral infarctions to be visible.

### Further Management Plan/Results

| | |
|---|---|
| Repeat CT of head 3 days later | Middle cerebral artery distribution infarction |
| EKG | Normal sinus rhythm |
| Echocardiogram—TTE and TEE | No thrombus |
| Carotid Doppler | Negative |
| 24-hr ambulatory EKG | Multiple episodes of a-fib |

### Treatment Plan

Tissue plasminogen activator (tPA) for those who present <3 hours from symptom onset, have persistent/disabling deficits, have no bleeding, and meet the inclusion/exclusion criteria

- Heparin, in the presence of a-fib (however, it may cause bleeding in those with acute stroke and a-fib, and is controversial)
- Aspirin, in the absence of a-fib and symptoms persist >3 hours
- Coumadin for long-term anticoagulation in those with a-fib
- Clopidogrel if stroke occurs while patient is on aspirin
- Digoxin, beta blockers, or diltiazem for rate control in those with arrhythmia
- Physical therapy and speech therapy

### Discussion

As more centers start to utilize neuromuscular intervention in ischemic stroke, tPA therapy indications will change. About 80% of strokes are caused by cerebral ischemia, either from embolus or thrombus. About 20% are hemorrhagic.

Thrombotic strokes are preceded by TIA about 50–75% of the time.

**Exclusion criteria for TPA** are the following:

1. Previous stroke or serious head trauma in the last 3 months
2. BP >185/110 mm Hg (despite Rx)
3. Recent invasive surgical procedure in the last 2 weeks

4. PT >15 sec or INR >1.7
5. Increased PTT if heparin was given in the preceding 48 hours
6. GI or GU bleeding in prior 21 days
7. Platelets <10,000/mm$^3$
8. Coma or stupor

Knowledge of specific vascular areas prone to infarction in the brain and their associated symptoms is key for localizing infarctions and narrowing the diagnosis.

| **Artery** | **Deficits** |
|---|---|
| Internal carotid artery/ophthalmic artery | • Amaurosis fugax |
| Anterior cerebral artery | • Hemiplegia affecting foot and leg more than the arm<br>• Aboulia, confusion, incontinence, Babinski |
| Middle cerebral artery | • Hemiplegia affecting arm/face more than leg<br>• Aphasia<br>• Apraxia |
| Posterior cerebral artery | • Thalamic disturbances<br>• Contralateral hemisensory deficit<br>• Macular-sparing homonymous hemianopsia |
| Vertebral artery | • Wallenberg syndrome |
| Basilar artery | • Pinpoint pupils<br>• Cranial nerve abnormalities<br>• Cerebellar symptoms |
| Cerebellar artery | • Vertigo<br>• Nausea<br>• Nystagmus<br>• Ipsilateral ataxia |
| Lacunar infarct | • Pure hemiplegia plus hemianesthesia<br>• Dysarthria<br>• Clumsy hand |

The heart and atherosclerotic plaques in the carotid arteries are the most common sources of emboli. Mitral stenosis, ventricular mural thrombus, septal defects, valvular vegetations, and atrial myxoma can all lead to emboli.

Atrial fibrillation predisposes the material in the heart to break off and embolize. Emboli from the heart lodge in the middle cerebral artery 80% of the time. They rarely reach the anterior circulation. Paradoxical stroke can occur in patients with patent foramen ovale, which can be diagnosed with echocardiogram bubble studies.

After evaluation with echocardiogram, carotid Doppler, and electrocardiographic monitoring, the source will still not be found in as many as 40% of cases. Hypercoagulable states such as protein C and S deficiency, antithrombin III deficiency, and antiphospholipid syndromes may account for a small percent of these cases. Thrombolytic therapy is used in acute nonhemorrhagic stroke if the patient presents <3 hours of developing the defect.

### Final Diagnosis

Embolic stroke

### CLINICAL PEARL

In embolic stroke, the heart is the **most common** source of emboli.

- Mitral stenosis, ventricular mural thrombus, septal defects, valvular vegetations, and atrial myxoma can all lead to emboli
- Atrial fibrillation predisposes material in the heart to break off and embolize
- Emboli from heart lodge in the middle cerebral artery 80% of the time
- Atherosclerotic plaques in carotid arteries also give rise to emboli

# CASE 9

## Chief Complaint

"I feel very tired at the end of the day and have trouble reading."

## History and Physical Examination

A 32-year-old woman comes to the office complaining of fatigue that worsens during the day. She also complains of double vision which appears after reading magazines for some time in the afternoon. She also states that she has some difficulty swallowing dry foods. Prior medical history is non contributory. Family history is positive only for a sister with lupus.

Vital signs are within normal limits. The patient is alert and oriented. Bipalpebral ptosis and weak eye closure are noted, as well as difficulty tracking objects. Pupillary light reflexes and accommodation are intact. Deep tendon reflexes are 5/5. Muscle strength is 4/5 in all extremities, but diminishes to 2/5 upon repeat examination.

## Differential Diagnosis

1. Myasthenia gravis: presents with fluctuating weakness in ocular, bulbar, limb and respiratory muscles; symptoms commonly worse later in day; early characteristic symptoms include ocular symptoms of ptosis and/or diplopia
2. Lambert-Eaton syndrome: symptoms commonly present early in the day and can improve with exercise; autonomic dysfunction is frequent symptom, as is an underlying cancer, i.e., small cell lung cancer
3. Botulism: can be confused with myasthenia because it also affects bulbar and eye muscles; 50% present with pupillary paralysis, whereas pupillary function is spared in myasthenia; commonly has rapid progression of symptoms; patient may have history of ingestion of food contaminated by botulinum
4. Periodic paralysis: presents with painless muscle weakness, usually precipitated by heavy exercise or fasting (rare muscle disease called "channelopathy"); can be classified as hypokalemic, hyperkalemic, or thyrotoxic periodic paralysis

## Initial Management

**Setting:** outpatient

## Diagnostic/Therapeutic Plan

- Acetylcholine receptor (AChR) antibodies
- Electromyography (EMG)

## Test Results

- AChR-Ab: (+) positive
- EMG: decreasing response amplitude upon repetitive stimulation

### CLINICAL PEARL

The Tensilon (edrophonium) test is no longer administered; it was inferior to AChR-Ab serology in specificity and had patient safety issues (i.e., causing classical cholinergic side effects).

## Assessment

Positive AChR antibodies with characteristic EMG tracings should confirm the diagnosis of myasthenia gravis. Although weakness and diplopia are shared with other disorders affecting the neuromuscular junction, progressive weakness with activity that improves with rest is very specific to myasthenia gravis. Diplopia and ptosis are common initial presentations, being found in about 50% of patients, while the oculomotor nerve is affected in 90% of cases. Family history is also a contributing factor for myasthenia, as 30% have a maternal relative diagnosed with a connective tissue disease.

Lambert-Eaton syndrome has a similar immunologic etiology and is heavily associated with small cell lung cancer. It is sometimes described as "reverse myasthenia," because, although it shares the proximal weakness in an asymmetric pattern, the weakness subsides with repeated muscle contraction. This is seen both clinically and in EMG studies, which show increasing amplitude responses on repeated stimulation. The antibody causing Lambert-Eaton is specific for $Ca^{++}$ channels in the presynaptic membrane, which supports the disease's "reverse myasthenia" moniker since myasthenia has antibodies directed at the postsynaptic membrane.

Botulism also affects the presynaptic membrane in the neuromuscular junction, as the botulinum toxin impedes vesicle release. It also presents with the symptoms of weakness and diplopia. Clinically it can be excluded here because it affects tendon reflexes and also causes mydriasis. In the history presented, the patient is also lacking exposure to an offending agent.

### Basic Science Correlate

- Myasthenia gravis is an example of type II hypersensitivity, in the form of antibodies against acetylcholine receptors in the postsynaptic membrane of the neuromuscular junction.
- Acetylcholinesterase inhibitors increase the availability of acetylcholine to the remaining receptors in the postsynaptic membrane.
- Immunomodulators decrease the amount of Ab produced. If corticosteroids are used, patients should receive regular EMG monitoring since steroids may cause proximal muscle weakness and worsen the condition.
- Aminoglycosides should be avoided in myasthenia patients, as they inhibit ACh-release from the presynaptic neuron and may worsen symptoms.
- Thymic hyperplasia is found in about 65% of myasthenia patients. This condition is microscopically described as non-neoplastic follicular hyperplasia in the thymic medulla.
- Electron microscopy of the neuromuscular junction shows a shallow scarce postsynaptic membrane with diminished secondary synapses.

## Further Management Plan

- Chest CT: 65% of myasthenia patients will have thymic hyperplasia and 10–15% will have a thymoma
- Thyroid function test: 5% may have a condition known as thyrotoxicosis with periodic paralysis, a disease in which myasthenia and thyrotoxicosis are concomitant

For treatment, thymoma is a clear indication for thymectomy. In the absence of thymoma, medical therapy is as follows:

- Symptomatic treatments: acetylcholinesterase inhibitors such as pyridostigmine and neostigmine
- Chronic immunomodulating treatments: glucocorticoids and immunosuppressive drugs such as prednisone, azathioprine, mycophenolate, cyclosporine, cyclophosphamide
- Rapid immunomodulating treatments: plasma exchange and IV immune globulin
- Surgical treatment: consider thymectomy if patient age <60 with generalized myasthenia even without presence of thymoma

Myasthenic crisis is a life-threatening condition, which is characterized by neuromuscular respiratory failure. It is an indication for either plasmapheresis and/or IVIG. Note that if corticosteroids are used, EMG monitoring is warranted.

## Discussion

Myasthenia gravis is a neuroimmunologic disease in which the acetylcholine receptors in the postsynaptic membrane of the neuromuscular junction are targeted. The AChR antibodies both block the receptors and increase their cellular degradation, resulting in a decreased number of receptors. It is commonly associated with thymic hyperplasia in 65% of cases.

Epidemiology of this disease is as follows:

- Populations age <40, the female to male ratio for incidence is 3:1
- Populations age >50, the male to female ratio for incidence is 3:2 (older population also has highest incidence of thymoma)

The disease has been linked to a positive family history of connective tissue diseases and a non-insignificant amount of patients with positive ANA.

The typical presentation of cranial nerve weakness and specifically oculomotor involvement is due to the constant use of these muscles and their relatively lower density of receptors. Patients may also present with facial weakness and a sign known as "trident tongue," which is described as 1 central and 2 lateral longitudinal furrows of the tongue.

The most significant symptom is weakness occurring with exertion that rapidly improves upon rest. Diplopia is caused by asymmetric weakness of the extrinsic ocular muscles. Clinical severity is quite variable as well as the response to treatment.

## Follow-up Management and Prevention

- Regular clinical follow-up and monitoring with EMG
- Avoid aminoglycosides, magnesium, and succinylcholine, which can worsen the condition

## Final Diagnosis

Myasthenia gravis

# CASE 10

## Chief Complaint

"My wife was weak in her right hand and couldn't speak or write."

## History and Physical Examination

A 56-year-old woman with a history of smoking, adult-onset diabetes mellitus, and hypertension is brought to the emergency department by her husband, who became concerned when she dropped a plate on the floor. He explains that, although his wife is usually quite verbal, she had difficulty expressing her thoughts. The husband was unable to understand what she was saying, so he gave her a pen and pad, but she could only write a couple of words which didn't make much sense. He immediately brought her to the hospital, but her symptoms resolved on the way.

Her blood pressure is 180/100 mm Hg and pulse 100/min. Upon auscultation a loud bruit is heard over the left carotid artery. There are no murmurs, rubs, or bruits over the precordium. Pulses are present and symmetric, with normal rate and rhythm. Neurologic exam is nonfocal.

## Differential Diagnosis

1. Transient ischemic attack (TIA)
2. Thrombotic or embolic stroke
3. Subdural hematoma
4. Migraine
5. Seizure

## Initial Management

**Setting:** emergency department

## Diagnostic/Therapeutic Plan

- CT scan

## Test Results

- CT: normal

## Assessment

This patient has multiple risk factors for cardiovascular disease. Although hypertension has the strongest correlation with the risk of stroke, other risks include diabetes, smoking, and hyperlipidemia. This patient's deficit seems to have occurred in the left temporoparietal area because it was characterized by an expressive aphasia; Broca's area was likely involved. Because the deficit lasted only several hours at most, this is a TIA, defined as a deficit lasting <24 hours.

The CT shows no lesions, which is quite characteristic of TIA. Even if the deficit had persisted and a stroke had occurred, the initial CT is commonly normal. It usually takes 3–5 days for nonhemorrhagic strokes to become visible, though some can appear earlier.

This patient has a bruit over her left carotid artery, which might represent an atheromatous plaque that sent a small embolus to the brain. Even without a cardiac murmur, it is wise to obtain an echocardiogram, particularly if no other source can be found for an embolus.

## Further Management Plan/Results

| | |
|---|---|
| Carotid Doppler | >70% stenosis of the left internal carotid artery (LICA) |
| MRA | 75% stenosis LICA |
| 24-hour Holter monitor | No episodes of arrhythmia |
| Echocardiogram with bubble study | No valvular disease or evidence of thrombus |

## Treatment Plan

- Antiplatelet agents: aspirin + clopidogrel OR aspirin + dipyridamole
- Heparin bridge with warfarin if presumed cardioembolic origin
- Carotid endarterectomy if ipsilateral carotid stenosis >70%

## Discussion

TIA is considered the harbinger of stroke. Be aware of the ABCD score which stratifies risk of progression to stroke, which takes into account **A**ge, **B**P, **C**linical features, **D**iabetes, and **D**uration of symptoms.

Treatment options for TIA are limited. Antiplatelet agents are the only effective option.

- Aspirin is used most often, but in cases of aspirin intolerance, clopidogrel may be used.
- Other antiplatelet combinations are clopidogrel + aspirin or aspirin + dipyridamole.
- If multiple TIAs occur over several days or the initial deficit continues to worsen, heparin may prevent "completion" of the stroke, which would mean a permanent neurologic deficit. A worsening deficit is presumed to be a clot in formation, and this is why heparin is used.

Tissue plasminogen activating factor may be used within 3 hours of the symptom onset if there is no known risk of acute hemorrhage, blood pressure is controlled, and CT scan shows no bleeding. Although tissue plasminogen activating factor gets a lot of favorable press, few patients currently qualify for its administration as the risk is hemorrhage.

Also, there should be aggressive risk-factor management with BP <140/90 mm Hg (<130/80 in diabetics), LDL <100, and smoking cessation if the patient smokes.

In this patient who has a carotid bruit on examination and evidence of stenosis on Doppler and angiography, endarterectomy is a possibility. The indications for endarterectomy are becoming more limited; it seems to be effective only when the lesion is tightly stenotic (≥70%) in the presence of recurrent symptoms.

Note that patients with TIA are also more likely to have concurrent heart disease.

## Final Diagnosis

Transient ischemic attack

### CLINICAL PEARL

The neurologic deficits of a TIA typically last only 5–10 min. Patients often do not seek medical assistance because they lose the appreciation that something is wrong (anosognosia) and they are not in pain.

### CCS NOTE

Urgent evaluation with hospitalization of all patients who have TIA is justified, because there is a 10% risk of stroke in the first 3 months after a TIA. Most strokes occur in the first 48 hours.

### CLINICAL PEARL

TIA is a neurologic deficit lasting <24 hours.

- CT scan is typically normal
- Evaluate carotid arteries and heart
- Treat with antiplatelet agents and possible carotid endarterectomy

### CLINICAL PEARL

A subdural hematoma can sometimes give intermittent symptoms that mimic TIA; these are usually chronic subdurals found in an older patient population than this patient. CT scan should exclude this from the differential diagnosis.

# CASE 11

## Chief Complaint

"Both of my legs hurt."

## History and Physical Examination

A 65-year-old man with a history of hypertension comes to the office with complaints of progressive pain and paresthesia in the legs after walking about 4 city blocks. His exercise tolerance has some variability. The patient initially noted the onset of numbness and weakness in the legs while walking downhill. He has started to sit at bus stops waiting for the pain to resolve and then walks to the next bus stop where he stops again for a rest. He initially had symptoms in the left leg and later they spread to the right. The numbness and tingling increase with walking and are alleviated by sitting and lying on his side. The patient recalls only mild lower back pain over the last few years. There is no change in bowel, bladder, or sexual function.

On physical examination a palpation of the lumbar spine elicits no tenderness or palpable masses. You instruct the patient to lie on the exam table with the hips and knees flexed. When tested in the recumbent position, reflexes are absent. When the patient sits up and stoops forward, all reflexes are present in the lower extremities. Vibratory sensation below the knees is mildly diminished. The rest of the neurologic exam is nonfocal with normal strength and tone.

## Differential Diagnosis

1. Lumbar spinal stenosis
2. Tumor involving the cauda equina
3. Claudication from peripheral vascular disease
4. Herniated disc
5. Compression fracture
6. Spondylolisthesis (displaced vertebra)

## Initial Management

**Setting:** outpatient

## Diagnostic/Therapeutic Plan

- Ankle-brachial index
- Peripheral pulses

## Test Results

- Ankle-brachial index: normal (1.0)
- Peripheral pulses: normal

### Assessment

This patient's presentation is not entirely straightforward, and it may be difficult to distinguish the exertional leg pain from vascular disease, lumbar spinal stenosis, or a herniated disc.

Two common causes of claudication are ischemic and neurologic. Ischemic claudication is brought on by lack of adequate perfusion relative to a performed exercise; it is common in atherosclerosis of lower limb arteries. Ankle-brachial index is an excellent first test to determine if symptoms are caused by compromised blood supply. Normal values are 0.9–1.3.

This patient has several presenting features that are not seen with the claudication of vascular disease, e.g., abnormalities of the reflexes, paresthesias, and lower back pain. The peripheral pulses are normal with spinal stenosis but diminished with vascular disease. In addition, claudication is usually bilateral, and the pain and abnormalities on physical exam should have no relation to body position.

Also, pain due to "pseudo" claudication by lumbar spinal stenosis is often increased by walking downhill and relieved by walking uphill. Patients with lumbar spinal stenosis often describe relief from pain when walking flexed with a shopping cart. That is different from the pain associated with a herniated disc, which usually worsens with flexion and is linked to a history of chronic back pain. A displaced vertebra in spondylolisthesis may or may not be palpated on physical exam, but this differential can be ruled out with imaging.

Given these differences, the diagnosis is often not certain until vascular studies or MRI of the spine are obtained. Hence, spinal stenosis is also called "pseudo" claudication.

#### CLINICAL PEARL

- **Peripheral arterial disease:** symptoms of "claudication" that resolve within seconds of rest; occur at night when legs are horizontal
- **Lumbar stenosis:** symptoms of "claudication" (pseudoclaudication) that occur while walking downhill or stairs; take minutes to resolve with rest

### Further Management Plan/Results

| | |
|---|---|
| • MRI | Hypertrophy of the ligamentum flavum, osteophytic overgrowth, spur formation, and narrowed lumbar canal |
| • CT myelography is second-line test if patient cannot have MRI due to pacemaker, presence of other metallic objects, or claustrophobia | |

### Treatment Plan

- Rest and anti-inflammatory medication
- Physical therapy with flexion exercises
- Spinal or facet joint steroid injections
- Surgical decompression at the level of the stenosis with laminectomy (if symptoms persist after conservative management)

### Discussion

Spinal stenosis is a general term for compression of the spinal cord or adjacent nerve roots. It can result from narrowing of the disc space, osteophyte formation, subluxation of the vertebral bodies, hypertrophy of the spinal ligaments, or any combination of these. This can occur at any level of the spinal cord. These abnormalities normally increase with age, but most are asymptomatic.

Clinical history is recognizable by the alleviation of symptoms on flexion, which differentiates it from disc herniation. Neurogenic claudication pain may initiate unilaterally. Achilles tendon reflexes may be absent when the patient is symptomatic and can reappear after flexion.

In claudication, the exercise tolerance should be predictable and reproducible, whereas with spondylosis, the pain can be variable.

Know how to differentiate clinically between lumbar stenosis and vascular claudication.

### Lumbar Spinal Stenosis

- Symptoms worsen when standing for a prolonged period of time and while walking down the stairs. Symptoms of lumbar stenosis take time to resolve after rest. The so called 'shopping cart sign' describes a common posture of patients with lumbar stenosis who adopt a simian-like posture that opens up the spaces in the spinal canal and relieves nerve compression.
- Can result from narrowing of the disc space, osteophyte formation, subluxation of the vertebral bodies, hypertrophy of the spinal ligaments, or any combination of these. This can occur at any level of the spinal cord.

### Vascular Claudication

- Symptoms are similar to those of neurogenic claudication, but symptoms resolve very quickly after patient rests (intermittent claudication).
- Generally, there is evidence of severe peripheral vascular disease such as absent dorsalis pedis pulses, femoral bruits, and other evidence of vascular disease (i.e., coronary artery disease, carotid disease).

### Final Diagnosis

Lumbar spinal stenosis

# CASE 12

## Chief Complaint

"My legs are weak and tingly."

## History and Physical Examination

A 30-year-old woman comes to the office with a history of visual disturbances starting about 5 years ago when she had a decrease in vision in her right eye. She also had an episode of double vision 1 year ago, which resolved on its own. Over the past week, she noted an ascending numbness and tingling in her legs, followed by difficulties walking.

Physical examination shows a pale optic disc with color desaturation in the right eye. She is not able to adduct her left eye when asked to look to the right, but pupillary reflexes and convergence are intact. Tone is increased in the lower extremities with 4+/5 weakness in hip flexion and dorsiflexion. Sensory examination reveals dysesthesia at the level of T4. Reflexes are increased in the lower extremities with a positive Babinski response bilaterally.

## Differential Diagnosis

1. Multiple sclerosis (MS) with transverse myelitis
2. Viral myelitis
3. Tropical spastic paraparesis
4. Subacute combined degeneration due to vitamin B12 deficiency
5. Neuromyelitis optica (Devic's disease)
6. Acute disseminated encephalomyelitis (ADEM)
7. Lyme disease

## Initial Management

**Setting:** outpatient

## Diagnostic/Therapeutic Plan

- MRI of the brain
- MRI of the spine with gadolinium

## Test Results

- MRI of the brain: multiple hyperintense lesions on T2 weighted images in periventricular white matter
- MRI of the spine: hyperintense lesion at T4 level on T2 weighted images, which enhance with gadolinium

## Assessment

This patient presents with evidence of multiple neurologic deficits affecting different parts of her CNS over a prolonged period of time. Individually, these deficits could represent stroke, encephalitis, vasculitis, etc, but when viewed as a syndrome over time, they are clearly part of the condition MS.

### CLINICAL PEARL

With MS, neurologic symptoms are produced or exacerbated by an increase in core body temperature. During febrile illness, symptoms may worsen. Transient unilateral visual blurring or loss is common during a hot shower or physical activity.

**CLINICAL PEARL**

Internuclear ophthalmoplegia (INO) is a disorder of conjugate lateral gaze. It is caused by damage of the medial longitudinal fasciculus, a heavily-myelinated tract which allows conjugate eye movement by connecting the paramedian pontine reticular formation with the abducens nucleus complex of the contralateral side to the oculomotor nucleus of the ipsilateral side. The patient is not able to adduct the affected eye when trying to look at the contralateral side with the unaffected eye showing a corrective nystagmus. Patients with MS often present with bilateral INO.

**CLINICAL PEARL**

Lhermitte's sign is seen in some patients with MS. Evoked by neck flexion, it feels like an electric shock that radiates down the back and legs.

**CLINICAL PEARL**

Charcot's neurologic triad:

- Nystagmus
- Intention tremor
- Dysarthria

MS is defined by several neurologic deficits occurring at different sites of the CNS in a waxing and waning fashion over time. The findings of multiple hyper-intense lesions on MRI of the brain and spinal cord confirm the diagnosis.

MS is a disease exclusively of the CNS. Any site in the CNS may be affected, resulting in sensory, motor, cranial nerve, bowel, bladder, cerebellar, or sexual dysfunction.

The most common presentation is fatigue with focal sensory symptoms and gait disturbances. Optic neuritis can be the first demyelinating event (20% of cases), which often resolves spontaneously. This patient also presents with spinal cord symptoms corresponding with the diagnosis of a sensory level deficit at the level of T4, which is suggestive of MS complicated by acute transverse myelitis. A spinal MRI must be done to rule out mechanical compression of the spinal cord (tumor, infection, etc.).

### Further Management Plan/Results

| | |
|---|---|
| • Lumbar puncture; evaluate CSF | • Positive for oligoclonal bands (85–95% sensitive in clinically definitive MS)<br>• Elevated IgG/albumin ratio in CSF |
| • For severe acute exacerbation or fulminant MS, consider IV steroids, IVIG or emergent plasmapheresis | |
| • For mild or moderate acute exacerbation, consider high dose IV steroids (pulse dose methylprednisolone); if poor response, consider cytotoxic drugs such as azathioprine, cyclophosphamide, and cyclosporine | |
| • After remission of acute symptoms, start treatment to prevent relapse and to slow progression of disease with immunomodulatory therapy (disease-modifying agents) such as interferon or copolymer 1 (glatiramer acetate) | |

### Discussion

MS is a disease of unknown etiology but is presumably an autoimmune phenomenon mediated by autoreactive lymphocytes with a predominant TH1 (CD4+) response and activation of macrophages against antigens present in the myelin of the CNS axons. In addition to T cell response, B cells are involved in the pathogenesis. Activated B cells differentiate into plasma cells and start making polyclonal antibodies that can be detected in the CSF of patients with MS as oligoclonal bands.

Numerous infectious etiologies (particularly viral) have been studied as a possible trigger for MS, but nothing has been proven. Among all the viral infections, Epstein-Barr virus (EBV) has antigens with a similar structure to myelin basic protein, a major component of CNS myelin. T-cells directed against EBV antigens may be redirected to attack CNS myelin due to similarity between the antigens, a process termed molecular mimicry.

MS is twice as common in women than in men and is predominately found in Caucasians from Northern European countries. The disease is virtually unknown in Africa.

### Basic Science Correlate

MS is an autoimmune condition due to a type IV hypersensitivity reaction in which activated TH1 helper cells secrete gamma interferon to activate macrophages, which directly destroy the myelin causing inflammation and demyelination in the CNS.

A condition which resembles MS is Devic's disease (neuromyelitis optica), characterized by recurrent episodes of myelitis and optic neuritis, but usually has no evidence of the brain lesions typical of MS.

In patients who have MS, MRI can closely resemble that of acute disseminated encephalomyelitis (ADEM). Look for a history of recent viral infection or recent vaccination. Also, in acute disseminated encephalomyelitis, the multiple lesions develop simultaneously and there generally should be no recurrence.

Diagnostic criteria of ADEM have not been fully established, but at a minimum certain criteria are used to distinguish ADEM from MS, such as atypical symptoms for MS (eg, encephalopathy), gray matter involvement on brain MRI, and absence of oligoclonal bands in the CSF.

Lyme disease can also sometimes present with the neurologic symptoms of transverse myelitis. More commonly, however, the main presentation is associated with the rash of erythema migrans and bilateral facial nerve palsy. A history of having hiked in the woods or coming from an endemic area in United States of high Lyme prevalence would raise clinical suspicion in this patient; however, these findings are not consistent with the history in this case.

Because the best explanation for the disease is an autoimmune phenomenon, treatment is largely based on immune-modulating drugs, such as steroids, adrenocorticotrophic hormones, or disease-modifying agents. Steroids are generally used as initial therapy for the treatment of acute exacerbations. Disease-modifying agents are used for long-term therapy to prevent relapse and slow the progression of the disease.

The FDA has approved the following drugs for long-term therapy:

- Interferon beta (**best initial choice for prevention of relapse**)
- Glatiramer acetate (**best initial choice for prevention of relapse**)
- Natalizumab
- Mitoxantrone
- Fingolimod
- Teriflunomide
- Dimethyl fumarate

All the drugs require parenteral administration (IV, IM, or SC) with the exception of fingolimod and teriflunomide which are given by enteral route.

Cytotoxic agents such as cyclophosphamide, azathioprine, methotrexate, and mycophenolate mofetil are used to induce remission in resistant cases of MS or poor response to treatment, especially in acute exacerbations when pulse steroids are ineffective. IV immunoglobulin (IVIG) and plasmapheresis are also effective in resistant or severe cases of MS.

### CLINICAL PEARL

Treatment with natalizumab, an inhibitor of alpha-4 integrin, could be complicated with reactivation of a latent JC virus infection by the development of progressive multifocal leukoencephalopathy, which presents as a worsening of neurologic symptoms after treatment has started.

Symptomatic treatment is a keystone of management. The most prominent symptoms include:

- Fatigue: amantadine (off-label)
- Spasticity: baclofen, benzodiazepines, tizanidine, gabapentin, or intramuscular botulinum toxin
- Bladder problems
  - Neurogenic bladder: intermittent catheterization and alpha-1 receptor blockers (prazosin)
  - Spastic bladder: anticholinergic drugs (oxybutynin or tolterodine)
- Pain: tricyclic antidepressant or anticonvulsants (gabapentin, carbamazepine, phenytoin)
- Impaired ambulation: dalfampridine has been shown to improve walking ability in patients with MS; it is the only medication approved by the FDA for this indication.

### CLINICAL PEARL

Vitamin B12 deficiency can:

- Affect the spinal cord (subacute combined degeneration)
- Cause proprioceptive loss due to lesion of the posterior columns
- Cause weakness/spasticity due to lesion of the corticospinal tracts
- Cause visual loss centrally

Measurement of methylmalonic acid and homocysteine (both elevated) is more sensitive for detecting vitamin B12 deficiency compared with serum vitamin B12 level.

### Basic Science Correlate

Baclofen is a $GABA_B$ receptor agonist that inhibits synaptic transmission through spinal reflex arcs via hyperpolarization of primary afferent fiber terminals. This may result in muscle spasticity.

## Final Diagnosis

Multiple sclerosis

## CASE 13

### Chief Complaint

"My husband walks with a shuffle."

### History and Physical Examination

A 65-year-old man with no significant medical history comes to the clinic for evaluation of his gait. He and his significant other initially attributed his problem to the natural course of aging, but now he seems to be just generally slow. On further questioning, he admits to increasing difficulty with his writing, which has become increasingly harder to read.

Physical examination shows that the patient has little facial expression and a decrease in eye blink. There is a resting tremor, which resolves with movement, and cogwheel rigidity with paratonia. The patient has micrographia, a decrease in rapid alternating movements, and he walks with a shuffling gait. Profound retropulsion, but no sensory abnormalities, is noted.

### Differential Diagnosis

1. Parkinson's disease
2. Essential tremor
3. Multiple system atrophy (includes striatonigral degeneration)
4. Progressive supranuclear palsy
5. Normal pressure hydrocephalus
6. Huntington disease
7. Wilson disease
8. Secondary parkinsonism

### Initial Management

**Setting:** outpatient

### Diagnostic/Therapeutic Plan

- MRI

### Test Results

- MRI: normal for age

### Assessment

Parkinson's disease is diagnosed mainly based on clinical impression, as MRI changes may not be initially seen.

- Characterized by the tetrad of symptoms of bradykinesia, resting tremor, rigidity, and postural instability
- Onset age >50
- Associated with resting tremor

### CLINICAL PEARL

Essential tremor is the most common neurologic cause of action tremor.

- Occurs at all ages (may have onset age >50)
- Most often symmetric
- Family history of tremor
- Often suppressed by alcohol

- Almost always starts unilaterally
- Most cases are sporadic, with family history playing a limited role
- MRI may demonstrate hypodensity in the putamen in T2 weighted images; PET scan may show a decrease in glucose metabolism in the striatum

Important differential diagnoses include essential tremor, progressive supranuclear palsy, secondary parkinsonism and other neurodegenerative disorders. Essential tremor manifests as intention tremor and tends to be symmetric, usually affecting the upper body and limbs, while not affecting the patient's gait. Familial cases of essential tremor are not uncommon.

Progressive supranuclear palsy is characterized by patients presenting with rigidity and dystonic postures of the neck and shoulders and a tendency to topple while walking. Paralysis of vertical gaze and eventually, lateral gaze distinguishes it from Parkinson's disease.

Normal pressure hydrocephalus usually presents with the triad of urinary incontinence, shuffling gait similar to the gait disturbance seen in Parkinson's, and dementia. The hallmark findings on MRI for this disease show enlarged ventricles.

It is also important to consider drug-induced causes of parkinsonism, which can occur with classic and atypical antipsychotic agents, metoclopramide, prochlorperazine, and reserpine.

## Further Management Plan/Treatment

Patients should be followed closely for progression of disease and treatment adjusted accordingly.

| | |
|---|---|
| • Carbidopa/levodopa 25/100 | Escalate dose and frequency as needed, to provide dopamine precursor |
| • MAO B inhibitors such as selegiline and rasagiline may be useful in patients with early Parkinson's but only have modest benefit as monotherapy | |
| • Alternative treatment: begin a dopa-mine-agonist (pramipexole, ropinirole) with plans for carbidopa/levodopa institution when condition progresses | |
| • Centrally acting anticholinergic drug, such as benztropine; used for younger patients in whom tremor is predominant symptom | |
| • Amantadine, a weak anti-Parkinson drug, is used in early disease, when symptoms are mild.<br>• COMT inhibitors stop the metabolism of dopamine.<br>• Tolcapone and entacapone are useful as L-dopa extenders (both are ineffective when used alone) | |
| • For equivocal cases, serial clinical examinations are warranted | |

## Discussion

The standard treatment for Parkinson's disease is replacement of the neurotransmitter dopamine with the precursor L-dopa (L-hydroxyphenylalanine). This is given in the formulation carbidopa/levodopa. Bromocriptine works as a dopamine-agonist. Be careful when dosing older adult and demented patients, as excess levels of dopamine/agonists can cause psychiatric side effects such as hallucinations.

Anticholinergic agents such as trihexyphenidyl and benztropine mesylate are also used in secondary parkinsonism resulting from medications. The use of selegiline is still the subject of much debate and is thought to help prevent the progression of disease. Selegiline increases concentrations of dopamine by blocking metabolism via inhibition of the enzyme monoamine oxidase.

The onset of Parkinson's disease usually begins age 40–70, with peak incidence in the sixth decade. The cause is a loss of pigmented cells in the substantia nigra. The essential features are:

- Expressionless face
- Poverty/slowness of voluntary movement
- "Pill-rolling" 4-cycle/second tremor
- Stooped posture
- Rigidity
- Shuffling gait

Initially, the symptoms may be subtle. A thorough history will bring out important features of this syndrome long before the patient or spouse suspects that something is wrong.

- One subtle sign is a decrease in eye blink to 5–10/min (normal 20/min).
- Micrographia (small handwriting) can also be an early sign that can be brought out by history.
- Bradykinesia or slowness in both the initiation and execution of movement is also characteristic of this disease.

Complications of long-term levodopa are GI symptoms, tachycardia, and orthostatic hypotension. CNS side effects include psychosis and "on–off" phenomena. "On–off" phenomena is when patients alternate between periods of severe parkinsonian rigidity and hyperkinetic movement, including hemiballismus, dystonias, and dyskinesia. Up to 40% of patients with Parkinson's disease will develop major depression. Patients can also develop a subcortical type of dementia in late stages. Subcortical dementia results in loss of both recent and long-term memory.

## Final Diagnosis

Parkinson's disease

### CLINICAL PEARL

Levodopa treatment should not be stopped abruptly; sudden withdrawal has been rarely associated with a syndrome resembling neuroleptic malignant syndrome (referred to as parkinsonism-hyperpyrexia syndrome).

### CLINICAL PEARL

Normal pressure hydrocephalus (NPH) may mimic Parkinson's. NPH typically presents as a clinical triad of gait abnormalities, incontinence, and dementia. CT/MRI appearance of hydrocephalus should be diagnostic.

## Basic Science Correlate

### Biochemistry

Tyrosine hydroxylase is the rate-limiting enzyme for dopamine production. It may be found in decreased concentration in Parkinson's disease.

### Neuroanatomy

Bradykinesia is caused by loss of dopaminergic neurons in the substantia nigra pars compacta. These neurons would normally excite the direct pathway striatal neurons and inhibit the indirect pathway striatal neurons, which cause the lack of movement.

### Pathology

Parkinson's disease is listed among the tauopathies, neurodegenerative diseases associated with intraneuronal protein tangles classified as Lewy bodies in Parkinson's.

### Pharmacology

Loss of dopamine in the striatal pathway is the main factor driving Parkinson's symptoms, so treatment strategies focus on raising dopamine availability through different mechanisms.

- L-DOPA is a dopamine precursor, while carbidopa slows its breakdown in the periphery, similarly to entacapone.
- MAO inhibitors (sub B type) decrease dopamine metabolism within the synaptic cleft.
- Ropinirole and pramipexole are dopamine-agonists.

## CASE 14

### Chief Complaint

"I've had headaches all my life but this one is the worst."

### History and Physical Examination

A 20-year-old woman comes to the emergency department because of a severe headache. She describes a headache history that began when she was age 14. Her headaches typically occur every 3 months and are very severe. She describes visual symptoms that begin in the right field of vision and consist of bright, flashing lights. She has just finished a very challenging year in college, and when returning home to her parent's house, she noted the recurrence of this headache, accompanied by visual symptoms and nausea and vomiting. This headache is much worse than her previous headaches, so she decided to seek medical attention. She has recently started birth control pills and has taken up smoking cigarettes. Physical examination of the patient is non-focal.

### Differential Diagnosis

1. Migraine with aura (classic)
2. Migraine without aura (common)
3. Cluster headache
4. Tension-type headache
5. Temporal (giant cell) arteritis
6. Medication overuse headache
7. Pseudotumor cerebri
8. Seizure
9. Brain tumor
10. Arteriovenous malformation

### Initial Management Plan

**Setting:** emergency department

### Diagnostic/Therapeutic Plan

- MRI of the brain

### Test Results

- MRI: negative

### Assessment

This patient has a history characteristic for classic migraine headaches. In women, migraines usually occur after the onset of menses.

The 2 major categories of migraine are **classic** and **common**. The classic migraine includes the presence of a visual aura (often described as "fortification spectra" or flashing lights), while the common migraine does not.

- Migraine headaches usually affect one side of the head more than the other, and they are unilateral in 60–70% of cases.
- In 80% of cases, there is no associated aura.
- Nausea and vomiting can occur with any acute headache, but it is mostly characteristic of migraines.
- Oral contraceptives can exacerbate migraines.
- Patients with migraine and who smoke are at higher risk for stroke and heart attack.

With any type of headache in which the intensity, character, or frequency changes, one should do further evaluation with imaging to rule out a brain tumor or arterial-venous malformation. MRI or CT with contrast is helpful. Any neurologic deficit that is transient requires the consideration of possible seizure activity.

The following types of headaches **require evaluation and imaging**:

- Abnormal neurologic examination
- "Worst headache ever"
- First severe headache
- Fever and systemic signs
- Vomiting precedes headache
- Induced by cough or lifting
- Disturb sleep or occur upon awakening
- Onset age >50
- In the context of known systemic illness (cancer, HIV, etc.)

**CLINICAL PEARL**

- Once the migraine occurs, abortive drugs are the mainstay of treatment, with triptans being the first line of treatment for moderate to severe migraine.
- If the migraines occur repeatedly, consider preventive treatment with beta-adrenergic blockers, amitriptyline or topiramate (taken daily for at least a few years).

## Further Management Plan

- Abortive treatment: oral triptans (sumatriptan, naratriptan, zolmitriptan, rizatriptan, or almotriptan); dihydroergotamine; ergotamine tartrate; NSAIDs and acetaminophen for mild cases
- Prophylactic treatment: beta-blockers, topiramate, amitriptyline, calcium-channel blockers, venlafaxine, and valproic acid
- Oral therapy, rectal ergotamine, subcutaneous sumatriptan, or IV prochlorperazine for migraine with nausea and vomiting
- Methylsergide only for refractory cases (has risks of cardiac, retroperitoneal, and pulmonary fibrosis)

## Discussion

The birth control pills should be discontinued for this patient, and the patient should be strongly advised to stop smoking. Drinking coffee and eating chocolate should also be discouraged. Proper sleep hygiene must be advocated.

After removing any precipitating causes for the migraine, implement prophylactic therapy if:

- Patient has >3 migraine episodes in a month
- Headaches last >12 hours
- Significant disability is associated with the attacks

Beta-blockers and calcium-channel blockers are used to control vasomotor tone, which is thought to underlie the etiology of migraine headaches. The FDA has also approved topiramate, amitriptyline, and valproate for migraine prophylaxis.

Abortive treatment is used in the acute setting and includes sumatriptan, dihydroergotamine, and ergotamine tartrate, which work as serotonergic agonists to relieve the headaches.

Triptans should be avoided during pregnancy, in familial hemiplegic migraines, ischemic heart disease, and Prinzmetal angina secondary to their vasospastic effects. The same is true for ergotamine. Triptans can be given orally, intranasally, or even subcutaneously, depending on the severity of the headache.

The classification of headache has some prognostic significance and major importance in determining treatment:

- Migraines can be bilateral or localizing. Migraines have characteristic motor, sensory, or visual symptoms preceding them. The common migraine occurs far more frequently. They are provoked by menses, caffeine, chocolate, alcohol, and emotional stress. Photophobia may be present in 80% of cases, leading to confusion with other diagnoses. The terms *classic* and *common* have no particular relevancy.
- Cluster headaches are characterized by multiple episodes in a single day for several weeks, with pain-free intervals lasting ≥1 year. An almost 10:1 male:female predominance occurs. In a cluster headache, the pain peaks in 5 minutes, whereas with migraine it takes several hours to peak. Cluster headaches are strictly unilateral, with a red eye, nasal stuffiness, and lacrimation. Beta-blockers and tricyclic antidepressants (e.g., amitriptyline) seldom work.
  - Calcium-channel blockers (verapamil) for prophylaxis
  - Lithium, steroids, ergotamine, and valproate (second-line) are tried sequentially until one is found that works
  - Triptans or ergotamine to abort an acute attack; if contraindicated, try 100% oxygen inhalation
- **Tension headache,** described as "band-like" around the head (e.g., a belt being tightened around the head) is usually bilateral. It is often described as "throbbing." Treatment is analgesics.
- **Temporal (giant cell) arteritis** usually occurs age >50 (mean age 70). Blindness may occur in up to 50% of patients, if left untreated. There is marked scalp tenderness. Erythrocyte sedimentation rate is elevated in >90% of patients. Definitive diagnosis requires temporal artery biopsy, and treatment is steroids.
- **Medication overuse headache** usually occurs in patients who use pharmacologic therapy for headaches ≥2 days/week. Treatment is complex withdrawal of the medication of overuse.

- **Pseudotumor cerebri** usually occurs in premenopausal (age 20–44), obese women. It is also associated with steroid withdrawal, tetracycline, oral contraceptive use, and vitamin A toxicity. Symptoms include headache and horizontal diplopia. Examination often reveals papilledema, sixth nerve palsy, and peripheral visual field deficits. Normal CT/MRI of the head and CSF pressure >250 mm $H_2O$ is diagnostic. Treatment is weight loss plus a diuretic (acetazolamide, furosemide or topiramate) for mild symptoms; for severe cases, prednisone, ventriculoperitoneal or lumboperitoneal shunts, or optic nerve sheath fenestration is used.

### CLINICAL PEARL

Brain tumors tend to cause progressive neurologic symptoms, characterized by a fixed neurologic deficit (i.e., paresis). This patient's intermittent symptoms—with a normal exam between events—argue *against* a space-occupying lesion, especially given the history of intermittent symptoms over years.

## Final Diagnosis

Migraine

# PART II

# PSYCHIATRY

# Psychiatry 16

## CASE 1

### Chief Complaint

"Let's party."

### History and Physical Examination

Police are called to a 34-year-old woman's apartment after neighbors complain that she has been playing loud music all night for the past 10 days. They discover her pacing the floor in her brightly lit apartment at 2:00 a.m. Any attempts to talk to her result in her becoming irritable and abusive. She reportedly greets them cheerfully and invites them in for "a party." She then attempts to engage the officers in a political discussion, saying that she has discovered the solution to the "Middle East crisis" and has just been trying to buy a plane ticket to Washington so she can explain it to the president.

When the police bring her to the emergency department, the patient is angry and resistant. There is no history of trauma or significant medical illness. Physical examination is normal. However, the patient's mood is labile and expansive. She speaks in a pressured manner, revealing that she has felt very little need to sleep over the past week or so, that she was fired from her job for "inappropriate behavior," and that she has been unable to purchase her plane ticket because her credit card has reached its limit. The patient seems quite undisturbed by these events.

### Differential Diagnosis

1. Substance-induced mood disorder
2. Bipolar I disorder
3. Cyclothymic disorder
4. Psychotic disorder (e.g., schizoaffective disorder, schizophrenia)
5. Hyperthyroidism

### Initial Diagnostic Plan/Test Results

- Urine toxicology screen: negative
- Thyroid function tests: normal

## Assessment

The differential diagnosis between bipolar I disorder and a psychotic disorder is sometimes difficult. In the psychotic disorders, psychotic symptoms are usually present in the absence of mood symptoms during some periods. Bipolar II disorder is the occurrence of $\geq$1 major depressive episodes accompanied by at least 1 hypomanic episode.

## Further Diagnostic Plan/Test Results

- Past personal and family history: no history of psychotic illness, with the exception of 1 previous manic episode 1 year ago; responded to lithium; no previous depressive episodes
- Detailed interview with patient's relative, if available

## Treatment Plan

- Hospitalize
- Antipsychotics, initially
- Lithium, antipsychotics, lamotrigine, or valproic acid

## Discussion

This patient needs to be hospitalized until she is stable because she needs to be protected from the consequences of poor judgment, elevated mood, and grandiose delusions. Acutely, she should be treated with antipsychotics or benzodiazepines in a quiet setting with minimal stimuli and firm limits.

Once the patient has been stabilized, start maintenance therapy with a mood stabilizer such as lithium or lamotrigine. It is also important to enlist another person in the patient's life (e.g., a family member) to help monitor medication, because patients often become noncompliant with medications. Some begin to feel "normal" and stop taking it, whereas others feel "down" when they are not manic and wish to feel better.

Diagnostic criteria for bipolar I disorder include a manic episode that may have been preceded by and may be followed by hypomanic or major depressive episodes. A manic episode is a distinct period of abnormally and persistently elevated, expansive, or irritable mood and abnormally and persistently increased goal-directed activity or energy, lasting at least 1 week and present most of the day, nearly every day. Emotional lability is also seen. During mood disturbance, other symptoms may include increased self-esteem or grandiosity, decreased need for sleep, talkativeness, flight of ideas, distractibility, psychomotor agitation, or excessive involvement in pleasurable, high-risk activities.

- If there is only 1 manic episode with no history of major depressive episodes, the diagnosis is bipolar I disorder, single manic episode.
- If there has already been at least 1 manic or mixed episode, the diagnosis can be bipolar disorder, most recent episode mixed, or most recent episode depressed, depending on current symptomatology.
- Even with no history of depression or hypomania, the diagnosis of bipolar I is given.

An episode is hypomanic when it is not severe enough to cause marked impairment in social and occupational functioning, hospitalization is not necessary, and there are no psychotic features. Cyclothymic disorder is a chronic disorder of fluctuating mood disturbances involving hypomanic periods and depressive periods that do not meet criteria for major depression. The above patient's symptoms are too severe to be characterized as hypomanic.

### Basic Science Correlate

Lithium is commonly used as maintenance treatment for bipolar disorder. It prevents the recycling of inositol (decreasing PIP2) by blocking inositol monophosphatase and decreasing cAMP. Lithium has a relatively narrow therapeutic index that predisposes patients to toxicity, which can be acute or chronic.

- Acute toxicity is often initially associated with GI symptoms (nausea, vomiting, cramping), which can progress to tremulousness, hyperreflexia, ataxia, and potentially cardiac dysrhythmias (T-wave flattening).
- Chronic toxicity includes the development of nephrogenic DI (most severe renal manifestation), hypothyroidism, and a syndrome of irreversible lithium-effectuated neurotoxicity (SILENT) such as cognitive impairment, sensorimotor peripheral neuropathy, and cerebellar dysfunction.
  - Nephrogenic DI can occur with chronic lithium use since it inhibits the action of antidiuretic hormone (ADH) on the distal renal tubule, thereby impairing sodium and water reabsorption. This condition can be treated with amiloride.
  - Hypothyroidism can occur with chronic lithium use since it is rapidly taken up by thyroid cells. Lithium results in a blockade of thyroid hormone release from thyroglobulin, which inhibits adenylate cyclase and thus prevents TSH from stimulating thyroid cells via the TSH receptor. Lithium also inhibits the activity of 5' deiodinase.

## Final Diagnosis

Bipolar I disorder, single manic episode

## CASE 2

### Chief Complaint

"I'm having a heart attack!"

### History and Physical Examination

A 23-year-old graduate student comes to the student health care center because she feels she is "having a heart attack" about 1x week for the past 6–8 weeks. The episodes always occur "out of the blue." She describes an accompanying fear so intense that she thinks she is "going to die or go crazy." The patient visited the emergency department 3 weeks ago with a similar attack. An electrocardiogram was normal, and she was sent home. Because she has since then experienced more attacks, the patient is now afraid to drive. She has a family history of cardiac problems: Her 2 grandparents and her father died of myocardial infarctions.

Vital signs today are temperature 37.4 C (99.3 F), blood pressure 120/78 mm Hg, respirations 22/min, and pulse 88/min. Cardiovascular examination shows regular heart rate and rhythm with normal S1 and S2 and no murmurs. The lungs are clear to auscultation and the abdomen is benign.

### Differential Diagnosis

1. Hypoglycemia
2. Hyperthyroidism
3. Substance abuse (chronic sedative withdrawal, amphetamine use, caffeinism)
4. Panic disorder
5. Generalized anxiety disorder
6. Supraventricular tachycardia

### Initial Diagnostic Plan/Tests Results

- Electrocardiogram: normal
- Thyroid function tests: WNL
- CBC, chemical screen: normal
- Blood glucose: normal

### Further Diagnostic Plan/Test Results

- Detailed clinical interview: patient has no circumscribed fears, has no trouble leaving her home, and denies suicidal ideation, hallucinations, delusions, and use of substances; patient has no vegetative signs of depression (e.g., weight loss, insomnia, anhedonia)

### Treatment Plan

- Acute symptoms: benzodiazepines (e.g., alprazolam, lorazepam, clonazepam)
- Chronic first-line: SSRIs or SNRIs
  - Chronic second-line: tricyclic antidepressants or MAO inhibitors at low doses (lower than needed for antidepressant effects)
- Psychotherapy to address underlying issues

### Discussion

This patient most likely has panic disorder. Essential features are recurrent, unexpected panic attacks with persistent concern about future attacks; worry about the consequences of them; and behavioral changes related to the attacks. There is an abrupt surge of intense fear or intense discomfort that reaches a peak within minutes and during which $\geq$4 of the following occur:

- Palpitations
- Sweating
- Trembling
- Shortness of breath
- Feelings of choking
- Chest pain
- Nausea
- Dizziness
- Chills or heat sensations
- Paresthesias
- Derealization
- Fear of losing control
- Fear of dying

The frequency of attacks may vary widely.

Individuals often fear they are suffering from an undiagnosed, life-threatening condition or that their brain is not working correctly. Some individuals change their behaviors (i.e., quit a job) or develop avoidant behaviors. Transient tachycardia and moderate elevation of systolic blood pressure may occur during some attacks. Age of onset varies but is typically between late adolescence and mid-thirties. Women are 3x more likely to be diagnosed than men.

**CLINICAL PEARL**

Panic disorder and agoraphobia are unlinked in DSM-5 (i.e., they were previously linked). These diagnoses now have unique diagnostic criteria and codes.

### Final Diagnosis

Panic disorder

# CASE 3

## Chief Complaint

"He deserved to be punched for the way he was talking about me!"

## History and Physical Examination

A 28-year-old man is brought to the emergency department by police after he punched a man at the bus stop. The patient said he had to defend himself because the man was disrespecting him. When asked to explain, the patient insists that the man was talking about him and telling people that he had a terrible body odor. He has a history of 2 other arrests for assault in the past 2 years. He insists that none of these was warranted because the strangers he assaulted were the ones "out of line," usually by talking about him.

The patient today is dressed appropriately and does not emit any significant body odor. He is verbose, talking in a loud voice, and frequently circumstantial. He is angry, and his affect is blunted. He is obviously wary, and his eyes frequently dart between the window and door. He says he is angry because people are always talking about his life. He is unable to sleep at night except for when he has a kitchen knife on his bed stand because voices are saying that someone is going to hurt him. After a while, the patient refuses to respond to more questions, saying that the FBI is recording the interview.

## Differential Diagnosis

1. Schizophrenia
2. Delusional disorder
3. Brief psychotic disorder
4. Paranoid personality disorder
5. Substance-induced psychotic disorder

### CLINICAL PEARL

**Atypical antipsychotics**

- Risperidone: less sedation; more movement side effects
- Olanzapine: more weight gain; greater risk for diabetes
- Ziprasidone: possible cardiac conduction problems
- Quetiapine: fewer movement side effects

## Initial Diagnostic Plan/Test Results

- Urine toxicology screen: negative

## Treatment Plan

- Hospitalize any patient who is currently dangerous to others; this helps provide the structure that a psychotic person needs
- Stabilize with medications (atypical antipsychotics such as olanzapine, risperidone, quetiapine, aripiprazole, or ziprasidone)
- Identify social support, e.g., family members
- Provide adjunct psychosocial therapy (e.g., cognitive therapy to help identify and work through cognitive distortions and to learn to correct errors in judgment)

### Discussion

Schizophrenia is diagnosed if there are $\geq 2$ of the following 5 symptoms:

- Delusions
- Hallucinations
- Disorganized speech
- Disorganized or catatonic behavior
- Negative symptoms (flat affect, avolition, etc.)

AND $\geq 1$ of the following symptoms:

- Delusions
- Hallucinations
- Disorganized speech

For a significant portion of the time since the onset of disturbance, level of functioning in $\geq 1$ major area such as work, interpersonal relationships, and self-care is significantly below the level achieved prior to the onset of symptoms.

There must also be continuous signs of the disturbance for at least 6 months AND the 6-month period must include 1 month of symptoms that meet the diagnostic criteria.

Brief psychotic disorder may or may not have the same symptoms as schizophrenia; however, the duration is limited to <1 month but lasts at least 1 day. The disorder may be a response to a severe psychosocial stressor or a group of stressors.

Delusional disorder is differentiated from schizophrenia on the basis of 2 things:

- Delusion is non-bizarre or bizarre
- Absence of other symptoms of schizophrenia (hallucinations, flat affect, etc.)

Paranoid personality disorder is characterized by chronic suspiciousness and mistrust of people in general. Unlike schizophrenia, there is an absence of hallucinations or a formal thought disorder.

There is also an absence of fixed delusions, which differentiates it from delusional disorder.

Substance-induced psychotic disorder is the presence of psychotic symptoms (e.g., delusions or hallucinations) resulting from the use of psychoactive substances.

#### CLINICAL PEARL

**What to do?**

- **Movement disorders:** avoid risperidone; use quetiapine
- **Diabetes:** avoid olanzapine
- **Weight gain:** avoid olanzapine
- **Conduction defects:** avoid ziprasidone

#### CLINICAL PEARL

The DSM-IV-TR subtypes of schizophrenia (paranoid, disorganized, catatonic, undifferentiated, and residual types) have been eliminated in DSM-5 due to their limited diagnostic stability, low reliability, and poor validity. Furthermore, those subtypes were not associated with distinctive patterns of treatment measures.

### Basic Science Correlate

The exact cause of schizophrenia remains unknown; however, likely risk factors include genetic predisposition (risk is higher in biologic relatives), perinatal factors (malnourished women and/or viral illness), and undefined socioenvironmental factors. Also vitamin D deficiency has been linked to increased risk for schizophrenia.

Regarding the proposed pathophysiology of schizophrenia, anatomic, neurotransmitter, and immune system abnormalities have all been linked to this disorder.

- **Anatomic abnormalities**: Patients with schizophrenia may have decreased brain volume in the medial temporal areas as well as alterations in the hippocampus. MRI studies have also shown abnormalities in a network of neocortical and limbic regions and interconnecting white-matter tracts.
- **Neurotransmitter abnormalities**: Hyperdopaminergic activity in the mesolimbic system is believed to be the primary underlying defect. However, other neurotransmitter systems, such as norepinephrine, serotonin, and gamma-aminobutyric acid (GABA), are likely involved. Researchers are also currently investigating the N-methyl-D-aspartate (NMDA) subclass of glutamate receptors.
- **Immune system abnormalities**: Overactivation of the immune system (either pre- or postnatal) may cause an overexpression of inflammatory cytokines leading to an abnormal change of brain structure and function.

### Final Diagnosis

Schizophrenia

# CASE 4

## Chief Complaint

Nausea and muscle cramps 2 days after surgery

## History and Physical Examination

A 35-year-old actor is referred by his surgeon 2 days post-op. He has become irritable, is suffering from diarrhea, complains of muscle cramps, and is nauseated. He acknowledges occasional heroin use but denies that he is "hooked on it." His temperature is 37.9 C (100.2 F), pulse is 90/min, and blood pressure is 150/90 mm Hg. His pupils are dilated but are equal and reactive to light. He is restless and irritable but coherent and oriented. He denies psychotic symptoms. He repeatedly verbalizes that he needs to go home and that the hospital is making him sick.

## Differential Diagnosis

1. Opioid withdrawal
2. Opioid use disorder

## Initial Diagnostic Plan/Test Results

- Toxicology screen: positive for opiates

## Treatment Plan

- Clonidine, buprenorphine/naloxone or methadone
- Supportive treatment for other symptoms
- Refer to rehab once detox complete (drug rehabilitation is usually 28 days or more)

## Discussion

Opiate withdrawal occurs as a result of either cessation (or reduction) in heavy opioid use or the administration of an opioid antagonist after a period of opioid use; within minutes to several days, $\geq$3 of the following will occur:

- Dysphoric mood
- Nausea or vomiting
- Muscle aches
- Diarrhea
- Rhinorrhea or lacrimation
- Pupillary dilation
- Piloerection
- Sweating
- Yawning
- Fever
- Insomnia

**CLINICAL PEARL**

In DSM-5, substance abuse and substance dependence are combined into a single substance use disorder, which specifies each substance or drug class with a new "addictions and related disorders" category. Example substance/drug classes:

- Alcohol
- Opioid
- Sedative, hypnotic, or anxiolytic
- Stimulant
- Cannabis
- Other hallucinogen use disorders

Criteria are prepared for each substance use disorder, as well as for intoxication, withdrawal, substance/medication-induced disorder, and unspecified substance-induced disorder.

Also in DSM-5, "recurrent legal problems" is deleted and "craving or a strong desire or urge to use a substance" has been added to the diagnostic criteria. The threshold of the number of diagnostic criteria that must be met was also changed. For example, use disorder severity ranges from mild to severe AND is based on the number of criteria endorsed from a list of 11 different criteria.

- 2–3 symptoms indicate mild substance use disorder
- 4–5 symptoms indicate moderate substance use disorder
- 6+ symptoms indicate severe substance use disorder

Also, these signs and symptoms cause clinically significant distress or impairment in social, occupational, or other important areas of functioning AND cannot be attributable to another medical condition or better explained by another mental disorder.

Opioid use disorder is a problematic pattern of opioid use leading to clinically significant impairment or distress manifested by $\geq$2 of the following, occurring within a 12-month period:

1. Taking the opioid in larger amounts or for longer than intended
2. Wanting to decrease the amount or discontinue using the opioid but unsuccessful
3. Spending a lot of time getting, using, or recovering from use of the opioid
4. Cravings and urges to use the opioid
5. Usage resulting in failure to fulfill major obligations at work, home, or school
6. Continued usage, even when it causes problems in relationships
7. Giving up important social, occupational, or other activities because of opioid use
8. Continued usage in situations where it is physically hazardous
9. Continued usage even when aware that a physical or psychological problem could have been caused or made worse by the opioid
10. Needing more of the substance to attain desired effect (tolerance)
11. Development of withdrawal symptoms, which can be reversed by taking the substance

### Basic Science Correlate

The "oral" combination drug buprenorphine/naloxone is indicated for opioid use disorder as both induction and maintenance treatment. Buprenorphine is a mixed opioid agonist-antagonist that binds to various opioid receptors, producing agonism at delta receptors, partial agonism at mu receptors, and antagonism at kappa receptors. Since oral buprenorphine has a potential to be abused (by manipulating the formulation and injecting it intravenously), it is combined with naloxone, which is a pure opioid antagonist that exerts it, effect when administered by the IV/SC/IM routes.

- Effective for treatment of opioid use disorder since the patient can only administer the medication orally.
- When administered orally, only the buprenorphine will be absorbed into systemic circulation.
- Naloxone has very poor oral bioavailability; hence, it will not be absorbed.
- If, however, the patient manipulates the oral formulation and injects it intravenously, the effects of buprenorphine will be blocked by the full antagonistic effects of naloxone.

## Final Diagnosis

Opioid withdrawal

## CASE 5

### Chief Complaint

"I'm worried about the cleanliness and safety of my food."

### History and Physical Examination

A 30-year-old woman reports that for the past 2 years, following a bad case of diarrhea for which she was hospitalized for a week, she has been scared of being sick again and has become very meticulous about ensuring that the foods she eats are safe and clean. She says that it started with her washing vegetables and fruits at least 3 times before consuming. It then progressed to her having to sterilize the silverware she uses before meals to bringing her own silverware when she goes out to eat. She is worried that it's beginning to affect her relationships because she is now concerned about food that she did not personally prepare, and this has forced her to stay at home. She turns down invitations to hang out with friends or to go out on dates. Physical examination is essentially normal, except for dry and chapped skin on both hands.

### Differential Diagnosis

1. Obsessive-compulsive disorder (OCD)
2. Obsessive-compulsive personality disorder
3. Delusional disorder
4. Specific phobia

### Treatment Plan

- SSRI: fluoxetine, sertraline, paroxetine, or fluvoxamine; clomipramine if TCA-indicated
- Behavioral therapy for exposure and response prevention

### Discussion

OCD is described in DSM-5 as having one or both of the following, becoming severe enough to be time-consuming or cause marked distress or significant impairment.

- Recurring obsessions (intrusive thoughts, feelings, ideas, or sensations)
- Compulsions (conscious, recurring patterns of behavior like counting or checking)

People afflicted with OCD know that their reactions are irrational, and it impinges on their functions and relationships. **In DSM-5, one of the following specifiers should be added:** with good or fair insight, with poor insight, or with absent insight/delusional beliefs.

Obsessive-compulsive personality disorder is defined as a pervasive pattern of perfectionism and inflexibility. There is preoccupation with rules, details, and being in control of things and situations.

Delusional disorder is differentiated from OCD by the absence of insight. In OCD, patients are aware and anxious about their condition.

Phobias are differentiated from OCD by the absence of a relationship between the compulsion and the obsessive thought.

## Final Diagnosis

Obsessive-compulsive disorder

# CASE 6

## Chief Complaint

"I can no longer handle my difficult son."

## History and Physical Examination

The mother of an 11-year-old boy reports that she has "lost control" of her son and "can't take it anymore." He has always been difficult, and his acting out has always been severe for his age. Recently, the child was suspended from school for setting fire in the locker room. Past incidents in school have included frequent fighting, truancy, vandalism of school property, and threatening the principal. The boy has stolen money from his family many times and refuses to follow rules at home, including curfew. Physical examination is essentially normal.

## Differential Diagnosis

1. Conduct disorder
2. Oppositional defiant disorder
3. Manic episode
4. Adjustment disorder
5. Attention deficit hyperactivity disorder

## Initial Diagnostic Plan/Results

- Clinical interview with boy: child is angry and defiant; says he "doesn't care" why he's here and refuses to talk.
    - Denies having a problem
    - Negative for pressured speech, grandiosity, delusions, and hallucinations
- Interview with mother: bad conduct not episodic in nature but persistent
    - No onset of psychosocial stressor before behavioral problems.
    - "My son has been like this as long as I can remember."

## Treatment Plan

- Individual therapy: first, focus on the relationship and develop a therapeutic alliance
- When the child becomes invested in the therapy, a variety of techniques (behavior modification, cognitive restructuring, etc.) may be used to change behavior

### Discussion

Conduct disorder is a repetitive pattern of behavior which violates the basic rights of others or breaks age-appropriate societal norms. These behaviors fall in 4 categories:

- Aggression to people and animals (bullies or threatens others; initiates physical fights; uses weapons; is cruel to people or animals)
- Destruction of property (sets fires or uses other forms of destruction)
- Deceitfulness or theft (breaks into homes, cars; "cons" others; shoplifts)
- Serious rule violations (breaks rules regarding curfew and truancy; runs away)

At least 3 behaviors must have been present in the past year, and at least 1 must have been present in the last 6 months.

The disorder causes significant impairment in social and academic functioning and is usually present in a variety of settings. Onset is usually late childhood and rare after age 16. It is more common in boys.

The following specifiers have been added in DSM-5:

- Childhood-onset type
- Adolescent-onset type
- Unspecified onset

Also, individuals must show at least 1 symptom characteristic of conduct disorder prior to age 10. This diagnosis is usually given to children but can be given to those age >18 if antisocial personality disorder criteria are not met.

Conduct disorder is associated with early onset of sexual behavior, drinking, smoking, use of illegal substances, and risk taking. Behaviors sometimes lead to school dysfunction, poor work adjustment, sexually transmitted disease, unplanned pregnancy, and physical injury.

Oppositional defiant disorder includes disobedience and opposition to authority figures but does not include the persistent pattern of a more serious behavior. Irritability and conduct problems can arise during a manic episode, but these bouts are episodic in nature, and other criteria for mania must be met.

Adjustment disorder (with disturbance of conduct or with mixed disturbance of mood and conduct) is only diagnosed if behavioral changes are preceded by the onset of a psychological stressor occurring within the past 3 months.

**CLINICAL PEARL**

When patients with conduct disorder reach adulthood, the symptoms of aggression, property destruction, deceitfulness, and violence against others may be exhibited in the workplace or home. When these symptoms are present in an adult, consider a diagnosis of antisocial personality disorder.

### Final Diagnosis

Conduct disorder

# CASE 7

## Chief Complaint

"I can't sleep."

## History and Physical Examination

A 64-year-old man comes to your office because he has had trouble sleeping since his wife died 3 weeks ago. He thinks of his wife frequently, has been unable to go through her things, and is tearful when he speaks of her. There is a history of weight loss and depressed mood, though the patient claims his appetite and mood are improving. He also admits to feeling angry that his wife had refused to stop smoking cigarettes, a contributing factor in her death. Physical examination is essentially normal.

## Differential Diagnosis

1. Bereavement
2. Adjustment disorder
3. Major depression

## Initial Diagnostic Plan

- Thorough clinical interview of patient and family member if available to determine if suicidal ideation is present
- Evaluate vegetative signs of depression and determine level of functioning

## Results

Interview confirms an absence of suicidal ideation and generally high level of functioning and self-care. The patient denies loss of interest in normal activities and he is able to go about normal daily routine. Patient does not have hallucinations and delusions and denies use of drugs or alcohol. His appetite is improving, and his weight has stabilized. However, he complains of insomnia.

## Treatment Plan

- Supportive psychotherapy
- Medications not needed since symptoms are usually self-limited
- Discuss sleep hygiene techniques
- Behavioral modification techniques
- If wanting to treat insomnia with medications, use zolpidem or eszopiclone for short term

### Discussion

Bereavement is diagnosed when the primary problem is a reaction to the loss of a loved one. Some patients present with signs similar to a major depression, such as sadness, insomnia, weight loss, etc. Patients tend to see their feelings as "normal" but may seek help to relieve symptoms.

Normal grieving can include guilt about things that happened around the time of death, feelings that the individual should have died with the loved one or would be better off dead, and transient feelings of "seeing" or "hearing the voice" of the deceased person. If the patient meets the diagnostic criteria for major depressive disorder, a diagnosis can be made irrespective of the amount of time following the patient's loss of a loved one.

This patient's symptoms are distinguished from frank suicidal ideation, excessive guilt, and hallucinatory experiences, which are more characteristic of major depression. The presence of these symptoms or of marked psychomotor retardation or functional impairment is cause for greater concern.

Adjustment disorder does not apply in this case because there is no significant impairment in occupational functioning as a result of the stressor.

### Final Diagnosis

Bereavement

**CLINICAL PEARL**

DSM-5 has removed the bereavement exclusion for a major depressive episode formerly found in DSM-IV-TR. This was done for the following reasons:

- Removes the inference that bereavement generally lasts only 2 mos; it is currently accepted that the normal duration of bereavement can last 1-2 yrs.
- Bereavement is recognized as a severe psychosocial stressor that can precipitate a major depressive episode in susceptible patients, which may begin shortly after the loss. Also, if not properly treated, these patients are at an increased risk for increased suffering, suicidal ideation, and other depression-related manifestations.
- Bereavement-related depressive symptoms generally respond to the same psychosocial and medication therapies as major depressive disorder.

## CASE 8

### Chief Complaint

"I miss him so much."

### History and Physical Examination

A mother brings her teenage daughter to the office because of a marked deterioration of her daughter's mood and behavior over the past 2 months. She has been depressed and anxious. The child has also begun to get detention notices at school for cutting classes and being disrespectful to teachers. Her schoolwork has begun to suffer. The patient reports that she had broken up with her long-time boyfriend 2 months ago and misses him deeply. Before this, the child was reportedly a B student with a good social life and no history of trouble at school or with law-enforcement authorities. Physical examination is essentially normal.

### Differential Diagnosis

1. Major depression
2. Generalized anxiety disorder
3. Adjustment disorder

### Initial Diagnostic Plan/Test Results

- Urine toxicology: negative

### Further Diagnostic Plan/Tests Results

- Clinical interview: patient denies use of substances; no vegetative signs of depression (e.g., weight loss, insomnia); some anxiety, but not predominant symptom; patient denies suicidal ideation

### Treatment Plan

- Short-term supportive therapy
- Consult with parents regarding ways in which they may support their daughter in reestablishing an appropriate social network

### Discussion

Adjustment disorder is diagnosed when there is the development of emotional and/or behavioral symptoms in response to an identified social stressor(s) occurring within 3 months of the onset of the stressor(s). The reaction is significant when it is out of proportion to what may be expected or when it involves an impairment of occupational or academic functioning.

Symptoms must be in response to a stressor that occurred <3 months of the onset of the stressor and must not persist >6 months. Distress is associated with an increased risk in suicide potential.

There are 6 subtypes or specifiers:

1. With depressed mood
2. With anxiety
3. With mixed anxiety and depressed mood
4. With disturbance of conduct
5. With mixed disturbance of emotions and conduct
6. Unspecified, depending on the predominant symptoms (used when maladaptive behaviors are not classifiable in another category)

The disorder can occur at any age, and both sexes are equally affected.

Adjustment disorder is used only when individuals do not meet criteria for another diagnosis such as major depression. PTSD and acute stress disorder (ASD) both require the presence of a psychosocial stressor but do not fit in this case.

- In PTSD, the stressor must have been of life-threatening severity and the reaction is more extreme.
- In ASD, the individual experiences dissociative symptoms.
- In both disorders, the traumatic event is persistently reexperienced.

Bereavement is diagnosed when the adjustment reaction is consistent with one that might be expected with the loss of a loved one. Adjustment disorder might be appropriate if the reaction is out of proportion or prolonged. When symptoms recur >6 mos, the adjustment disorder may also continue to be present and become a persistent form.

The use of pharmacologic agents for treatment of adjustment disorder is directed toward improving the debilitating symptoms (insomnia, anxiety, and panic attacks) rather than treatment of the disorder itself. Benzodiazepines (alprazolam, lorazepam) and antidepressants (SSRIs) are the most commonly used agents when pharmacotherapy is indicated.

Antidepressants may be used in those with minor or major depressive disorders who have not responded to psychotherapy or other supportive interventions for ≥3 mos.

## Final Diagnosis

Adjustment disorder

# CASE 9

## Chief Complaint

"My son just freaked out!"

## History and Physical Examination

A mother brings in her 18-year-old son after his screaming woke her up. She reports that this is his second night home on his holiday break from college, where he is in his freshman year. She says that since he came home, he is irritable, restless, and chain smoking. According to the patient, he had been "okay" until about 3 months ago after he "survived" his fraternity initiations. He had told his parents that he was not really ready for the "rituals" and at some point was afraid he wasn't going to live through it. The mother says that she was shocked herself when she got a call from the hospital following the initiations for loss of consciousness. When she arrived, she saw bruises on various parts of his body. Since then he said that he has not been sleeping well because of nightmares. He also said that he had been thinking of dropping out altogether because every time he sees members of the frat, he is suddenly "brought back" to the frat house and events prior to his loss of consciousness.

Except for a pulse of 100/min, the physical examination today is unremarkable. The patient is appropriately dressed but his shirt is drenched in sweat. His affect is appropriate and his mood is anxious. There are no psychotic symptoms elicited. Cognitive functions are intact. The patient says he can't stand what's going on and is afraid he will go crazy if the nightmares persist.

## Differential Diagnosis

1. Posttraumatic stress disorder (PTSD)
2. Acute stress disorder
3. Malingering

## Treatment Plan

- Crisis intervention
- Antidepressant medication (SSRIs, first-line)
- Psychotherapy (trauma-focused CBT)

## Discussion

PTSD is characterized by the presence of the following:

- Exposure to a traumatic event where the person is confronted with an actual or threatened injury or risk of death, accompanied by an overwhelming sense of helplessness; persistent reexperiencing of the event (e.g., nightmares)
- Persistent avoidance of the stimuli and numbing of general responsiveness
- Persistent symptoms of hyperarousal

The duration of the disturbance is >1 month and causes significant distress or impairment in social, occupational, or other important areas of functioning.

Acute stress disorder is very similar to PTSD but the symptoms occur only within 3 days to 1 month of the event (trauma exposure), and last from 3 days to 4 weeks. Onset may be immediate or delayed with a duration of up to 1 month.

Malingering is characterized by the voluntary production or false presentation of a physical or psychological illness. There is always an identifiable motivation for the production of such symptoms that may fall under any one of the following: the avoidance of responsibility, punishment, or difficult situations; receiving compensation, drugs, and other material things; or retaliating or "getting back" at someone.

### Final Diagnosis

Posttraumatic stress disorder

# CASE 10

## Chief Complaint

"I don't want to do anything anymore."

## History and Physical Examination

A 66-year-old man is brought to the office by his daughter, who is visiting from out of town. For the past 3 weeks he has felt depressed most of the day, nearly every day. He has had a markedly diminished interest in things that used to be enjoyable. He has lost weight and has difficulty concentrating and remembering things. He frequently thinks of death and suicide. The patient retired 8 months ago. He was treated for depression twice before and responded to antidepressant medication.

Physical examination is normal. The patient is oriented to time, place, and person, but is slow to respond to questions. He says he "just wants to go home and rest."

## Differential Diagnosis

1. Major depressive disorder
2. Persistent depressive disorder (dysthymia)
3. Hypothyroidism
4. Bipolar disorder

## Initial Diagnostic Plan/Test Results

- Thyroid function tests: normal

## Further Diagnostic Plan/Test Results

- Detailed interview/history: no previous manic episodes; no delusions or hallucinations
- Evaluate suicide potential: patient thinks that if he decided to kill himself, he would close all the windows in his apartment (so as not to disturb anyone) and use his handgun

## Treatment Plan

- Hospitalize: this patient is a suicide risk. He thinks of it often, has a plan, and the means to implement his plan are readily available. He does not appear to have any support nearby. He is also not caring for himself well.
- Treat with SSRIs or SNRIs (first-line) or tricyclic antidepressants (second-line) or MAO inhibitors (third-line).
  - SSRIs are always first-line treatment (fluoxetine, paroxetine, sertraline, citalopram, or escitalopram).
  - If SSRIs are not present, consider bupropion, venlafaxine, or duloxetine.
- If medication fails, electroconvulsive therapy may be initiated (often effective in older patients).
- After discharge, outpatient supportive psychotherapy is indicated.

### Discussion

Major depressive disorder is diagnosed when there is a period of 2 wks of depression or loss of pleasure in nearly all activities. The individual must also experience at least 4 additional symptoms from the following:

- Change in appetite or weight
- Change in sleep patterns (insomnia or hypersomnia)
- Psychomotor agitation or retardation
- Decreased energy or fatigue
- Feelings of guilt or worthlessness
- Difficulty thinking or concentrating
- Recurrent thoughts of death or suicide plans or attempts

The episode is accompanied by significant impairment in functioning. In most cases, symptoms persist for ≥6 mos and remit. In some individuals, only partial remission is noted. Episodes often recur.

If there has been a history of mania, the diagnosis of bipolar disorder, most recent episode depressed, is given.

Persistent depressive disorder (dysthymia) is a less severe state of chronic depression diagnosed after a minimum of 2 years of depressed mood.

**CLINICAL PEARL**

- When differentiating grief/bereavement from major depressive disorder, consider that in grief the predominant affect is a feeling of emptiness and loss.
- In major depressive disorder, there is an inability to anticipate happiness or pleasure.
- Also, the dysphoria associated with grief tends to diminish in intensity over a period of weeks and may also occur in waves.

### Final Diagnosis

Major depressive disorder

## CASE 11

### Chief Complaint

Heart is skipping beats.

### History and Physical Examination

A mother reports that her teenage daughter engages in recurrent binge-eating. She has heard her "throwing up" in the bathroom frequently. Additionally, the girl exercises daily to the point of exhaustion. There has been no recent weight loss. She is 5' 5" tall, 118 lb, with blood pressure 80/52 mm Hg.

Physical examination shows poor dentition with a loss of enamel. Her teeth are chipped and ragged, and the parotid gland is enlarged. The lungs are clear. The heart is tachycardiac with frequent, skipped beats. Calluses on the dorsal surface of the left hand are noted.

### Differential Diagnosis

1. Bulimia nervosa
2. Anorexia nervosa, binge-eating, purging type
3. Binge-eating disorder

### Initial Diagnostic Plan/Test Results

- Sodium: 132 mEq/L (normal 135–145)
- Potassium: 2.8 mEq/L (normal 3.5–5.2)
- BUN, creatinine: 40 mg/dL (normal 8–18); 1.3 mg/dL (normal 0.6–1.2)
- Glucose: 65 mg/dL (normal 80–120)
- Electrocardiogram rate 110 sinus rhythm

### Further Diagnostic Plan/Test Results

- Detailed clinical interview:
  - Girl reports being depressed about her inability to control her eating
  - Says she "must maintain her weight" and seems to base her self-evaluation solely on body weight
  - Denies abuse of laxatives
- Beck depression inventory: does not meet criteria for major depression

### Treatment Plan

- Initial hospitalization to prevent life-threatening complications
- Individual and family therapy with behavioral modification upon discharge
- Antidepressants such as SSRIs may help if major depressive disorder or OCD is also present

## Discussion

Eating disorders are characterized by severe disturbances in eating behavior. There is a characteristic distortion of body image and an obsession about weight.

**Bulimia** is characterized by repeated episodes of binge-eating, followed by inappropriate compensatory behaviors to ensure the maintenance of normal weight. **Anorexia nervosa** can include these symptoms but additionally necessitates a refusal to maintain a normal body weight. This patient has a BMI of 19.6 (normal 18.5–24.9) and has had no recent weight loss, which contributes to a diagnosis of bulimia nervosa.

- Both disorders are most common in adolescent women, with bulimia being seen more frequently.
- Both disorders can be associated with physical problems.
- Anorexia nervosa can be of the **restricting type** (no binge/purge behavior) or the **binge-eating/purging type**.
- Recurrent vomiting often leads to poor dentition, enlargement of the salivary glands, and calluses on hands.
- Abuse of laxatives or diuretics can lead to GI problems.
- Menstrual irregularity is often reported (but no longer a diagnostic criteria in DSM-5).
- Electrolyte disturbances are often severe enough to cause serious medical problems.

Binge-eating disorder has recurrent binge-eating in common with bulimia nervosa; however, it differs in the following ways:

- The recurrent inappropriate compensatory behavior found in bulimia is not present in binge-eating disorder.
- In binge-eating disorder, there is not a marked dietary restriction designed to influence body weight and shape between binge-eating episodes.
- Treatment measures tend to be more successful with binge-eating disorder.

### Basic Science Correlate

Many of the complications of anorexia nervosa are related to starvation and nutrient deficiency. Consequently, there can be disruptions of multiple organ systems.

- Endocrine: delayed puberty, amenorrhea, increased growth hormone, hypercortisolism, low estrogen states
- Metabolic: acidosis, decreased antidiuretic hormone, osteoporosis, hypothermia, hypokalemia, hyponatremia, hypoglycemia
- Cardiovascular: cardiomyopathy, supraventricular and ventricular dysrhythmias, long QT syndrome, bradycardia, heart failure
- Renal: decreased GFR, elevated BUN, electrolyte disturbances, edema, renal calculi
- Integumentary: dry skin and hair, alopecia, other hair loss, lanugo body hair
- Hematologic: anemia, leukopenia, thrombocytopenia
- Neurologic: peripheral neuropathy

## Final Diagnosis

Bulimia nervosa

## CASE 12

### Chief Complaint

"Please help us."

### History and Physical Examination

The parents of a 7-year-old boy arrive at your office in tears. The mother reports that she does not know what to do with her son. His behavior, she states, has continued to escalate over the last few years. At home he is often explosive and irritable. He has frequent accidents and cannot sit still. At school he is oppositional and unable to sit in class. His teacher tried to seat him at the front of the class to see if his behavior improved but it did not help. He fights frequently with others and believes that the teacher "picks" on him. His grades are poor and he is failing the second grade. He is the middle child with one sister and one brother, and he routinely picks on them.

While in the first grade he was evaluated by a psychologist and given an IQ test. He scored 110 and did well on the subtests. He was also evaluated by the school counselor who believed he had poor self-esteem.

### Differential Diagnosis

1. Specific learning disorder
2. Oppositional defiant disorder
3. Attention-deficit hyperactivity disorder
4. Conduct disorder

### Treatment Plan

- Methylphenidate, atomoxetine, or clonidine
- Family therapy
- Supportive therapy

### Discussion

The treatment of attention-deficit hyperactivity disorder (ADHD) must include the use of psychostimulants. These include methylphenidate and amphetamine salts.

- In children with tics, methylphenidate can worsen the tics.
- Methylphenidate can cause growth hormone suppression.

Another option is atomoxetine. Common side effects include headaches, insomnia, and GI problems.

### Final Diagnosis

Attention deficit hyperactivity disorder

# CASE 13

## Chief Complaint

"Please take me home!"

## History and Physical Examination

A 32-year-old female G3P3 is taken to the emergency department by her husband due to bizarre behavior and recent weight loss of approximately 15 pounds since the birth of their youngest son 3 weeks ago. She denies that anything is wrong and believes her husband is "exaggerating." Her husband reports that she has been isolative and has not been interacting with others, including her children. At home he has been the main caretaker since she has not shown any interest in them.

When asked about this, she responds that she is "tired" but will "snap out of it." She has had periods of emotional lability and cries frequently. During the last few days, she has become concerned that her son has an "abnormality." She believes that the baby is defective and so frequently stays up at night watching him sleep. Her husband has heard her whispering to herself and when asked what she is doing, she quickly becomes quiet. Last night her husband found her holding a knife over the baby's crib while whispering, "You are not normal." He quickly took the knife away and took her to the bedroom. While there, she appeared suspicious and appeared dazed and confused as to what had just happened.

## Differential Diagnosis

1. Bipolar disorder
2. Brief psychotic disorder with postpartum onset
3. Major depressive disorder with psychotic features
4. Hypothyroidism
5. Major depressive disorder with peripartum onset
6. Substance-induced psychotic disorder

## Initial Diagnostic Plan/Test Results

| | |
|---|---|
| • Urine toxicology screen | Negative |
| • Thyroid function tests | Normal |

## Further Diagnostic Plan/Test Results

- Past personal and family history:
  - Prior history of bipolar disorder
  - Interview with patient relative if available
  - Patient had responded well to lithium and olanzapine

### Treatment Plan

- Hospitalize
- Behavioral therapy
- Antipsychotics and/or lithium therapy (if appropriate)

### Discussion

Brief psychotic disorder with postpartum onset is considered a psychiatric emergency. The patient should be placed in a safe environment to ensure she will not harm herself or the baby. If she wishes to have contact with the baby, the visits must be supervised to assure the baby's safety.

No pharmacologic agents should be prescribed to a mother who is breast-feeding so patient must assure you she will not breast-feed her baby since she is on medications.

### Final Diagnosis

Brief psychotic disorder with postpartum onset

# CASE 14

## Chief Complaint

"He started it!"

## History and Physical Examination

A 14-year-old boy is brought to the emergency department due to disruptive behavior at school. According to the teacher, he assaulted another boy while in the cafeteria. He has a history of compulsively doing things such as grabbing others. You notice that he frequently blinks his eyes and continuously clears his throat. When you begin to ask him questions, he begins to bark and you are unable to continue. Upon interviewing his mother, she reports that he has been in special education since the age of 8. In school, he does not get along with the other children since he fights with them when they laugh at him. He cannot follow rules and is a sore loser. She reports that his first tics began at the age of 7 when he started to blink his eyes, though this lasted for more than a year unnoticed.

## Differential Diagnosis

1. Obsessive compulsive disorder (OCD)
2. Attention deficit hyperactivity disorder (ADHD)
3. Tourette's disorder

## Treatment Plan

- Antipsychotic medications to help control the tics
- Family therapy
- Behavioral therapy

## Discussion

Pharmacotherapy is the most effective treatment for Tourette's disorder. However, patients with mild symptoms may not need treatment. Antipsychotic agents (risperidone, olanzapine, haloperidol, and pimozide) are considered to be the treatment of choice. Alternative therapies include alpha-2 adrenergic agonists (clonidine and guanfacine) and the presynaptic dopamine-depleting agent tetrabenazine.

Psychotherapy, although effective in helping the patient deal with the symptoms of the disorder, is not first-line for Tourette's. Behavioral therapy will help control the tics but studies have shown it to be less effective than the use of psychostimulants. It is imperative to assess if there are symptoms of depression since many patients also have problems with self-esteem.

There is a high comorbidity with ADHD and OCD.

- If ADHD is also present, consider the use of an antidepressant to treat the disorder since the psychostimulants will increase the tics when given to treat the ADHD.
- If OCD is also present, consider the use of SSRIs and psychostimulants.

## Final Diagnosis

Tourette's disorder

## CASE 15

### Chief Complaint

"We cannot get him to say anything."

### History and Physical Examination

A 4-year-old boy is referred for an evaluation by his pre-school teacher because he cannot follow directions. In class, he does not communicate with the other children or the teacher. At times he is noted to be aggressive and hyperactive. The teacher informed the parents that while at the playground, the boy frequently pushes other boys and bites them on the legs.

His parents state that there were no abnormalities during his birth. He is their second child. As a baby, he seemed a happy boy who laughed frequently with others. His parents became concerned that he did not speak much or even babble a lot. However, his pediatrician assured them that he was normal and that sometimes boys develop language at a much later age than girls. His parents have also observed that he does not turn when his name is called and shows great interest in the sound of the washer and dryer. At times, he can be found standing next to them while rocking back and forth.

### Differential Diagnosis

1. Autism spectrum disorder
2. Schizophrenia, childhood type
3. Deafness

### Initial Diagnostic Plan/Test Results

- IQ test: score of 55
- Audiogram: normal hearing

### Treatment Plan

1. Antipsychotic medication (only if accompanied by continued disruptive or harmful behavior)
2. Behavioral therapy
3. Family therapy

### Discussion

Autism spectrum disorders (ASDs) are characterized by social-interaction difficulties, communication challenges, and a tendency to engage in repetitive behaviors. Symptoms of ASD and their severity vary widely across these 3 core areas:

- Deficits in social-emotional reciprocity
- Deficits in nonverbal communicative behaviors used for social interaction
- Deficits in developing, maintaining, and understanding relationships

**CLINICAL PEARL**

DSM-5 merges 4 former DSM-IV-TR disorders:

- Autistic disorder
- Asperger's disorder
- Childhood disintegrative disorder
- 'Catch-all diagnosis' of pervasive developmental disorder not otherwise specified

Taken together, they may result in relatively mild challenges for someone on the high functioning end of the autism spectrum. For others, symptoms may be more severe, as when repetitive behaviors and lack of spoken language interfere with everyday life.

The goal of treatment for autism spectrum disorder is to increase prosocial behavior and decrease the aggressive behavior. Another goal is to improve the development of both verbal and nonverbal communication.

Given the patient's likely diagnosis of intellectual disability (intellectual developmental disorder) as well, he would benefit from simple behavioral interventions to encourage the use of language and self-care skills. The parents would also benefit from support and counseling. If not aggressive, educational and behavioral therapy would be the treatment of choice.

### Final Diagnosis

Autism spectrum disorder

## CASE 16

### Chief Complaint

"I can't see."

### History and Physical Examination

A 25-year-old woman comes to the clinic with reports that she woke up from a nap 2 days ago and was unable to see. There is no history of head trauma, headache, or dizziness prior to this. There are no other accompanying symptoms. Further history-taking reveals that 1 day prior to the loss of vision, the patient caught her boyfriend in bed with another woman. The patient says that although she was very upset about that, she did not want to lose him. The sister accompanying her today reports that, despite the blindness, the patient was able to negotiate her way between her room and the bathroom without hurting herself. Vital signs and physical examination are normal.

Neurologic examination is essentially normal. Both pupils are briskly reactive to direct and consensual light stimuli. There are no lateralizing signs. The patient is calm and pleasant throughout the interview and evaluation. Her mood is euthymic, and her affect is appropriate and full. She does not appear anxious or worried about her sudden blindness. The responses are appropriate, and there are no psychotic symptoms elicited. Cognitive functions are intact.

### Differential Diagnosis

1. Conversion disorder (functional neurologic symptom disorder)
2. Ophthalmologic problems
3. Malingering
4. Somatic symptom disorder

### Initial Diagnostic Plan/Test Results

| | |
|---|---|
| • Refer to ophthalmology and neurology | • Normal |
| • Cortical-evoked potential | • Normal |

### Treatment Plan

Resolution is usually spontaneous but may be helped by insight-oriented supportive or behavioral therapy, with emphasis on issues of stress and coping.

### Discussion

Conversion disorder (functional neurological symptom disorder) is characterized by the presence of one or more neurologic symptoms that cannot be explained by a known neurologic or medical disorder. There may or may not be a psychological factor associated with the onset or exacerbation of symptoms. The production of symptoms is not voluntary and causes clinically significant distress or impairment in social, occupational, or other important areas of functioning.

If true ophthalmologic problems are present, the patient will usually have findings on a neurologic/ophthalmologic examination.

Malingering is characterized by the voluntary production or false presentation of a physical or psychological illness. There is always an identifiable motivation for the production of such symptoms, which may fall under one of the following categories:

- To avoid responsibility, punishment, or a difficult situation
- To receive compensation, drugs, and another material thing
- To retaliate or "get back" at someone

### Final Diagnosis

Conversion disorder (functional neurological symptom disorder)

# PART III

# ETHICS

# Ethics 17

## CASE 1

### Ethical Issue

Informed consent/refusal; exceptions

### History and Physical Examination

A 22-year-old woman is brought to the emergency department by a friend because of a sudden onset of headache, stiff neck, vomiting, photophobia, and fever 38.8 C (102.0 F). A lumbar puncture is performed, and Gram stain of the cerebrospinal fluid reveals gram-positive cocci in pairs, CSF protein 1.5 g/L, and CSF glucose 23 mg/dL. The physician prescribes immediate antibiotics. As the nurse is hanging the intravenous medication, the patient—who appears confused—screams that she won't have the medicine because the nurse is trying to poison her. She tries to pull out her IV.

### Preliminary Questions

1. What are the medical indications for treatment?
2. Is this a life-threatening emergency?
3. What goals of medicine can be achieved in this case?

### Ethical Considerations

- Does this patient have the capacity to make medical decisions for herself? If not, who should make decisions on her behalf?
- Should the patient's refusal of treatment be respected?
- Do these circumstances warrant an exception to the legal and ethical doctrine of informed consent or refusal?

### Basic Ethics Correlate

Competence is a legal issue, not a medical one. Only a court can decide if a patient is incompetent. From an ethical and legal standpoint, all adult patients are considered competent unless specifically proven otherwise.

Any physician—not just a psychiatrist—can determine whether or not a patient has the capacity to understand medical and treatment issues. That determination by the physician is based on whether there is, for example, an organic delirium due to a medical condition. Is there alcohol/drug intoxication? Is there meningitis (as seen in this case)? Does the patient have a psychiatric disorder? The conclusions of the physician are based primarily on neurologic exams and assessment of the patient's comprehension, memory, judgment, and reasoning skills.

A physician should always assume that **patients have capacity** to make their own decisions unless there is clear behavioral evidence that indicates otherwise. There are 3 primary examples that **show lack of capacity**:

1. Attempted suicide
2. Grossly psychotic and dysfunctional behavior
3. Physical or mental state in the patient that prevents simple communication, including emergency situations in which patient is unconscious or delirious

## Discussion

A patient is presumed by law to be competent unless there has been judicial determination of legal incompetence. In this case, the patient appears to lack the mental and emotional capacity to refuse treatment. Her belief that the nurse is trying to poison her seems delusional and may be related to her clinical condition.

Based on the patient's presentation, age, and lab findings, the diagnosis is likely *Streptococcus pneumoniae* meningitis. Adults with bacterial meningitis commonly present with both altered mental status and confusion. Given this diagnosis, the patient does not have the mental capacity to make an informed decision, and her refusal of treatment should be overridden.

If a patient's condition is life-threatening and the physician believes that the patient lacks the capacity to decide, emergency facilities typically have a policy to override refusals of life-saving therapy by incapacitated patients. In other words, the most appropriate immediate action for a physician in this emergency situation is to administer appropriate medical care.

One might also consider whether the patient in this case has a mental disorder (brought on by the infection) that makes her dangerous to herself. Involuntary treatment for the mental disorder may also be justified after appropriate treatment measures for meningitis have been instituted and the patient has been stabilized.

If a patient is legally competent and has the capacity to make medical decisions, even life-saving therapy may be refused. Physicians may, however, try to persuade patients whose refusal of treatment seems irrational to accept treatment.

This patient did not have an advance directive or a legally appointed agent authorized to make health-care decisions for her. Steps should be taken to save her life and restore her capacity to make decisions for herself (if possible). One might even challenge a refusal of treatment by a surrogate decision-maker in this case. Although involuntary treatment seems justified here, efforts should be made to contact the patient's relatives.

## EXAMPLE CASE

A 22-year-old woman is diagnosed with bacterial meningitis. The physician prescribes antibiotics and the patient refuses therapy. The patient expresses irrational thoughts and removes her IV line.

- Because altered mental status and confusion are commonly seen in adults with bacterial meningitis, the health care providers should conclude that the patient does not have the mental capacity to make an informed decision.
- Therefore, her refusal of treatment should be overridden and the antibiotics should be administered in this life-threatening situation.

### Management Plan

1. Clarify involuntary treatment situations when a patient refuses recommended treatment. *Refusal of treatment* is not sufficient to determine that a patient lacks capacity to decide.
    - When a patient does not have a life-threatening disease or injury, it may be necessary to seek judicial determination of competency or to locate family members who may help to persuade a patient to accept medically indicated treatment.
    - In this case, the indications for treatment and the case for making an exception to the usual informed consent requirements are strong. Examples should be given to illustrate circumstances when a refusal of treatment, even in an emergency facility, should be respected.
2. Explore the legal and ethical doctrine of informed consent or refusal. Patients must have the capacity to take in and process information about their medical condition.
    - Physicians should explain the diagnosis, prognosis, treatment options, and benefits/risks of treatment, including the consequences of no treatment.
    - A patient's consent or refusal may not be coerced or manipulated, but physicians should recommend and even try to persuade the best treatment option.

### Resolution

Emergency exception to informed refusal of therapy

# CASE 2

## Ethical Issue

Brain death; declaration of death

## History and Physical Examination

A 62-year-old woman with a history of hypertension is brought to the hospital after allegedly placing her hand on the back of her head, complaining of a terrible headache, and collapsing. Paramedics were called and transported her rapidly to the hospital.

In the emergency room the patient is found to be without spontaneous respiration and movement or response to painful stimuli. Her pupils are fixed and dilated. Corneal, oculovestibular, gag, cough, and oculocephalic reflexes are all absent. Spontaneous respirations are also absent. The patient is intubated and admitted to the ICU. She is placed under the care of a family physician who is newly in practice and who is seeing emergency-room patients who have no attendings at this hospital. The resident staff approach and ask this physician to declare the patient brain dead so that her organs can be harvested, if possible.

## Preliminary Questions

1. Should this physician declare this patient brain dead?
2. If not this physician, then who should do so?
3. What is the process for declaring brain death?

## Ethical Considerations

- If the patient is declared dead and has a valid donor card, organs can be taken for transplantation. All 50 states have adopted the Uniform Anatomical Gift Act, which records individuals' desire to donate their viable organs upon their death.
- If the patient is dead but does not have a donor card, next of kin may be asked for consent to donate the organs of their family member. Some states require the hospitals to have a protocol to ask family members to donate organs of a deceased relative.
- Although the patient's desire to donate organs is sufficient under the law, it is common practice to ask available family members as well. This may be based on consideration of family sentiments or mistaken concern about legal authority. If family members object, physicians or hospitals sometimes disregard the patient's legally valid intent to donate organs. Doing so is technically illegal but is sometimes rationalized as a way of avoiding conflict, bad publicity, and the like.
- Declaration of death, especially if organs are being harvested, should closely follow institutional protocol.

### Basic Ethics Correlate

The 2 primary methods of defining death are **termination of heartbeat** and **brain death**.

- The patient is considered legally dead if the heart is still beating but the patient is brain dead.
- A determination of brain death is made only if the physician has excluded all other potential causes of dramatically decreased brainstem and respiratory function.
- Appropriate determination of brain death is essential before patient organs can be harvested for donation.

## Discussion

Most generalist physicians, especially new doctors, are not adept at diagnosing brain death. The diagnosis should be made by one skilled and familiar with the manifestations of brain death, such as a neurologist, neurosurgeon, or intensivist.

Brain death is defined as the total, irreversible loss of total brain functioning (that is, function of cerebral hemispheres and brainstem). Examination for the declaration of brain death must demonstrate both these elements: **total** and **irreversible**. Several questions must be answered and findings demonstrated:

- Reason for patient's brain death must be known
- Confounding factors (i.e., conditions generating a clinical picture that looks like brain death but is not) must be ruled out, including drug overdose (particularly barbiturates) and hypothermia
- Neurologic exam must show total lack of functioning of the cerebrum and brainstem, including **absence of all the following**:
  - Awareness of the environment
  - Spontaneous movements or response to stimuli
  - Pupillary response
  - Doll's eyes maneuver to both head movement and cold calorics
  - Spontaneous respirations to formal apnea testing (formal apnea testing has a specific protocol)
  - On rare occasions, spinal reflexes may remain functional
- Exam results must remain consistent for a period of time, generally not <6 hrs. When ancillary tests are not available, formal exams should be spaced no closer than 24 hrs.
- Ancillary tests may include ≥1 of the following: brain flow studies (**best**), evoked potentials, and EEG. There are strict criteria for the use of these tests in the diagnosis of brain death. The physician must be familiar with the particular hospital policy. While these tests can provide evidence of the brain death, they **do not take the place of the exam**. Furthermore, ancillary tests are not performed when the etiology of the brain death is clear and the exam is consistent with brain death.

| Management Plan | Results |
| --- | --- |
| CT scan (noninfused) to evaluate for cerebral hemorrhage (suspected on basis of history) | Massive pontine hemorrhage |
| Temperature (rectal) checked | 37.2 C (99.0 F) (rectal); hypothermia ruled out |
| Blood work to include toxicology screen; if history supports a possibility of poisoning or other motor paralysis, check for that as well | No evidence of toxins/overdose |
| Consultation with physician adept in evaluating brain death | Physician adept in brain death evaluation consulted |

| Further Evaluation | Results |
| --- | --- |
| Neurologic exam | • Complete absence of any evidence of cerebral or brainstem functioning<br>• Unresponsive<br>• Absent pupillary reflexes, corneal reflexes, doll's eyes (to cold water and movement), spontaneous movements, and movements in response to painful stimuli<br>• No spontaneous respirations, even to formal apnea testing |
| Physician orders blood flow study | Total absence of blood flow to the brain over 10 min of study |
| Second neurologic exam | Done immediately after blood flow study and about 3 hrs after first exam: unchanged |

The checklists below are adapted from the **American Academy of Neurology: Determining Brain Death in Adults** and the **Checklist for Determination of Brain Death.**

**Prerequisites** (all must be checked)

- Coma, irreversible and cause known
- Neuroimaging explains coma
- CNS depressant drug effect absent (if indicated toxicology screen; if barbiturates given, serum level <10 μg/mL)
- No evidence of residual paralytics (electrical stimulation if paralytics used)
- Absence of severe acid-base, electrolyte, endocrine abnormality
- Normothermia or mild hypothermia (core temperature >36 C)
- Systolic BP ≥100 mm Hg
- No spontaneous respirations

**Apnea testing** (all must be checked or apnea test is aborted)

- Patient is hemodynamically stable
- Ventilator adjusted to provide normocarbia ($PaCO_2$ 35–45 mm Hg)

- Patient preoxygenated with 100% $FiO_2$ for >10 min to $PaO_2$ > 200 mm Hg
- Patient well-oxygenated with PEEP of 5 cm water
- Provide oxygen via a suction catheter to the level of the carina at 6 L/min or attach T-piece with CPAP at 10 cm $H_2O$
- Disconnect ventilator
- Spontaneous respirations absent
- Arterial blood gas drawn at 8–10 min, patient reconnected to ventilator
- $PCO_2$ ≥60 mm Hg, or 20 mm Hg rise from normal baseline value

**Examination** (all must be checked)

- Pupils nonreactive to bright light
- Corneal reflex absent
- Oculocephalic reflex absent (tested only if C-spine integrity ensured)
- Oculovestibular reflex absent
- No facial movement to noxious stimuli at supraorbital nerve, temporomandibular joint
- Gag reflex absent
- Cough reflex absent to tracheal suctioning
- Absence of motor response to noxious stimuli in all 4 limbs (spine-mediated reflexes are permissible)

**Ancillary testing** (only 1 needs to be performed) (to be ordered only if patient factors prohibit clinical examination from being fully performed or if apnea testing is inconclusive or aborted)

- Cerebral angiogram
- HMPAO SPECT
- EEG
- TCD

## EXAMPLE CASE

A 62-year-old woman is brought to the hospital after reporting a horrible headache and then collapsing. In the emergency department, the patient is unresponsive and has no apparent brainstem function. She is placed under the care of a new physician, and a resident asks that the patient be declared brain dead so that her organs can be harvested.

- The new physician cannot declare brain death; the diagnosis of brain death should be made by a skilled and experienced physician.
- A number of tests must be performed and show specific results before a diagnosis of brain death can be made.

### Management Plan

At this point, the patient should be spoken of as "dead," even if the patient remains on life support for organ perfusion for a time.

- The patient's family should understand that the patient is dead.
- Termination of support systems should be done as soon as feasible.
- If the family wishes to say goodbye to their relative, time should be given.
- It is most honest and kind to explain the situation to the family in clear terms.

### Resolution

Diagnosis of brain death

# CASE 3

## Ethical Issue

Confidentiality

## History and Physical Examination

A basic scientist is admitted to the hospital for pneumonia. Both the physician assigned to this patient and the physician's best friend were students under the patient, who was a professor at their medical school. At that time, the physician observed this man behaving bizarrely on several occasions and frequently noticed alcohol on his breath while he was teaching. It was a standing class joke that he had a bad alcohol abuse problem.

The physician and the physician's friend are having lunch together in the cafeteria when the friend remarks on seeing the physician's name on this patient's chart. She asks, "Well, were we right back then in medical school? How much of a lush is he?"

## Preliminary Questions

1. Is the physician's friend involved in the care of this patient?
2. If she is, is this information relevant to this case?
3. If yes, can it be disclosed in this environment without breaching confidentiality?

## Discussion

The physician's friend is not involved in this man's care. Hence, the physician cannot answer her question. If she were involved, the physician would have to judge the relevance of the information requested. If it were deemed relevant, the physician must then consider whether it can be disclosed and in what setting. Cafeteria discussions of this sort, though common, are inappropriate.

The physician has a patient-physician relationship with this man. As a result, the physician is ethically obliged not to disclose personal, sensitive information, including both medical information and any social information that might arise as a result of caring for him. To enter into any discussion of the patient with a friend would be inappropriate.

### Basic Ethics Correlate

Apart from certain ethical exceptions, patient confidentiality is absolute. There are several patient confidentiality laws designed to protect patient privacy and autonomy. Breaching patient confidentiality is an ethical violation with potential legal consequences. In this case, only clinicians who are directly involved in the care of the patient should have access to the patient's medical information.

Exceptions to patient confidentiality include the following:

- Duty to warn and duty to protect (Tarasoff case)
- The patient is a threat to himself/herself (suicide) or others (homicide, abuse)
- Specific situations for infectious diseases and STDs

In certain rare instances, physicians may be obliged to breach patient confidentiality. These instances occur when the patient poses a serious, immediate threat to himself or another individual. In such circumstances, the physician is advised to consult with another trusted colleague or legal counsel prior to disclosing otherwise confidential information.

### EXAMPLE CASE

A former medical school instructor is admitted to the hospital for pneumonia, and placed under the care of a physician who was once his student. Based on interactions from prior years, the physician suspects that the instructor is abusing alcohol. While at lunch, a former classmate and personal friend asks the physician if their former instructor is an alcoholic.

### Resolution

The physician cannot answer the friend's question about the drinking habits of their former instructor. In fact, he cannot even acknowledge that the former instructor is his patient. Except in rare cases where the patient may be harmful to self or others, the physician must keep patient confidentiality—even from another colleague.

# CASE 4

## Ethical Issue

Do-not-resuscitate orders; futility of therapy

## History and Physical Examination

A 64-year-old Hispanic woman with known metastatic ovarian carcinoma is admitted to the hospital. She is very ill but competent. She states, "I want everything done in the event of an emergency." She is admitted to the floor, and therapy is initiated for her current problem.

Her medical records show that discussion about do-not-resuscitate (DNR) status took place during previous admissions, the most recent of which were 4 wks ago and 2 wks ago. The patient was briefly made DNR when hospitalized 4 wks ago, but the DNR order was revoked during that hospitalization. During the hospitalization 2 wks ago, the patient refused a DNR order. Although she appears relatively stable today, her disease is very advanced: She could code during this hospitalization. This patient's medical condition is such that cardiopulmonary resuscitation seems a futile therapy. Discussion about DNR is again raised with the patient, who reiterates that she wants everything done. She says, "I know that once patients are made DNR, nobody pays attention to them anymore."

## Preliminary Questions

1. Is the patient in an advanced stage of her disease?
2. Is there possible impending cardiac arrest?
3. Is there patient-physician disagreement about DNR status?
4. What action should be taken if the patient goes into cardiac arrest?

### Basic Ethics Correlate

Patients should always be given the chance to establish DNR orders, and the physician should follow them. These discussions should occur early in treatment, and the decision on DNR status should be made by a competent patient or the patient's surrogate.

- DNR orders refer only to cardiopulmonary resuscitation.
- If the patient "codes," all the other ongoing treatments should continue.
- In the event of a cardiopulmonary arrest, there is an implied consent on the part of the patient unless the patient has specifically refused in advance.

The following **misperceptions about DNR orders** are common. Be prepared to correct such errors of understanding through discussion with the patient:

- DNR means that the patient is "terminal" and about to die.
- DNR orders prevent all treatment measures, not just cardiopulmonary resuscitation.
- DNR orders mean that the patient will receive a lower standard of care in all treatment measures.
- Once a DNR order is instituted, it cannot be revoked.

### Discussion

Cardiopulmonary resuscitation (CPR) was designed as an intervention to prevent sudden, unexpected cardiac death, but today it is used much more widely. The Joint Commission on Accreditation of Healthcare Organizations mandates that all hospitals have a DNR policy. Policies differ among hospitals; it is critical that physicians know the policy of the hospital where they work. In this case, the hospital's policy states that CPR is to be performed unless a DNR order is affirmatively recorded in the patient's chart. The basis for this policy is the special status of CPR as a medical intervention for preventing unanticipated death.

The patient may have many reasons for refusing a DNR order, including fear that nothing will be done for her or fear that she will be abandoned by medical providers if she is made DNR. Literature supports her concerns: Patients often receive less "caring" and attention once a DNR order is entered. It is important to elicit from the patient what led her to establish and then revoke the previous DNR order. The patient's reasons should be identified, not invalidated. The physician must help her reach the most appropriate decision regarding CPR. The most appropriate decision may be to perform CPR, even if medically it seems unwise.

A helpful Jonsen, Siegler, and Winslade definition of medical futility is "an effort to achieve a result that is remotely possible, but that reasoning and experience suggest is highly improbable, and that cannot be systematically reproduced." Patients' views must be considered before determining that therapy is futile. Even if the predicted chance of success is small, that chance is of great importance to the patient. It is not clear at this time that DNR would be futile therapy in this patient. Even if it were, the hospital policy does not permit not doing CPR unless a DNR order is entered in the chart.

| Management Plan | Results |
|---|---|
| Explore patient's reasons for not wanting DNR | • Patient is afraid of abandonment by the medical and nursing staff<br>• Physician attempts to reassure her that this will not occur<br>• The chaplains and others talk with her, and the patient continues to want CPR<br>• A colleague of the physician suggests, "Just do a slow code when it happens" |

### Additional History

Three days later the patient has a cardiac arrest.

#### EXAMPLE CASE

A 64-year-old woman with known metastatic ovarian carcinoma is admitted to the hospital and deemed competent. She states that she wants "everything done in the event of an emergency." Her past medical history shows that she was previously made a DNR but then revoked the DNR order. The patient reiterates that she wants "everything done." The physician believes that cardiopulmonary resuscitation would be a futile therapy in this patient.

### Management Plan

The physician is obliged to do a full code on this patient. It is clear that the patient understands what is involved with CPR. Although her medical team might not agree with her reasons, that is not the most relevant matter in this setting. It does not matter whether the physician agrees with the patient's refusal of a DNR order. It would be dishonest to the patient and to the broader society to act counter to the patient's wishes regarding resuscitation.

At the same time, the physician is not obliged to run the code longer in this patient than would be done in another patient with similar medical problems. If the patient survives the arrest, the physician may then consider other aspects of her case management, including discontinuation of therapies, if appropriate.

### Resolution

CPR is done in the absence of a DNR order.

# CASE 5

## Ethical Issue

Refusal of blood products on religious grounds; informed consent/refusal

## History and Physical Examination

A 54-year-old man comes to the office for his first visit since he moved to this area. He has a known history of hypertension and bleeding esophageal varices. Physical examination reveals no acute mental problems.

During conversation, this patient says, "Doctor, I know I have problems that you might usually treat with blood. But you can't with me. I'm a practicing Jehovah's Witness. If you give me blood, it's a horrible offense to Jehovah's law and to me. Even if it means that I might die someday, you cannot give me blood."

## Preliminary Question

1. Is this a competent or incompetent refusal of potentially life-saving therapy?

## Ethical Considerations

- Is the patient legally competent?
- Is the patient clinically competent?
- Does the patient understand implications of his request?
- Can the physician meet the patient's demands?

### Basic Ethics Correlate

A competent patient has the right to refuse any treatment including life-saving measures, such as blood products, for any reason. However, parents cannot withhold life- or limb-saving treatment from their children, regardless of religious beliefs. Clinically, if a child needs blood to save their life, the health care provider must administer the blood. Withholding life-saving (or limb-saving) therapy for a child is comparable to child abuse.

If parents refuse permission to treat their child, the following rules should be applied:

- If immediate emergency, go ahead and treat.
- If not immediate, but still critical (e.g., type 1 diabetes), generally the child is declared a ward of the court and the court grants permission.
- If not life- or limb-threatening (e.g., child needs minor stitches), listen to the parents.

## Discussion

This patient is an adult and presumed legally competent unless formally adjudicated as incompetent. He appears to be clinically competent and to understand his medical condition, the potential need and benefits of receiving blood, and the potential problems if he does not get blood.

Although the patient appears to understand, it is appropriate for the physician to specifically ask if the patient knows that his position might result in death in some emergency settings. The physician should explain that this condition places him at high risk for needing blood products and for potential death if they are not provided.

Responding to a patient's refusal of treatment is highly individual. Physicians must be certain that they can comply with the patient's request. If they can, they should inform the patient and document the chart. If they cannot comply, they should inform the patient and recommend that a new physician be found. The physician should never lie about promising compliance that will not happen. Ideally, there should be other clinicians present during these types of discussions.

## EXAMPLE CASE

A 54-year-old man with a history of hypertension and bleeding esophageal varices comes to the physician. The patient appears competent. During the interview, the patient indicates that he is a practicing Jehovah's Witness and cannot receive blood products. The patient indicates that he understands that he may die if he does not receive blood products and continues to maintain his request that no blood products be administered under any circumstance.

### Management Plan

The physician should regularly do both of the following:

- Confirm that the patient continues to competently express this belief
- Determine whether the physician can continue to manage the patient's case with this restriction on care

In general, competent patients are able to refuse medical interventions, even if that refusal will result in death. Jehovah's Witnesses have a longstanding, well-recognized history of refusing certain blood products on the basis of their interpretation of the Bible. Imposing blood products on these patients against their will is unethical.

Note that this case does not deal with a juvenile patient or with an adult patient who appears to be coerced or otherwise incompetent.

The physician is generally not required to accept a patient who places restrictions or demands on care that the physician finds ethically untenable. However, the physician should not abandon the patient. If the physician is unable to fulfill the patient's request, care should be taken to help identify alternate health care providers.

The physician should regularly confirm (1) that the patient continues to competently express this belief, and (2) that the physician himself/herself can manage the patient's case with this restriction on care.

### Resolution

Physician accepts refusal of blood products by a competent Jehovah's Witness.

# CASE 6

## Ethical Issue

Medical error

## History and Physical Examination

While on call in the hospital, the physician is summoned to deal with a patient who is very agitated. The patient is a 34-year-old woman who is screaming, "I'm being killed! The hospital wants to poison me!" The patient states that the nurse gave her the wrong medication, and she demands that the physician take action. "I'm sure I'm going to die. Please help me." The patient was given aripiprazole 20 mg instead of ziprasidone 20 mg. The patient says she was hesitant when given the wrong pill but eventually took it after the nurse assured her "The doctor ordered it." Later that day, the patient's doctor told the patient that her medication order had not changed.

In conversation with the physician, the nurse confides that the patient was given another patient's medication. "Please don't tell anyone. I'm sure I'll be fired, and I can't lose my job because I am a single parent with 2 small children." The nurse continues, "I am sorry for the mistake. The good news is that the medication the patient received is in the same drug class. She is not likely to experience any adverse effects."

## Preliminary Questions

1. Does the patient have the right to know about the mistake?
2. If she does, when should you tell her about the mistake?
3. Should you respect the nurse's wishes not to tell anyone?

### Basic Ethics Correlate

In this case study, the physician did not make the error. However, it is still his responsibility to take care of the patient and ensure that she is fully informed.

When a physician makes a mistake, the physician should immediately inform the patient of the error. It is the physician's ethical duty to take responsibility for the error. When an error is discovered, the physician should first ensure that the patient receives proper care and attention. Then the physician should discuss the error in detail with the patient.

The physician should never place blame for an error on a nurse or medical resident. From a malpractice standpoint, every prescription that leaves a physician's office and every step taken in a surgical procedure is the responsibility of that physician.

## Discussion

The patient has the right to know about the medical error; it is the physician's duty to inform her of the mistake even if it means that the physician or nurse will get in trouble. While job loss would be unfortunate for the nurse who is a parent with small children, the physician's primary concern is always the patient. Furthermore, the patient has a right to know that an error has occurred even though the incorrect medication has the same drug class and a similar side effect profile as the correct medication.

It is the physician's responsibility to ensure that the patient is always fully informed about her medical condition. The damage to the physician–patient relationship would be irrevocable if the physician does not tell the truth. The physician cannot honor the nurse's wishes: It is the physician's duty to be honest with the patient.

It would be appropriate to tell the patient about the error in her room or with family members. She is now agitated; the physician should take care to inform her of the error in a way that is least likely to escalate the situation. It is possible that the patient will be calmed by learning that the new medication is in the same class as the intended medication and therefore should not cause a medical problem.

## EXAMPLE CASE

A patient is profoundly agitated that she was administered the wrong medication by a hospital nurse. The patient insists that something be done about the error. The nurse admits giving the patient aripiprazole 20 mg instead of ziprasidone 20 mg but asks the physician to not tell anyone about the error. The nurse, who is a single parent with 2 small children, expresses concern about job loss if the error is known. She emphasizes that no harm is likely to come to the patient because the medication given was in the same drug class as the medication that had been prescribed.

### Resolution

The physician tells the patient about the error. The news calms the patient, who realizes it is unlikely that she will experience any adverse effects.

# CASE 7

## Ethical Issue

Partial emancipation

## History and Physical Examination

A 16-year-old girl comes to the community clinic asking for birth control pills. She states that she has been sexually active for 3 years and would like to use oral birth control to avoid pregnancy. She does not want her parents to know, and she asks the clinic staff not to tell them.

The physician seeing this patient is a volunteer at the clinic who finds contraception of any kind morally reprehensible. The physician also considers it inappropriate to withhold any medical information about a minor child from the child's parents.

## Preliminary Questions

- Can a physician treat a patient who is a minor without parental consent?
- Should the physician tell the parents of the patient's sexual activity and request for birth control?
- Should the physician provide birth control pills despite the physician's personal beliefs?
- What should the physician do regarding the physician's personal belief that the patient should not be taking birth control pills?

### Basic Ethics Correlate

Children age <18 are considered to be legally incompetent. Children (minors) cannot make a health-related decision for themselves. Thus they cannot give "informed consent" to authorize a medical procedure or treatment measure. Unless there is an exception, a parent or guardian must give informed consent for all health-related decisions.

Exceptions to the requirement to obtain parental or guardian consent for a minor occur in cases of emancipated minors and partially emancipated minors. Examples of an emancipated minor are:

- Patient age >13 and taking care of self
- Patient who is married
- Patient who is serving in military

Partial emancipation or temporary competence is granted to minors in the cases of:

- Substance and drug-abuse treatment
- Prenatal care
- Sexually transmitted diseases
- Birth control (as seen in this case)

### Discussion

This patient meets the criteria for partial emancipation. Partially emancipated minors are minors who do not need parental consent for treatment of sexually transmitted diseases, prenatal care, contraception, HIV, or substance abuse. The laws were designed to allow the minor to make these decisions without parental consent since access to treatment is a better choice than no possibility of receiving treatment.

A physician does not have to provide services or treatment that the physician finds morally reprehensible. However, the physician must find another doctor who can provide those services. It is the physician's duty to treat the patient. In this case, although the physician may opt to avoid personally providing contraception to the patient, the physician must find an alternative physician for the patient.

**EXAMPLE CASE**

A 16-year-old girl comes to the clinic requesting birth control pills. She does not want her parents informed about the visit or the use of oral contraceptives. The clinic physician finds any type of contraception morally reprehensible.

### Resolution

No treatment is provided by the physician who feels uncomfortable with the request. Instead, the physician finds another doctor who prescribes birth control pills to the patient and does not notify the patient's parents.

# CASE 8

## Ethical Issue

Impaired physician

## History and Physical Examination

A third-year surgical resident finds that he is frequently asked to assist more than usual in the cases and that the attending surgeon is forgetful. Yesterday the attending seemed confused and somewhat disoriented; he had forgotten both the date and the fact that he had a surgery scheduled later that day. The attending is age 69 and, to the resident, appears to have some cognitive decline. When the resident expresses concern on this point, the attending becomes upset and threatens his subordinate with possible termination of the residency.

## Preliminary Questions

1. Is the attending surgeon an impaired physician?
2. If he is, what should the resident do?
3. If the resident reports the attending, can the attending fire the resident from the department?
4. Can the resident lose his/her license for reporting the attending?

### Basic Ethics Correlate

If a health care professional poses a danger to his patients, he must be immediately removed from his duties to prevent patient harm. Examples include using illegal substances, being incompetent, and having selected infectious diseases.

## Discussion

Impairment in a physician may stem from a medical disorder, psychiatric disorder, or substance abuse disorder. Laws vary from state to state but the ethical guidelines are the same: **The impaired physician should be reported to the appropriate authorities, and the reporting physician is expected to follow certain hospital, state, and legal procedures.** The physician who does the reporting is not the one responsible for monitoring the physician. In fact, the monitoring should be done by an independent physician who has no conflict of interest.

It is every physician's duty to report an impaired physician. In this case, it is very clear that the attending surgeon is suffering from cognitive decline, which is affecting patient care: The attending has trouble with memory and appears disoriented. He may be suffering from Alzheimer's dementia or some other disorder.

Reports of impairment usually go to the person's direct supervisor.

- An impaired medical student should be reported to the dean or course director.
- An impaired resident should be reported to the residency director or program chair.
- An impaired attending should be reported to the department chair.
- An impaired physician in the community must be reported to the state board.

In this case, if the resident reports this physician, the resident's job is not in jeopardy. In fact, the resident will be doing the right thing by making the report and preventing further harm. A health care provider cannot be fired for doing the right thing, nor is their license in jeopardy from reporting of any kind. In fact, reporting the attending might ensure that the reported individual receives proper treatment.

## EXAMPLE CASE

A third-year surgical resident encounters a 69-year-old attending physician with apparent cognitive decline. The attending physician is forgetful and frequently asks for more than the usual assistance in cases. After the resident expresses concern, the physician threatens possible termination of the resident.

### Resolution

The resident goes to the director of the department and reports the attending. The department head meets with the attending and compels him to undergo a thorough evaluation. The attending is diagnosed with Alzheimer's disease and started on medication to slow the cognitive decline. The attending's spouse encourages him to retire from the hospital and give up his practice.

# CASE 9

## Ethical Issue

Abortion

## History and Physical Examination

A psychiatrist is called to evaluate a 25-year-old woman who is 9 weeks pregnant. The patient wants an abortion because she is convinced that her baby is "the devil." She believes that her baby is possessed, and thus she wants it terminated: She does not want to be responsible for bringing evil into the world. The patient's husband informs you that he is her decision-maker and that he wants the abortion as well.

## Preliminary Questions

1. Does this patient have the capacity to make this decision?
2. If not, should her decision be granted?
3. Does the husband have the right to authorize an abortion?
4. Should the health care provider follow the husband's decision to grant the abortion?

### Basic Ethics Correlate

Informed consent is a complete discussion of proper information related to a treatment or procedure between a physician and their "competent" patient in which the patient voluntarily agrees to the plan of care and is free of coercion. Full, informed consent requires that the patient has received and understood the following 5 pieces of information:

- Nature of the procedure
- Purpose or rationale
- Risks of the treatment regimen
- Benefits of the treatment regimen
- Alternatives to the recommended treatment regimen

There are times that a physician does not need to obtain informed consent from a patient in order to perform a procedure or administer another form of treatment. These 4 exceptions to informed consent are as follows:

- Emergency situation
- Waiver by the patient
- Patient lacks capacity (as seen in this case) (when they are unconscious, have attempted suicide, are in a grossly psychotic or dysfunctional state, are intoxicated, or are in a physical/mental state that prevents simple communication)
- Therapeutic privilege

### Discussion

The patient clearly does not have the capacity to make decisions at this time: She is suffering from delusions, which diminish her ability to give informed consent. Thus this patient meets the criteria for exceptions to informed consent. (She lacks the capacity to give informed consent.) She should be evaluated and treated with medication to reduce her delusions.

The psychiatrist must act quickly: The patient is in her first trimester, and an abortion, if performed, must occur before the pregnancy reaches the second or third trimester. Some states restrict second-trimester abortions. Third-trimester abortions are not usually done unless the life of the mother is in imminent danger.

In this case, the patient's husband agrees with her wishes for the abortion. However, a woman does not need a husband's consent for abortion. The fetus is considered part of the woman's body, and therefore the husband does not have the authority to make any decision regarding the fetus.

## EXAMPLE CASE

The psychiatrist is summoned to evaluate a 25-year-old woman who is 9 weeks pregnant. The patient is convinced that her baby is the "devil" and is requesting an abortion. The patient's husband states that he is her decision-maker and that he wants the abortion as well.

### Resolution

The psychiatrist begins treatment with antipsychotic medication, and within 3 wks the patient's symptoms have subsided. She is now 12 wks pregnant, and she still wants the abortion. The patient is not delusional and does not believe the fetus is possessed.

The health care provider in this case is the psychiatrist, not the obstetrician, so would not perform any abortions. However, if the patient wanted to abort her pregnancy, she would be able to do so because the pregnancy is still in its first trimester.

## PART IV

# HIGH-YIELD IMAGES

## Dermatology, Radiology, and Ophthalmology

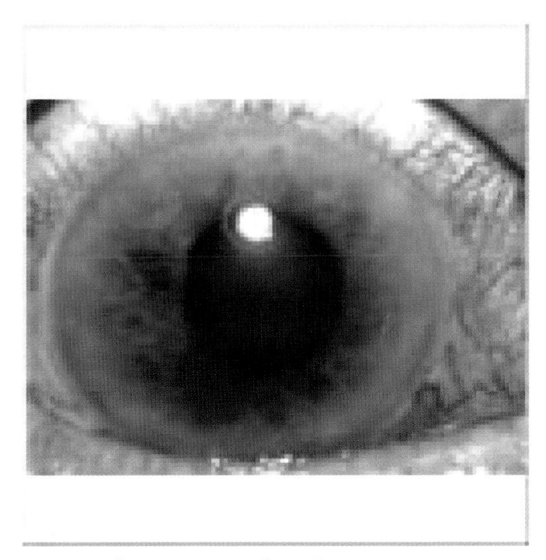

**Acute angle glaucoma**

Reproduced with permission from
International Council of Ophthalmology

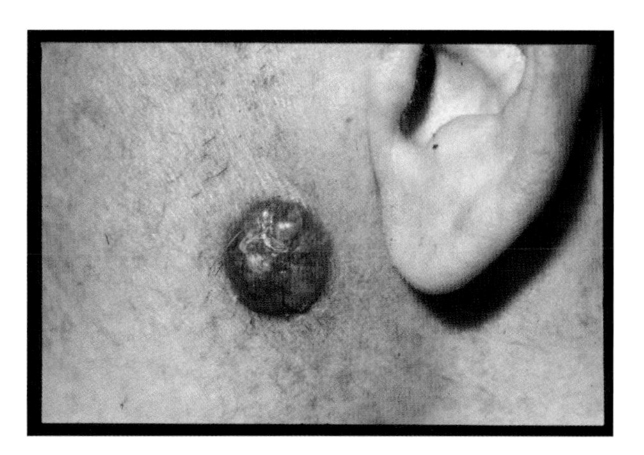

**Basal cell carcinoma**

Reproduced with permission from
DxR Development Group © 2008

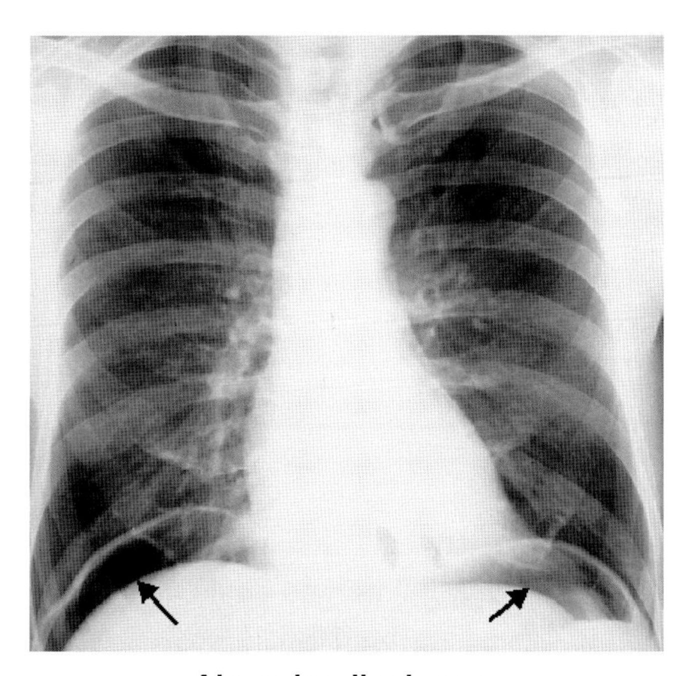

**Air under diaphragm**

Reproduced with permission from
University of Szeged, Faculty of Medicine

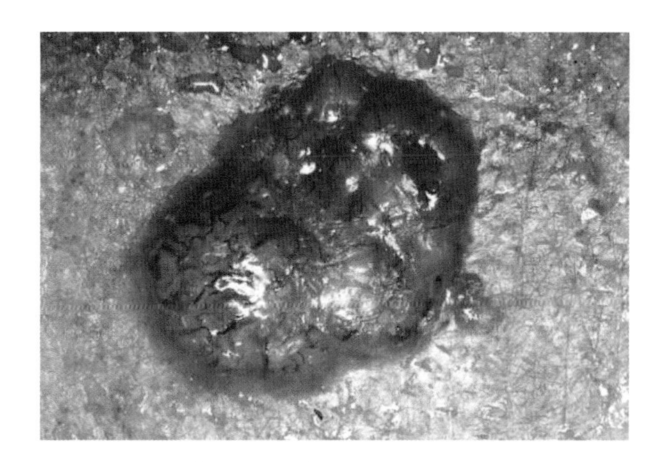

**Basal cell carcinoma**

Reproduced with permission from
John Hendrix, MD

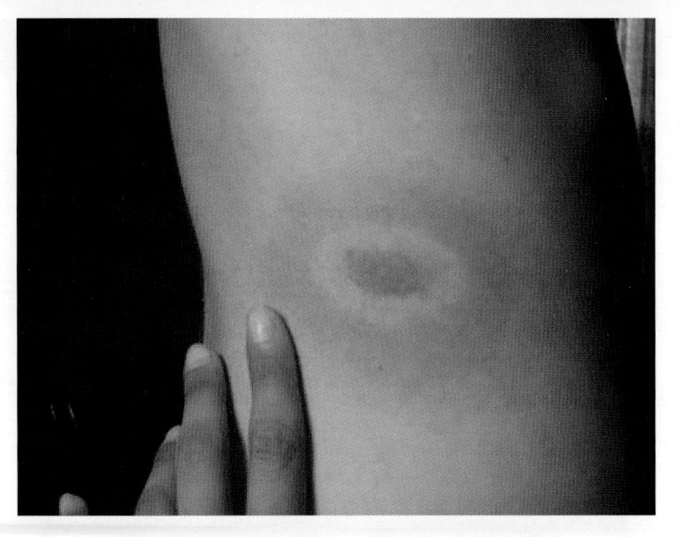

**Bulls-eye Lyme disease rash**

Reproduced with permission from Hannah Garrison (public domain image obtained from wikipedia.com)

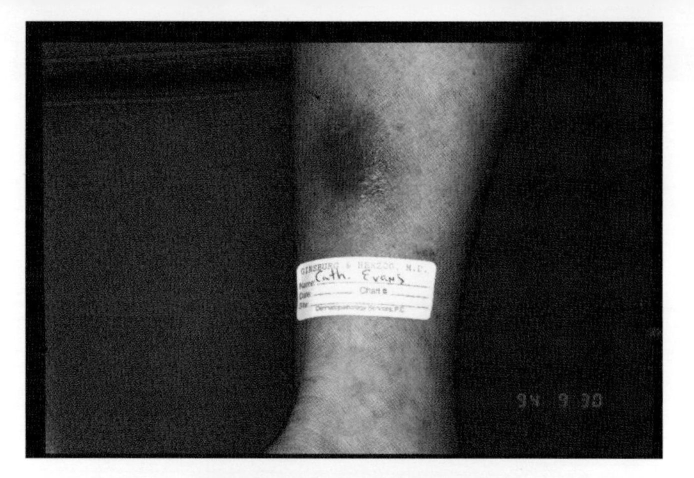

**Erythema nodosum**

Reproduced with permission from DxR Development Group © 2008

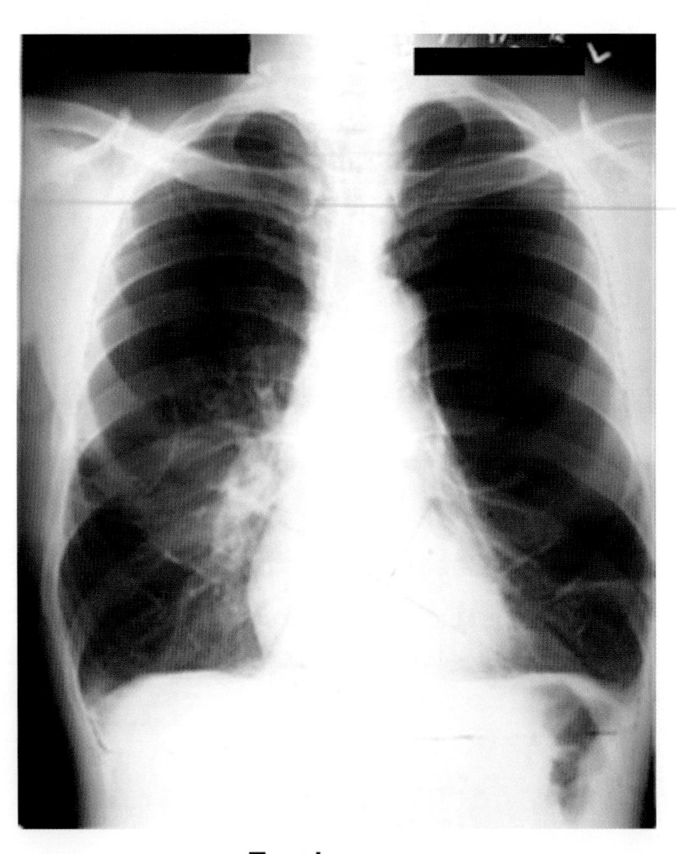

**Emphysema**

Reproduced with permission from wikipedia.org (public domain)

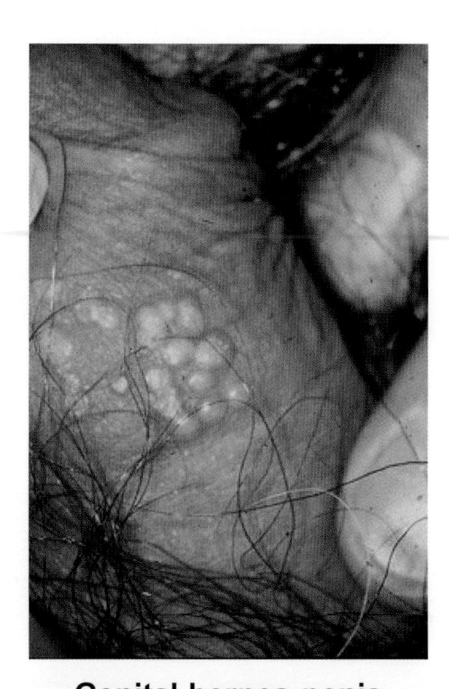

**Genital herpes-penis**

Reproduced with permission from herpes-simplex.org

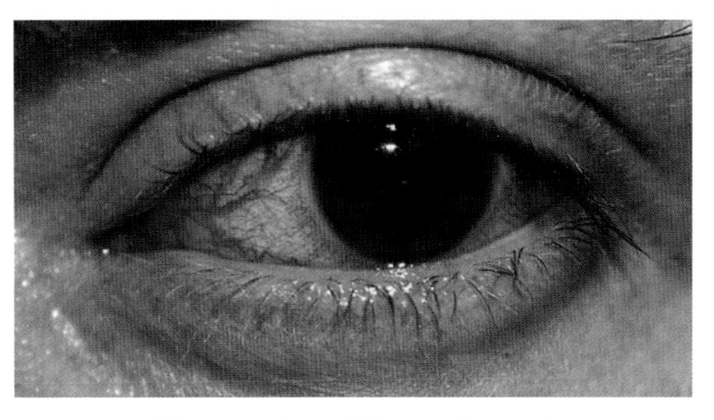

**Herpes keratitis–external**

Reproduced with permission from wikipedia.org (public domain)

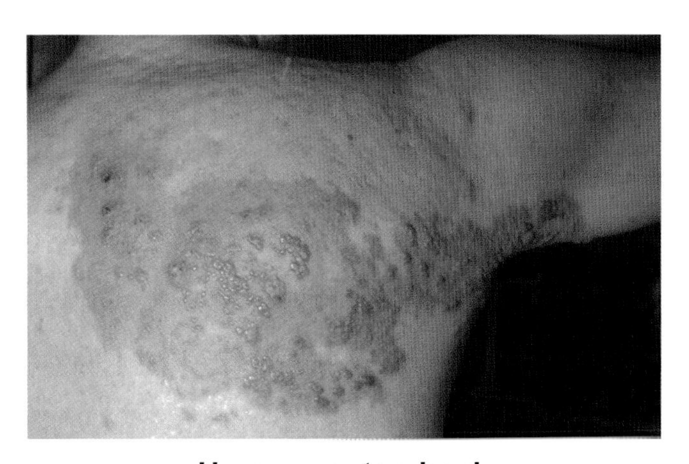

**Herpes zoster–back**

Reproduced with permission from wikipedia.org (public domain)

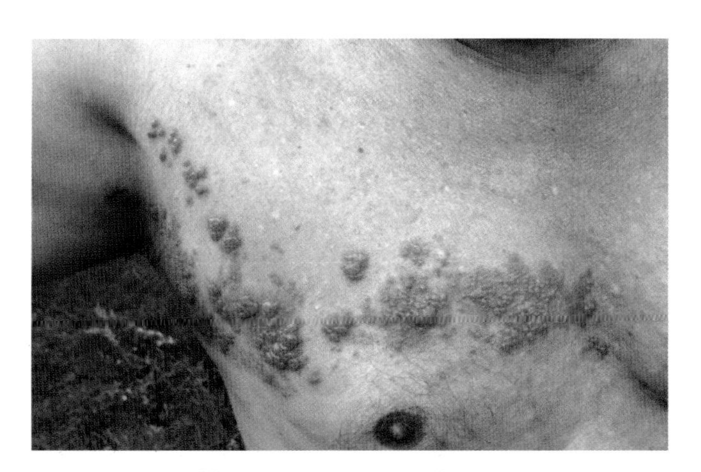

**Herpes zoster–chest**

Reproduced with permission from wikipedia.org (public domain)

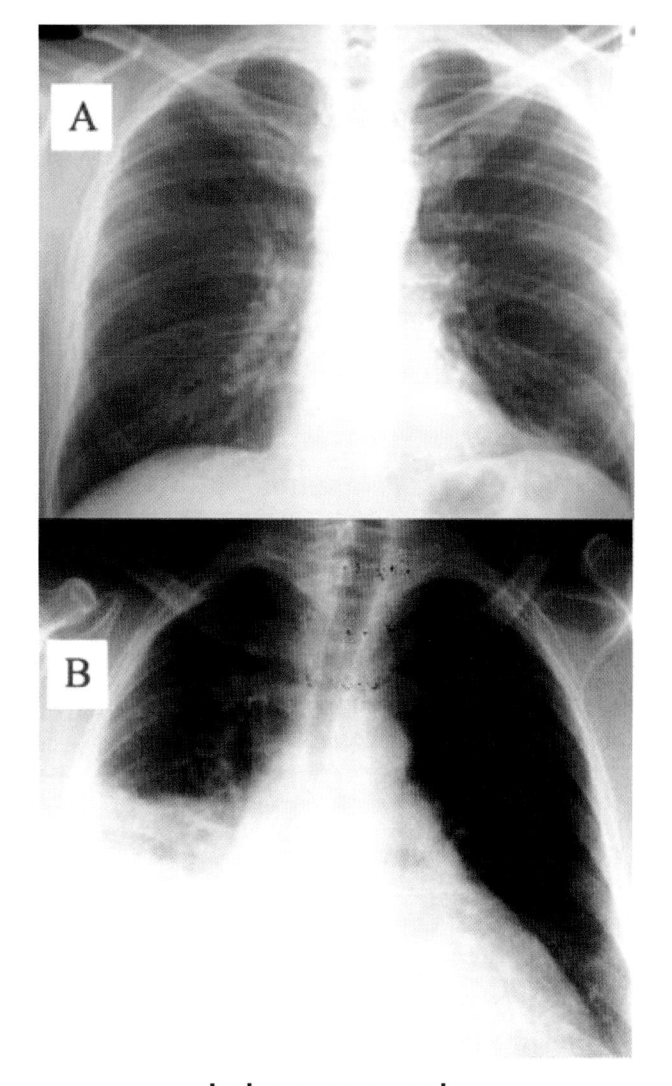


**Lobar pneumonia**

Reproduced with permission from wikipedia.org (public domain)

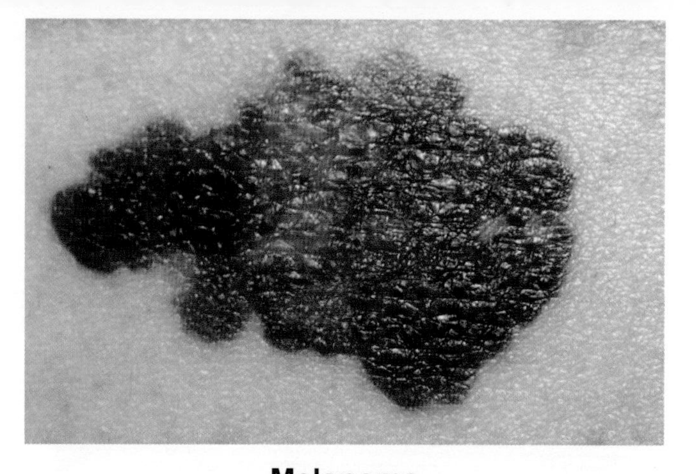

**Melanoma**

Reproduced with permission from National Cancer Institute (public domain)

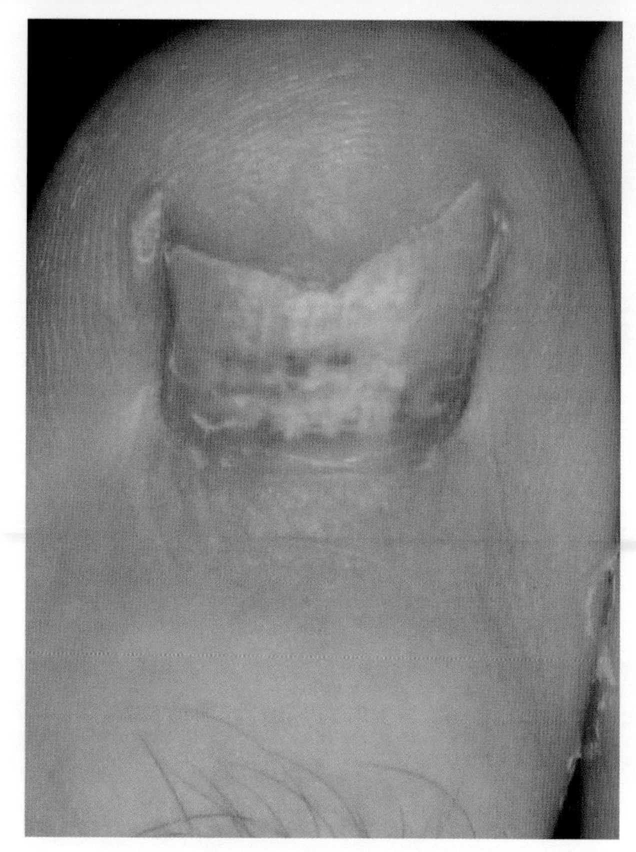

**Onychomycosis**

Reproduced with permission from wikipedia.org (public domain)

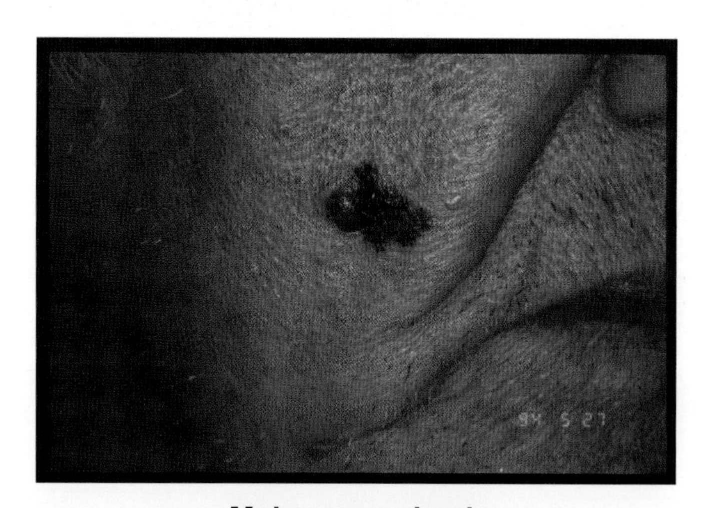

**Melanoma–cheek**

Reproduced with permission from DxR Development Group © 2008

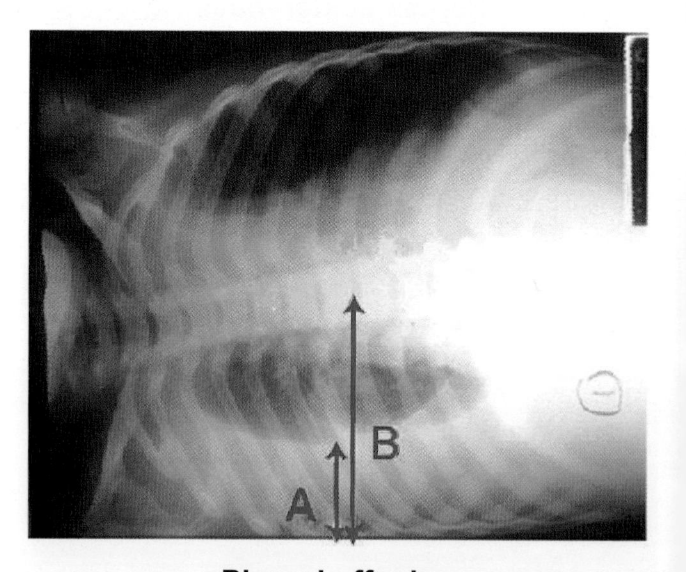


**Pleural effusion**

Reproduced with permission from wikipedia.org (public domain)

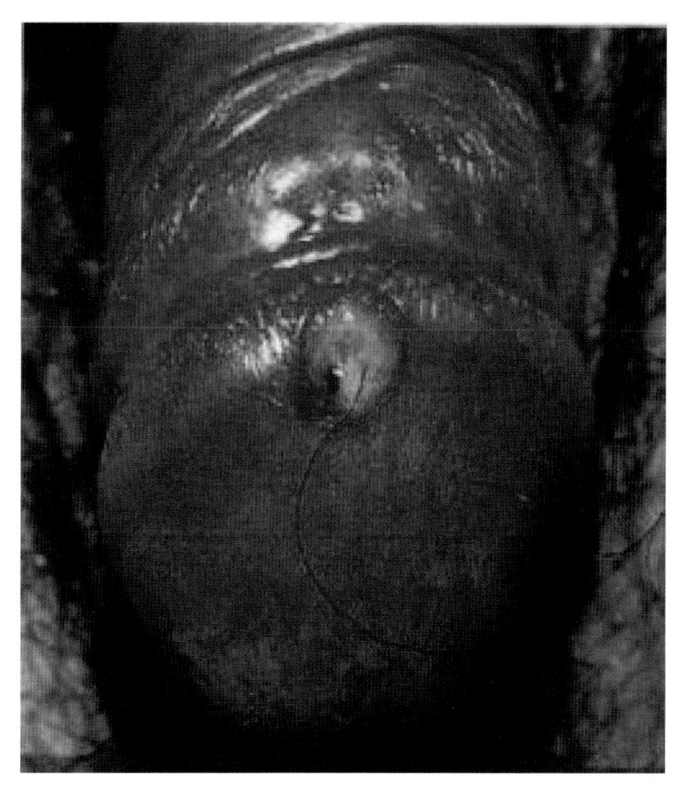

**Primary syphilis**

Reproduced with permission from
gettestedchicago.com

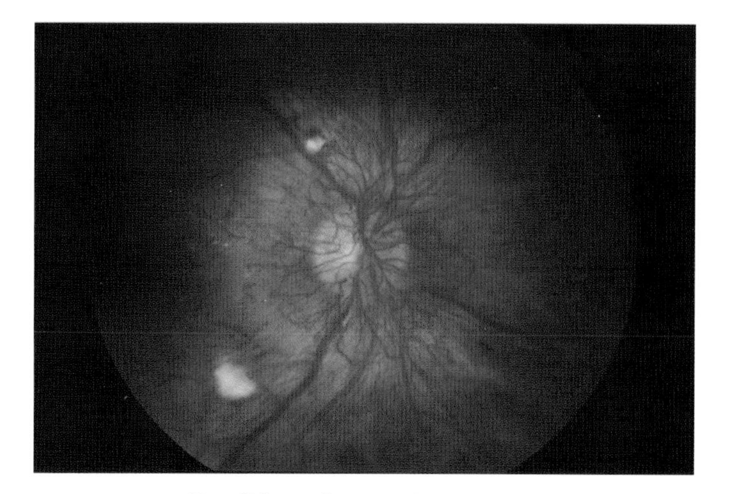

**Proliferative retinopathy**

Reproduced with permission from
National Eye Institute, National Institutes of Health

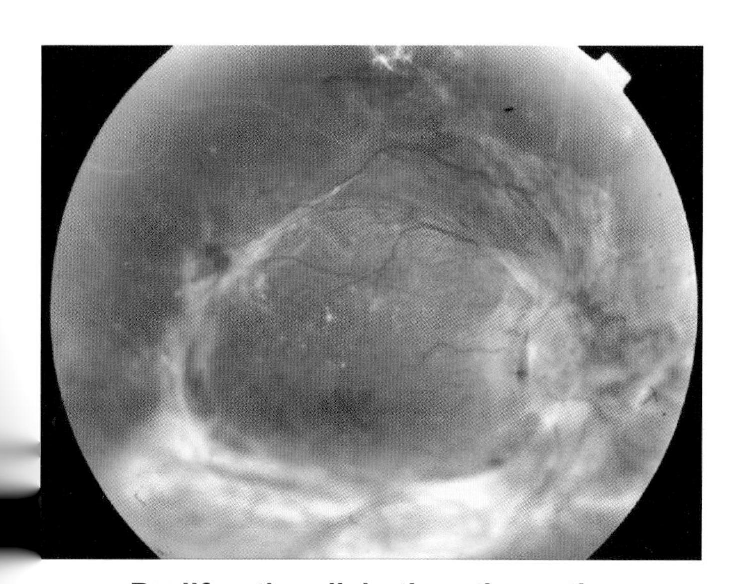

**Proliferative diabetic retinopathy**

Reproduced with permission from
retinacarecenter.com

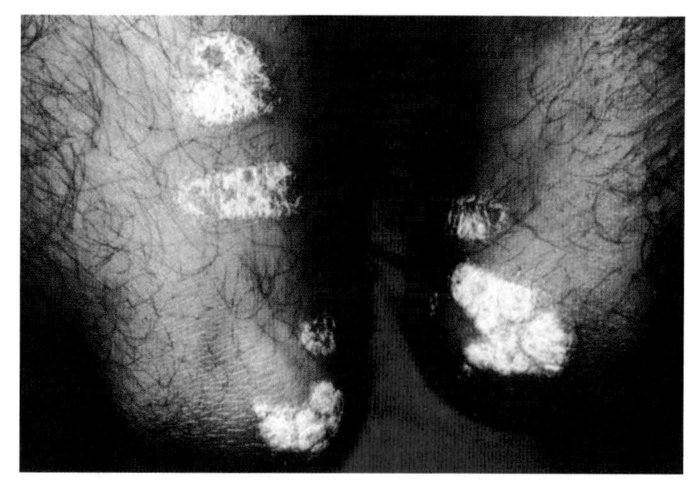

**Psoriasis of elbows**

Reproduced with permission from
DxR Development Group © 2008

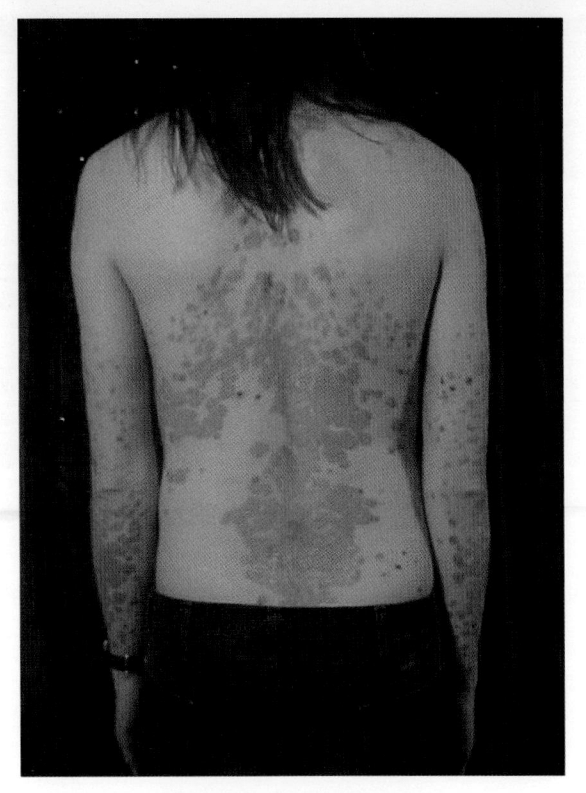

**Psoriasis of back**

Reproduced with permission from wikipedia.org

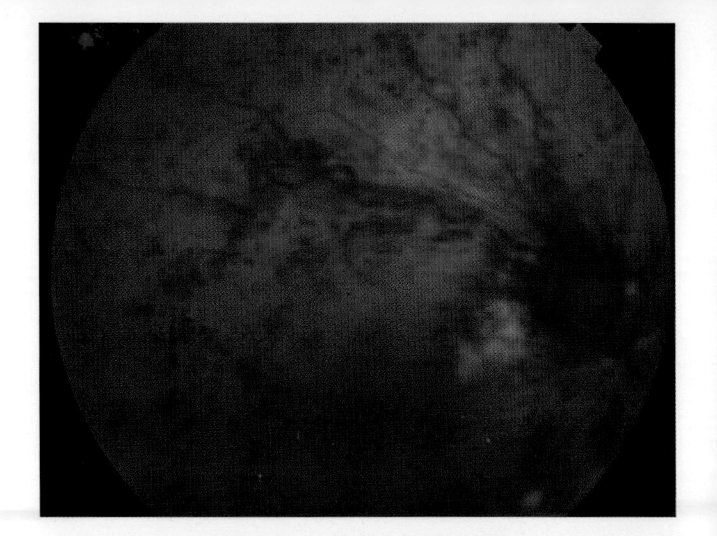

**Retinal vein occlusion**

Reproduced with permission from retinacarecenter.com

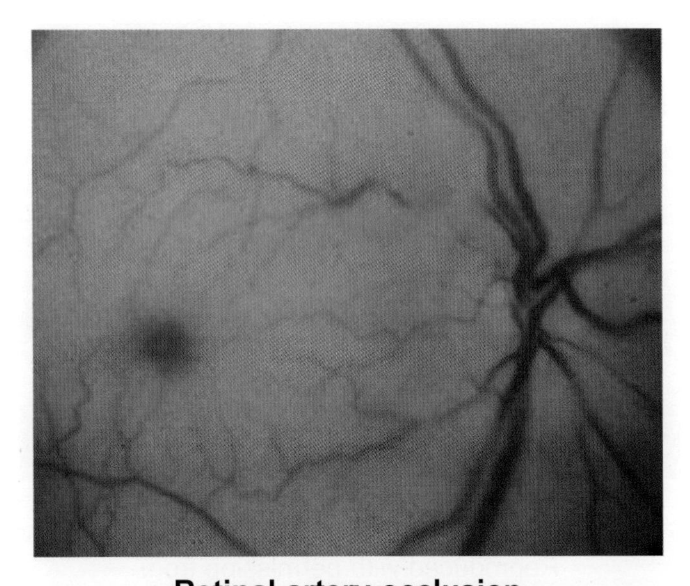

**Retinal artery occlusion**

Reproduced with permission from retinacarecenter.com

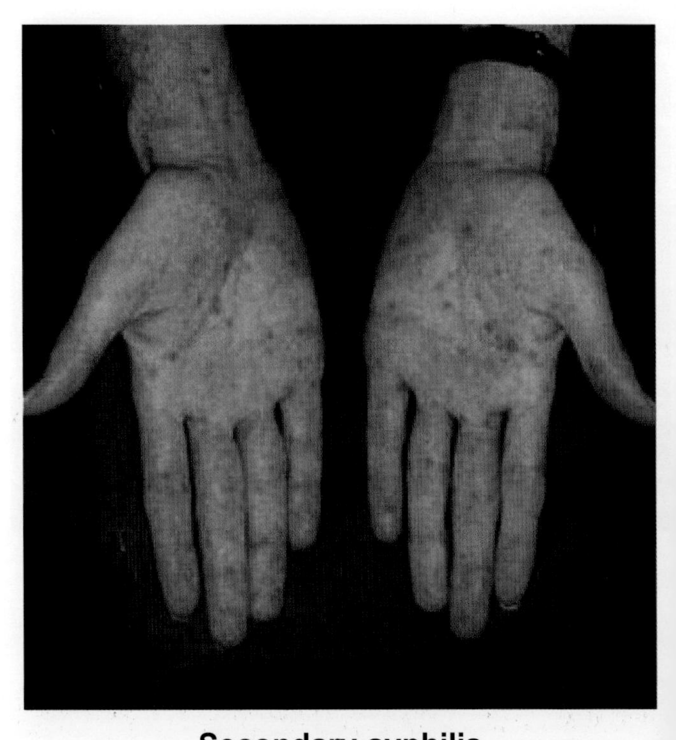

**Secondary syphilis**

Reproduced with permission from nlm.nih.gov

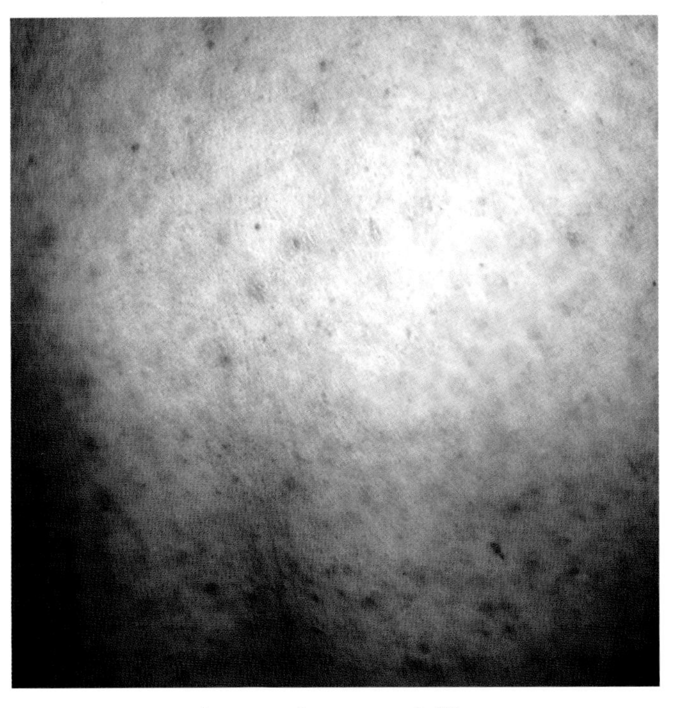

**Secondary syphilis**

Reproduced with permission from
Dr. Charles Goldberg and Jan Thompson
http://medicine.ucsd.edu/clinicalimg/browse.htm

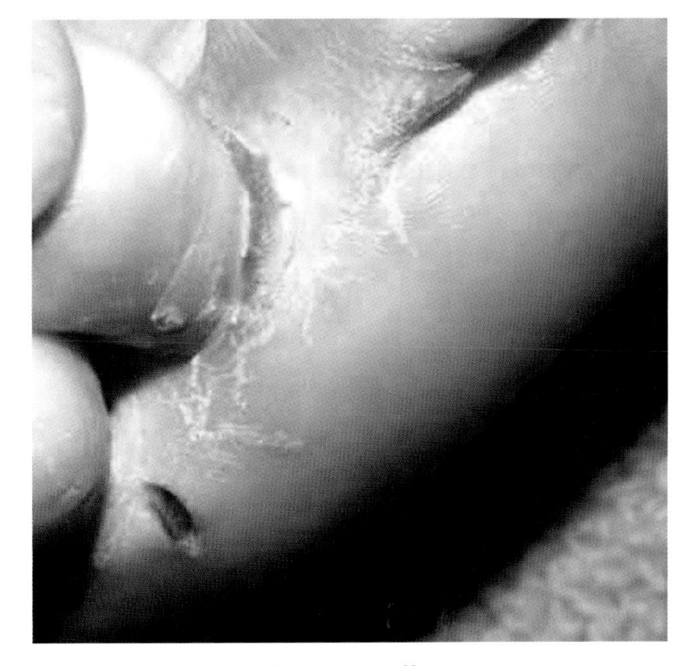

**Tinea pedis**

Reproduced with permission from
wikipedia.org

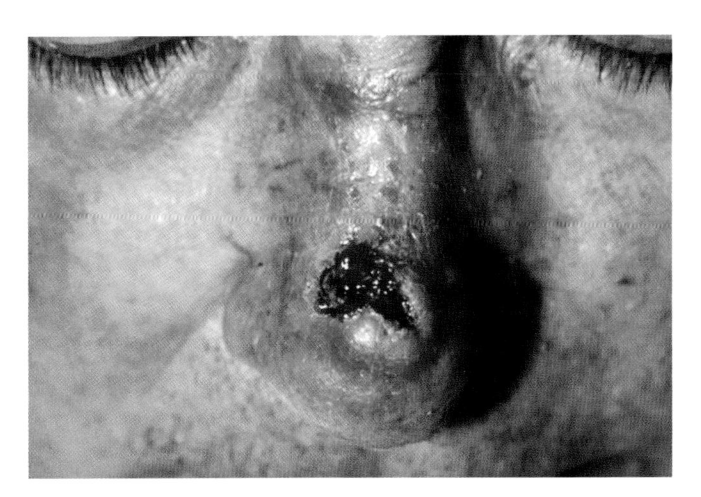

**Squamous cell carcinoma–nose**

Reproduced with permission from
National Cancer Institute (public domain)

**Tinea versicolor**

Reproduced with permission from
DxR Development Group © 2008

# PART V

# MEDICAL ABBREVIATIONS

# Medical Abbreviations 18

| | |
|---|---|
| 4Q | 4 quadrants |
| yo or y/o | year old |
| m | male |
| f | female |
| b | black |
| w | white |
| L | left |
| R | right |
| Hx | history |
| h/o | history of |
| c/o | complaining/complaints of |
| c | with |
| NL | normal limits |
| r/o | rule out |
| s | without |
| w/ | with |
| WNL | within normal limits |
| Ø | without or no |
| + | positive |
| – | negative |
| | |
| A&0x3 | alert & oriented to person, place, and time |
| AA | Alcoholics Anonymous |
| AAA | abdominal aortic aneurysm |
| abd | abdomen |

| | |
|---|---|
| ABG | arterial blood gas |
| AC | abdominal circumference |
| ACE | angiotensin-converting enzyme |
| ACTH | adrenocorticotropic hormone |
| ADH | antidiuretic hormone |
| AFB | acid-fast bacilli |
| AFI | amniotic fluid index |
| afib | atrial fibrillation |
| AIDS | acquired immune deficiency syndrome |
| Alb | albumin |
| ALP | alkaline phosphatase |
| ALS | amyotrophic lateral sclerosis |
| ANS | autonomic nervous system |
| ant | anterior |
| A&P | auscultation and percussion |
| ARDS | acute respiratory distress syndrome |
| AV | arteriovenous |
| AP | anteroposterior |
| ASA | aspirin |
| AST | aspartate transaminase |
| ALT | alanine transaminase |
| ANS | autonomic nervous system |
| | |
| b/l | bilateral |
| BID | twice a day |
| BM | bowel movement |
| BMI | body mass index |
| BP | blood pressure |
| BPD | biparietal diameter |
| BPH | benign prostatic hypertrophy |
| BPP | biophysical profile |

| | |
|---|---|
| BSA | body surface area |
| BUN | blood urea nitrogen |
| | |
| Ca | calcium |
| CA | cancer |
| CABG | coronary artery bypass grafting |
| CAD | coronary artery disease |
| CAP | community-acquired pneumonia |
| cath | catheterization |
| CBC | complete blood count |
| cc | chief complaint |
| CCB | calcium channel blocker |
| CCU | cardiac care unit |
| CEA | carcinoembryonic antigen |
| CF | cystic fibrosis |
| chemo | chemotherapy |
| CHF | congestive heart failure |
| chol | cholesterol |
| Cl | chloride |
| CLL | chronic lymphocytic leukemia |
| CML | chronic myelogenous leukemia |
| CMV | cytomegalovirus |
| CN | cranial nerve |
| CNS | central nervous system |
| COPD | chronic obstructive pulmonary disease |
| CPAP | continuous positive airway pressure |
| CPK | creatine phosphokinase |
| CPR | cardiopulmonary resuscitation |
| Cr | creatinine |
| C&S, C/S | culture and sensitivity |
| CSF | cerebrospinal fluid |
| CST | contraction stress test |

| | |
|---|---|
| CT | computed tomography |
| CTA | clear to auscultation |
| CVA | cerebrovascular accident |
| CVP | central venous pressure |
| Cx | cervix |
| CXR | chest x-ray |
| | |
| D&C | dilatation and curettage |
| DI | diabetes insipidus |
| DM | diabetes mellitus |
| DSRP | daily record of severity of problems |
| DTR | deep tendon reflexes |
| DVT | deep vein thrombosis |
| dx | diagnosis |
| | |
| ECC | endocervical curettage |
| EKG/ECG | electrocardiogram |
| EEG | electroencephalogram |
| ED | emergency department |
| EGD | esophagogastroduodenoscopy |
| EMG | electromyogram |
| ENT | ears, nose, and throat |
| EOMI | extraocular muscles intact |
| ERCP | endoscopic retrograde cholangiopancreatography |
| ESR | erythrocyte sedimentation rate |
| EtOH | alcohol |
| ext | extremities |
| | |
| FBS | fasting blood sugar |
| Fe | iron |

| | |
|---|---|
| fFN | fetal fibronectin |
| FSH | follicle stimulating hormone |
| FH | family history |
| FUO | fever of unknown origin |
| Fx | fracture |
| | |
| GA | general appearance |
| GERD | gastroesophageal reflux disorder |
| GI | gastrointestinal |
| Glu | glucose |
| GnRH | gonadotropin-releasing hormone |
| GTT | glucose tolerance test |
| GU | genitourinary |
| | |
| HA | headache |
| HBsAg | hepatitis B surface antigen |
| HC | head circumference |
| Hct | hematocrit |
| HDN | hemolytic disease of the newborn |
| HEENT | head, eyes, ears, nose, and throat |
| Hgb | hemoglobin |
| HIV | human immunodeficiency virus |
| HOCM | hypertrophic cardiomyopathy |
| HRT | hormone replacement therapy |
| HPI | history of present illness |
| HR | heart rate |
| HSM | hepatosplenomegaly |
| HTN | hypertension |
| | |
| IBD | inflammatory bowel disease |
| IBS | irritable bowel syndrome |
| ICU | intensive care unit |
| IDDM | insulin-dependent diabetes mellitus |

| | |
|---|---|
| IM | intramuscularly |
| INR | international ratio |
| IUD | intrauterine device |
| IV | intravenously |
| | |
| JVD | jugular venous distension |
| JVP | jugular venous pressure |
| | |
| K | potassium |
| KUB | kidney, ureter, and bladder |
| | |
| LAD | lymphadenopathy or left anterior descending |
| LDH | lactate dehydrogenase |
| LE | lower extremity |
| LFTs | liver function tests |
| LH | luteinizing hormone |
| LLL | left lower lobe |
| LLQ | left lower quadrant |
| LMP | last menstrual period |
| loc | loss of consciousness |
| LP | lumbar puncture |
| LUL | left upper lobe |
| LUQ | left upper quadrant |
| | |
| M, R, G | murmurs, rubs, or gallops |
| mets | metastases |
| MI | myocardial infarction |
| MRI | magnetic resonance imaging |
| MRSA | methicillin-resistant *Staphylococcus aureus* |
| MS | multiple sclerosis |
| MVP | mitral valve prolapse (cardiology) or maximum vertical pocket (obstetrics) |
| | |

| | |
|---|---|
| Na | sodium |
| NC/AT | normocephalic atraumatic |
| neuro | neurologic |
| NIDDM | non–insulin-dependent diabetes mellitus |
| NKA | no known allergies |
| NKDA | no known drug allergy |
| NPH | normal pressure hydrocephalus |
| NSR | normal sinus rhythm |
| NST | non-stress test |
| NSVD | normal spontaneous vaginal delivery |
| N/V | nausea and vomiting |
| | |
| occ | occasional |
| OCP | oral contraceptive pills |
| OD | right eye |
| OS | left eye |
| OTC | over-the-counter |
| | |
| PA | posteroanterior |
| PAN | polyarteritis nodosa |
| PCP | primary care provider |
| PCP | *Pneumocystis carinii* pneumonia |
| PE | physical examination |
| PE | pulmonary embolus |
| PEEP | positive end-expiratory pressure |
| PERRLA | pupils are equal, round, and reactive to light and accommodation |
| PET | positron emission tomography |
| PFTs | pulmonary function tests |
| PID | pelvic inflammatory disease |

| | |
|---|---|
| PMI | point of maximum impulse |
| po | orally |
| POC | products of conception |
| pos | positive |
| PPD | packs per day |
| PPD | purified protein derivative |
| PRN | as needed |
| PSA | prostatic specific antigen |
| PT | prothrombin time |
| PTSD | post-traumatic stress disorder |
| PTT | partial prothrombin time |
| PUD | peptic ulcer disease |
| PVD | peripheral vascular disease |
| | |
| RA | rheumatoid arthritis |
| RBC | red blood cells |
| RDS | respiratory distress syndrome |
| RLL | right lower lobe |
| RLQ | right lower quadrant |
| RMG | rubs, murmurs, or gallops |
| ROM | range of motion |
| RR | respiratory rate |
| RRR | regular rate and rhythm |
| RUL | right upper lobe |
| RUQ | right upper quadrant |
| | |
| SBO | small bowel obstruction |
| SCFE | slipped capital femoral epiphysis |
| SERM | selective estrogen receptor modulator |
| SH | social history |
| SLE | systemic lupus erythematosus |

| SLR | straight leg raising |
|---|---|
| sob | shortness of breath |
| SQ | subcutaneous |
| Staph | *Staphylococcus* |
| STD | sexually transmitted disease |
| Strep | *Streptococcus* |
| SAB | subarachnoid bleed |
| | |
| T | temperature |
| T1DM | type 1 diabetes mellitus |
| T2DM | type 2 diabetes mellitus |
| TB | tuberculosis |
| TIA | transient ischemic attack |
| TSH | thyroid stimulating hormone |
| TURP | transurethral prostatectomy |
| TVF | tactile vocal fremitus |
| | |
| U/A | urinalysis |
| UE | upper extremity |
| UGI | upper gastrointestinal |
| URI | upper respiratory tract infection |
| U/S | ultrasound |
| UTI | urinary tract infection |
| | |
| vag | vaginal |
| VAS | vibroacoustic stimulation (vibration and sound) |
| VCUG | voiding cystourethrogram |
| VDRL | Venereal Disease Research Laboratory |
| vs | vital signs |
| | |
| WBC | white blood cells |
| wks | weeks |
| WNL | within normal limits |
| wt | weight |